THE
Detox
BOOK

How to Detoxify Your Body to Improve Your Health, Stop Disease and Reverse Aging

Bruce Fife, N.D.

Revised Second Edition

Piccadilly Books, Ltd.
Colorado Springs, Colorado

Acknowledgements
Grateful acknowledgement is given to the publishers of following
materials for use of information in the preparation of this book:
Understanding Normal and Clinical Nutrition, West Publishing
Company; *Alternative Medicine*, Future Medicine Publishing;
American Journal of Natural Medicine, IMPAKT Communications;
Nutrition Action Healthletter, Center for Science in the Public Interest;
Diet for A New America, Stillpoint Publishing; *The 120-Year Diet*,
Simon & Schuster; *Newsweek*; *Your Health, Your Choice*, Lifetime
Books; *The Miracle of Fasting*, Health Science; *Oxygen Therapies*,
Energy Publications; *The New Miracles of Rebound Exercise*, AIR;
Stress-Proofing Your Child, Bantam Books.

Cover design by Michael Donahue

Revised Second Edition

Piccadilly Books, Ltd.
P.O. Box 25203
Colorado Springs, CO 80936

Library of Congress Cataloging-in-Publication Data

Fife, Bruce, 1952-
      The detox book : how to detoxify your body to improve your health,
   stop disease, and reverse aging / Bruce Fife.
         p.   cm.
      Includes bibliographical references and index.
      ISBN 0-941599-32-9 (pbk.)
      1. Toxicology--Popular works. 2. Toxins. 3. Health. 4. Longevity.
   I. Title.
   RA1213.F48   1997
   615.9--dc21   97-14627

Simultaneously Published in Australia, UK, and USA
Printed in the United States of America

TABLE OF CONTENTS

Chapter 1

TOXIC TIME BOMB

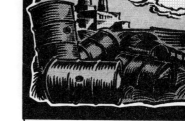

DEGENERATIVE DISEASE: A Modern Epidemic

Carrie* was every parent's dream: At 26, she was bright, energetic, self-supporting. "She was my cheerleader," says her mother, Sophie. "She even taught me to swim."

In 1989, Carrie's future looked bright. She worked as a youth counselor in Denver, where she had scores of friends. Then one day she called home with panic in her voice.

"Mom," she said, "I have leukemia, and the doctor wants me to go to the hospital right away."

"At that moment," says Sophie, "my whole world fell apart."

Carrie was told that her only chance was to undergo a bone marrow transplant. But no one in her immediate family was a good match. Because of her Hispanic heritage, the odds that a stranger would match were 1 in 20,000. The future looked dim.

Carrie was informed that unless a donor could be found, she could die in a matter of months. A frantic search for a donor was instigated. As she waited, she was given the standard medical treatments for leukemia which included chemotherapy. Despite the side effects of these treatments she had hope that the disfigurement and pain she had to endure were only temporary.

While waiting for a donor, time ran out for Carrie. She died a few months later, bald and bloated from cancer-fighting drugs.

"With everything that medical science can do, I wasn't able to save my daughter," Sophie said, choking back tears.

Neva, 21, was pregnant with her first child when a burning feeling in her right leg began to nag her. It was centered near a rubbery lump that had formed on the front of the ankle after she bruised it some years earlier doing gymnastics. The lump had never gone away and now it was growing larger and firmer. She ignored it.

One night, soon after the baby was born, Neva was watching TV when a terrifying feeling came over her. Numbness struck her hands and arms, then traveled up her neck to her face. The room began spinning. When she tried to tell her husband what was happening to her, she couldn't form the words. He rushed her to the local hospital. Nurses there began pumping blood thinners and other

The frog does not drink up the pond in which he lives.
— *Buddhist Proverb*

---

* Names of some of the people used in the case histories of this book have been changed to protect privacy.

medications into her, trying to bring her out of what the doctors had diagnosed as a transient ischemic attack—or "mini-stroke" as it is sometimes described. Neva's ankle also hurt more than ever during this whole episode.

Her ankle hurt so much and was so stiff that her doctor eventually ordered a bone biopsy. The biopsy revealed cancer. "To stop the spread of cancer," the doctor told her, "we're gong to have to amputate a part of your leg, right below the knee."

Shocked, Neva asked, "Isn't there something else you can do?"

"I'm sorry," he said, "but there's no other way out. It has to be done."

Neva underwent chemotherapy to kill the tumor before going in for surgery. She underwent a four-hour operation during which her entire leg below the knee was removed. More chemotherapy followed to prevent any stray cancer cells from moving to her lungs. The pathologist reported that there was no more cancer in her. Her tumor hadn't spread beyond the ankle, which increased her odds for survival. The surgery and chemotherapy were apparently successful. Everything looked bright for Neva.

She endured five months of treatment, including chemotherapy and two surgeries. Chemotherapy, however, took its toll. Neva's hair fell out in clumps, her throat became raw, and some mornings she was so nauseous that she couldn't climb out of bed. But it was a small price to pay to remove the cancer that would have killed her.

After the surgery, life went on with the hope of a brighter future. It took some time to adjust to the use of an artificial leg, but she managed and was able to spend time with her baby.

A year passed when Neva felt a nagging soreness near the middle of her back. At first, she thought she had pulled a muscle. Despite hot baths and medications the pain persisted. Breathing became labored and when she started coughing up blood, she knew something serious was wrong.

It was discovered that the cancer had returned and settled in her lungs. Over the next two years she underwent three more surgeries, removing all of one lung and portions of the other. As with many other cancer patients who survive surgery, radiation, and chemotherapy, cancer often returns. Repeated chemotherapy treatments left her weak and ill. Her health gradually deteriorated.

She used to ask, "Why me?" But now her attitude is, "Whatever happens, happens. You just learn to live with it." What other option is there?

When Rick, age 38, was diagnosed with terminal cancer, he was devastated. "How could this happen to me," he wondered. "I'm too young for this type of thing." This is something that happens to others, not to young, seemingly healthy, people. Rick had a loving wife and three healthy children. His career was successful and he was anticipating an important promotion. He and his wife were making plans for buying a new, bigger home. It seemed that Rick's lifelong dreams were being fulfilled. Cancer changed all of that.

There was nothing that could be done to help Rick, his condition was considered incurable and he was told that he had less than a year to live. As Rick's condition worsened, his physician referred him to the local hospice to help make his last days as comfortable as possible. With the help of the hospice nurses and physicians Rick received the medications he needed to help control the pain and discomfort as the disease slowly devoured his body. Since his condition was considered irreversible, no attempt was made to preserve his life. Six months later Rick was dead.

Doris was a 66-year-old diabetic with clogged arteries. The seriousness of her condition had been driven home a week earlier by a sudden heart attack. She was now wheeled into an operating room at the local medical center. For the next eight hours her life was in the hands of a team of nurses, physician-assistants, anesthesiologists, and surgeons. They cut veins out of her legs, sawed her sternum in half, spread her ribs, than sewed the veins from her leg onto her heart to bypass the clogged artery.

The surgery was a success and Doris was soon home again. With the aid of blood thinning medications and other drugs she pursued life pretty much as usual. Her diabetes required daily injections of insulin. Her lifestyle and eating habits did not change.

It wasn't long, however, before she was suffering from badly swollen legs which gave her pain and caused her to remain inactive most of the time. She gradually lost the ability to hold the contents of her bladder and colon. This necessitated the use of adult diapers which she hated and removed at every opportunity. She was in need of constant care as Alzheimer's disease progressed from a minor nuisance to a major disability. She continued to suffer with these conditions, spending the majority of her retirement income for health care and medications until she died. The last nine years of her life were spent as a near invalid—demented, medicated, and in pain.

The stories of Carrie, Neva, Rick, and Doris are all too typical in today's society. Degenerative diseases like cancer, arthritis, osteoporosis, heart disease, emphysema, and a host of others are occurring in epidemic proportions. Modern medicine has been powerless to stop it. We hear of the great advances in medicine, but the disease rate continues to rise to an alarming level. Despite the fact that medicine has made great advances, there is more sickness now than a century ago. Infectious diseases like small pox and tuberculosis have been, for the most part, successfully controlled, but degenerative diseases that were once rare or nonexistent are now at epidemic levels. It is estimated that nearly 92 percent of the population in Western countries will succumb to one or more of these degenerative conditions before they die. Often it will be the cause of their death. If not, then the drugs, radiation, and surgery used to treat them will further weaken the body, causing the death.

This is not true in Third World countries where such diseases are relatively rare. They suffer more from infectious diseases and malnutrition than from degenerative disease. Where food is plentiful and nutritional deficiencies absent, the people in the less civilized areas of the world live full healthy lives without suffering prolonged illnesses caused by degenerative or nutritional diseases. Degenerative disease, for the most part, is a product of modern society.

Over the past decade, hundreds of studies have demonstrated the dangers to health from toxins in the environment. Toxic accumulation manifests itself in a variety of ways, including decreased immune function, autoimmune disease, enzyme dysfunction, hormonal imbalances, psychological disturbances, altered metabolism, nutritional deficiencies, and even cancer. Toxic accumulation is the underlying cause for most all degenerative disease. Bad genes aren't the problem, old age isn't the problem, nor are germs the problem. All these things may be involved, but the real problem is excess toxins in the body. Toxins build up faster than they can be removed, and disease results.

OUR TOXIC WORLD

"There are no healthy kids here," laments Yury, a resident of Karabash, Russia. Yury has two children both of which are continually sick. The people of Karabash are being poisoned. Every year a local factory spews out 162,000 tons of pollutants into the air—9 tons for every man, woman, and child living there.

In a study performed in Mexico City, Dr. Margarita Castillejos found that even in a wealthy area of the city, the children were sick four days out of five. "To be sick has for them become normal," she observed. One of the main culprits, she says, is the pervasive smog produced by the thousands of vehicles that clog city streets.

In many cities in the United States, smog gets so bad that schools keep children indoors during recess to keep exposure to a minimum. But staying indoors can be just as dangerous, if not more so, because of fumes and particles from paints, solvents, cleansers, asbestos, bacteria, and other pollutants. Everywhere you turn, people are getting sick from exposure to man-made toxins in our environment.

There is an ominous pattern behind the increasing epidemic of degenerative sickness around the world, particularly in industrialized countries where pollution has become a critical problem. As industry increases, so does degenerative disease. Degenerative diseases that were rare or even unheard of a few decades ago are running rampant now. Lester Brown, president of the Worldwatch Institute, stated recently that "the overwhelming threat to our future is not military aggression but the environmental degradation of the planet." The places hit worse are the places with the best medical care and facilities—industrialized Western countries. Third World countries, particularly those that have limited contact with Western influences, are relatively free of the degenerative diseases that are rampaging across the civilized world. The common thread between industrialization and disease is pollution—air, water, and food pollution. We are slowly poisoning our environment in a sea of deadly toxins.

In the state of New York there is a waterway near Niagara Falls known as the Love Canal. The area around the canal was, at one time, described as "charming." Now warning signs are posted and people are kept out by a fence. In the late 1940s and early 1950s, the Hooker Chemical Company disposed of its chemical wastes near the Love Canal. Years later it was discovered that the incidence of cancer and birth defects among people living in the area was unusually high. Investigators found the area still highly contaminated and that wildlife was being affected. Small field mice, for example, living around the canal were found to have a reduced life expectancy. The closer the mice live to the canal the younger they die. Those living nearest to the canal show liver damage and high tissue levels of chemicals that were discarded in the area decades ago. People no longer live near the Love Canal.

In recent history, mankind has drastically changed the chemistry of the environment in which we live. Since the end of World War II, the world has been flooded with tens of thousands of synthetic chemicals. Today, approximately 60,000 different chemicals are in common use, and many of these are highly toxic.

Every year more than 1,000,000,000 pounds of these chemicals are released into the ground worldwide, threatening a portion of the soil in which we grow our food and the natural underground water tables that supply our drinking and irrigation water. Over 188,000,000 pounds of chemicals are also discharged into surface waters such as lakes and rivers. More than 2,400,000,000 pounds of chemical emissions are pumped into the air we breathe. A grand total of 5,705,670,380 pounds of chemical pollutants are released into our environment. And this amount is increasing every year. It's as if a toxic time bomb has exploded, spreading poisons throughout the world. We all are suffering the effects of it.

Water has become dangerously polluted. Over 20 chemicals—including fluoride, chlorine, and aluminum—are intentionally added to our drinking water. Groundwater and reservoirs collect more poisons from runoff which contains pesticides, chemical fertilizers, and industrial waste. Contaminated water is used to irrigate crops and for livestock which in turn are used for food. Water can be further contaminated with toxic heavy metals, such as cadmium and lead, from pipes.

Our atmosphere is a sea of pollution. Millions of tons of pollutants are released into the air we breathe. When these pollutants accumulate in urban areas, they interact with oxygen and sunlight to produce smog and acid rain.

Industry and leaded gasoline* pollute the atmosphere and water with hundreds of thousands of tons of lead. We also get lead from the solder in canned foods, cadmium and lead from cigarette smoke (even second-hand smoke), mercury from dental fillings, and aluminum from antacids, baking powder, and cookware.

Our foods are packed with preservatives, artificial colorings, sugars, and flavor enhancers and other chemical additives. Solvents, bacteria, fungi, pesticides, herbicides, heavy metals, and packaging materials all contaminate the foods sold at grocery stores and in restaurants.

We are exposed to an endless variety of toxins in the air we breathe and the foods we eat. We are also exposed to toxic chemicals in items we come into contact with every day such as synthetic carpets, paints, hair spray, cosmetics, furniture polish, toothpaste, detergents, household cleaning aids, fertilizers, gasoline, etc. The list can go on and on.

Harmful chemicals and pathogenic microorganisms are swarming around us 24 hours a day. We cannot prevent contact with all harmful substances. Nor can we stop all toxins from entering our bodies. In fact, it is normal for the body to contain some toxins. But our bodies were designed to neutralize and eliminate these toxic substances as quickly as possible to maintain good health. The immune system, liver, kidneys, and other organs work together to remove harmful substances from the body.

Toxins are also created inside all of us as a natural byproduct of cellular metabolism and as cells deteriorate

*Some countries still use leaded gasoline and those that have stopped its use still have lead in the environment.

or die. This debris is quickly gathered up and removed from the body. If it were not removed, this waste would poison and kill other cells and lead to massive cellular degeneration, excessive stress on organs and tissues throughout the body, and eventually death. The body is fully capable of handling the cleanup and removal of all naturally occurring toxins. It has enough reserve strength to fight off infections from microorganisms without serious complications.

However, when toxins are being assimilated or created faster than they can be eliminated, the toxic accumulations create an environment in which "dis-ease" will develop. Dis-ease is defined as any form of discomfort caused by cellular or tissue malfunction, sickness, or feelings of ill health which put the body or mind at dis-ease.

FOOD CONTAMINATION

Toxins are created in the body from metabolic waste and free-radical formation. They also enter the body through our lungs, skin, and mouth. The most destructive toxins or poisons in our bodies usually enter through the mouth. They are hidden in our everyday foods and drinks. These toxins include biological contaminants (bacteria, fungi, viruses, etc.) and industrial contaminants (preservatives, solvents, chemical food additives, heavy metals, etc.). Pollutants from industry are a major concern because they can find their way into our food from animal products we eat, crops we grow, and water we drink.

In 1953, a number of people in Minamata, Japan, became ill with a disease no one had seen before. By 1960, 121 cases had been reported, including 23 infants. Forty-six died. Many more cases went unreported. Symptoms included progressive blindness, deafness, incoordination, and intellectual deterioration. The cause was ultimately revealed to be methylmercury contamination from fish taken out of the bay these people lived on. The infants who contracted the disease had not eaten any fish, but their mothers had, and even though the mothers exhibited no symptoms during their pregnancies, the poison had been affecting their unborn babies. Manufacturing plants in the region were dumping mercury into the bay and the fish were accumulating this poison in their bodies. Some of the people who were affected had been eating fish from the bay nearly every day.

The incident in Japan was a natural consequence of industrial pollution, something that is going on all around us. Toxic chemicals often get into our food supply by accidents, many of which may go unnoticed. Some are purposely kept secret so that companies can sell

Our Daily Dose Of Lead

At nine months, Joey crawled about, exploring the world around him—touching and tasting everything, as all babies do. At two, his parents proudly watched as he began to toddle about. At four, he amused his parents when he'd chase after balls tossed his way. At five, he exhibited remarkable carefulness, holding tightly to the stair railings with both hands as he slowly climbed up or down.

Although his parents didn't notice it, Joey's health was gradually deteriorating. Joey was late in walking, and rarely caught a ball or skipped and jumped at the playground like other kids his age. His small size was another clue that something was wrong, as was his clinging to the stair railings. The kindergarten teacher reported that Joey had some difficulty hearing and that his progress was slower than expected, but each clue was easily dismissed with a comment that "children progress at different paces." No one expected lead toxicity was the problem.

The signs of mild lead poisoning include diarrhea, irritability, and lethargy. With higher levels of lead, the symptoms become more pronounced, yet are still difficult to pinpoint to a cause. Children lose their sense of balance and their general cognitive, verbal, and perceptual abilities, developing learning disabilities and behavior problems. Even more worrisome is that only one year of exposure can permanently impair the brain, nervous system, and psychological functioning. Recent experiments have shown that the effects occur with lower doses than had been thought in the past. The Public Health Service has singled out lead poisoning as the worst environmental threat to children.

Lead aggressively attacks fetuses, infants, and children, because the body absorbs lead most efficiently during times of rapid growth. Lead readily transfers across the placenta, inflicting severe damage on the developing fetal nervous system. Infants and young children absorb five to ten times as much lead as adults do. *One out of every six children between the ages of six months and five years, and one out of every nine fetuses, are exposed to threatening levels of lead!* Lead absorption increases when the diet lacks adequate nutrition. Since many of the foods

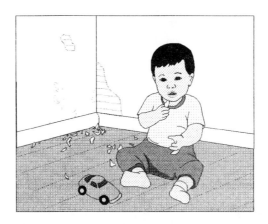

children eat nowadays are nutrient deficient, lead absorption is a problem to be seriously concerned about.

All foods contain some lead. Much, perhaps all, of it is from industrial pollution. People are exposed to lead in gasoline, paint, newspaper ink, batteries, water pipes, tin cans, and pesticides, as well as in industrial pollution that is released into our air and water. Lead works its way through rainfall and soil and then into plants and animals that people use for food. Lead also enters food from food containers such as tin cans sealed with lead solder and old or imported pottery decorated with lead glazes. Paint in old homes and apartments contains lead. Many children have become deathly ill and died from nibbling on paint chips. People taking baths in painted bathtubs have become seriously sick from lead poisoning. Although residential paint no longer contains lead, paint used for other purposes, such as playground equipment, sometimes does. Pipelines with lead solder joints also release lead into bathing and drinking water. Lead in water is the country's most significant contaminant.

—Adapted from *Understanding Normal and Clinical Nutrition* by Eleanor Noss Whitney, Ph.D., R.D., et al.

contaminated products without suffering a loss. People who eat these products may get sick and simply blame it on the weather or a "bug" that is going around. When contamination is serious enough to cause widespread sickness and death, the cause is often investigated.

In Michigan in 1973 a half a ton of polybrominated biphenyl (PBB), a toxic chemical, was accidentally mixed into some livestock feed that was distributed throughout the state. Millions of contaminated animals went to market and the chemical was passed to people who ate the meat. The seriousness of the accident began to come to light when dairy farmers reported their cows' going dry, aborting their calves, and developing abnormal growths. Although more than 30,000 cattle, sheep, and swine, and more than a million chickens were eventually destroyed, people were still affected. By 1982, it was estimated that 97 percent of Michigan's residents had been contaminated with PBB.

In the late 1980s more than 1,500 people in the United States contracted an unknown disease eventually called eosinophiliamyalgia syndrome (EMS). One-third of the people were hospitalized and dozens died. This disease was traced to a batch of contaminated tryptophan. Tryptophan is an essential amino acid that was commonly sold as a dietary supplement.

Pesticides are another contaminant which are intentionally added to our environment. Pesticides have caused birth defects, sterility, tumors, organ damage, and central nervous system impairment. We cannot usually see or taste pesticides in our food, so it is nearly impossible to detect them. Government agencies regulate tolerances for pesticide residues in foods. Regulations differ from country to country, some being very lenient; consequently, imported foods contain both higher concentrations of pesticides than domestic foods and also contain pesticides that have been banned in this country.

Pesticides are not only a potential contaminant in produce but also in animal products. Pesticide residues concentrate in animals' fat. Fat is intermingled within muscle fibers. So when we eat meat, even lean cuts, we not only consume cholesterol and saturated fat but pesticide residue.

Toxins are intentionally added to foods in the form of food additives. Artificial additives include synthetic vitamins, colors, flavors, flavor enhancers, preservatives,

Some Major Heavy Metal Contaminants

Metal	Sources	Toxic Effects
Aluminum	Used to manufacture or process foods, cosmetics, and medicines; a food additive, to purify water.	Spinal cord and brain disease, skeletal pain
Cadmium	Used in industrial processes, including electroplating, plastics, batteries, vapor lamps, alloys, pigments, and as a substitute for tin in solder; present in cigarette smoke.	Emphysema, fatigue, headache, vomiting, anemia, loss of smell, kidney failure
Chromium	Used in car manufacturing	Lung cancer, kidney damage
Lead	Used in solder, gasoline, newspaper ink, batteries, and some nonresidential paints	Damage to the nervous system, the blood-forming system, the kidneys, the reproductive system, the endocrine system
Mercury	Widely dispersed in gases from the earth's crust; local high concentrations from industry, electrical equipment, paints, pesticides	Damage to the nervous system causing emotional disturbances, including excitability and quick-tempered behavior, lack of concentration, loss of memory, depression, fatigue, weakness, headache, stomach and intestinal disorders

Adapted from R. W. Miller, The metal in our mettle, *FDA Consumer*, December 1988-January 1989.

emulsifiers, sweeteners, etc. Some additives are relatively harmless, such as ascorbate (vitamin C); others are very dangerous, such as saccharin which is a known carcinogen. Chemical additives that are known to cause health problems are usually controlled so that only a small portion is allowed in the food. Some are not, like monosodium glutamate (MSG), which is a flavor enhancer, known to cause health problems. MSG is widely used in restaurants and convenience foods. MSG, which is commonly used in Asian restaurants, received notoriety because it produces immediate adverse reactions in some people called the Chinese restaurant syndrome. Symptoms include: burning sensations, chest and facial flushing or pain, and throbbing headaches.

Preservatives are poisons added to foods to prevent oxidation and to kill or inhibit the growth of microorganisms. Sulfites are commonly used in may processed foods, beverages, and drugs. The use of sulfites on salad bars to keep raw fruits and vegetables looking fresh has been banned in the United States. The ban came after sulfites caused adverse reactions in some people with asthma. These reactions were sometimes serious, and for a few, deadly. Sulfites also destroy some vitamins in foods. Sulfites are still used on dried fruits and other foods. Numerous other chemical preservatives and food additives have serious health consequences.

Incidental food contaminants are substances that find their way into food as the result of some phase of harvesting, production, processing, storage, or packaging. Examples include: animal hairs, rat droppings, tiny bits of plastic, glass, paper, tin, and other substances from packages as well as chemicals such as the solvents used in processing and cleaning. The migration of incidental food additives is considered to be generally unavoidable and government allows certain measurable amounts of these substances to be in foods.

With all the toxins that enter the food and water supplies from industrial pollution, pesticides, chemical additives, and incidental contaminants, it seems nearly impossible to avoid them.

While the daily intake of food additives and other contaminants may have only a minute effect on body organs and their functions, their repeated effects are accumulative. Decades of exposure to dietary toxins exert a gradual, but serious, impact on our health that begins to manifest itself as we age. By the time you're 65, you will have consumed about 100,000 pounds of food, including nearly 10,000 pounds of food additives and incidental contaminants! Consumption of these noxious substances will certainly be reflected in the state of your health by age 65, if not long before.

WATER CONTAMINATION

In 1993 nearly a half a million people in the Milwaukee area became sick after drinking contaminated municipal water. More than 100 died. The culprit was cryptosporidium, a bacteria found in cattle feces. Cryptosporidium is resistant to chlorine. The Milwaukee incident was the largest outbreak of a water-born disease in United States history. Smaller outbreaks occur all the time. Just three months after the Milwaukee incident, the water of tens of thousands of New Yorkers was found to contain unhealthy levels of bacteria. At least six other states have also had major outbreaks of the bacteria. A recent report indicates that cryptosporidium may be present to some degree in every water supply in the country.

In an effort to make our drinking water safe, municipal water supplies are routinely treated with chlorine, aluminum, and other disinfectants to kill microorganisms. Water treatment has eliminated the danger of cholera, typhoid fever, and other deadly diseases that were prominent in the past. But is our water safe to drink?

Even though water is treated to remove most disease-causing microorganisms and parasites, it does not remove them all. Our household water, including our drinking water, comes to us from reservoirs by way of treatment plants. This water is replenished by streams, rain, and groundwater as well as household wastewater and drainage from lawns, streets, and sewers. All waste—including chemicals commonly used around the home, like pesticides, fertilizers, drain cleaners, soap, detergent, ammonia—that is flushed down the drain finds its way into the public water supply. Wastewater treatment plants are designed to remove organic human wastes, not man-made pesticides or other chemicals. When these chemicals pass through the plant, toxins remain in the stream flow. It also does not remove all industrial pollution, waste, chemical fertilizers, or pesticides. Recently the Environmental Protection Agency (EPA) issued warnings in eight Mid-Western states of contaminated water supplies due to high concentrations of herbicides. Water treatment itself contributes to contamination with the addition of dozens of chemicals including chlorine, aluminum, and fluoride all of which are highly poisonous. When we drink water from the tap we are, in fact, getting a chemical soup detrimental to health.

According to a Ralph Nader study, drinking water in the United States contains more than 2,100 toxic chemicals. Some of these include volatile organic chemicals, which are specifically regulated by the Environmental Protection Agency (EPA). Although the EPA has published maximum contaminant levels for these chemicals, it recommends a zero contamination level in drinking water for seven that are known or suspected to be highly toxic. Two of these,

Is Your Water Safe?

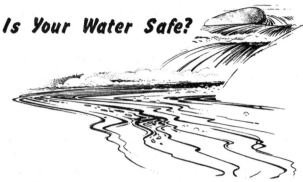

Water from rain and snow in the Rocky Mountains of North America flows either east or west of the continental divide. All the major rivers on the west side of the continental divide drain to the west and eventually into the Pacific Ocean. The rivers on the east flow toward the Mississippi River and Gulf Coast. It is from these rivers that water for drinking and agricultural use for most of the continent is derived.

The state of Colorado is bisected by the continental divide. Snows which accumulate in the Colorado peaks provide water for much of the United States. A recent study by the U.S. Geological Survey has reported that tributaries in Colorado contain as much as 30 different pesticides. The chemicals diazinon, alachlor, and cyanazine were found at levels above the safe drinking water limits. At least three herbicides—atrazine, simazine, and prometon—were detected year-round, regardless of the season or stream-flow volume. What's most alarming is that the headwaters in the Rocky Mountains are already dangerously polluted before they are even used for drinking or agriculture. The problem is compounded because the farther the waters flows toward the ocean, the more pollutants they pick up from runoff of pesticides, herbicides, and industrial waste. So the rest of the country which depends on this water is getting a heavily polluted soup. Fish from these waters, likewise, are contaminated.

Some people may feel protected because they use well water or eat crops irrigated from underground reservoirs. But they don't stop to think where this water comes from. Subsurface reservoirs are filled by penetrating surface water—the same polluted water in our streams and rivers.

Source: *Environmental Science & Technology*, vol. 30, no. 3, 1996

---

benzene and vinyl chloride, are known carcinogens.

The EPA recognizes three major contaminants in drinking water: (1) microbes (viruses, bacteria, parasites); (2) chemicals (inorganic, such as lead and nitrate, and organic, such as benzene); and (3) disinfection byproducts (what chlorine produces, for example, when it reacts with the residue of organic debris, such as leaves). The most common contaminants that are linked to health problems are bacteria, lead, nitrate, radium, and disinfection byproducts. The EPA does not consider chlorine and other harmful substances *purposely* added to water to be contaminants.

Herbicides, pesticides, and nitrates (from fertilizers) are toxic chemicals that enter our water supply through runoff of cultivated farmland, maintenance of golf courses and parks, as well as our own chemically treated lawns. In children under a year old, nitrates can cause "blue-baby syndrome," a potentially fatal blood disorder. These agricultural chemicals soak into the soil and into streams to contaminate groundwater, which in turn, contaminate water receivers used for drinking.

Toxic heavy metals such as lead, mercury, arsenic, and aluminum, and radioactive minerals from radium or uranium, can also be found at dangerously high levels. Some of these are removed in the filtration process, but the smaller microscopic particles are not. Lead is of particular concern because it can enter the water supply after water has left the filtration plant while traveling through service pipes to your house and through household plumbing. Lead might be leached from solder in your pipes or in the supply line leading to your house. The EPA recently identified excess levels of lead in 819 water systems that serve 30 million people. Identifying problems does not necessarily stop them. These people are still drinking contaminated water despite the fact that a problem was found. Lead interferes with brain development in children and damages the kidneys. It can also cause learning disorders and behavior problems.

Bacteria can infect water after it has left the filtration plant despite being treated with chemicals, as in the case of the cryptosporidium bacteria that caused the Milwaukee outbreak. Bacteria is the biggest concern as it can cause immediate health problems. For this reason chlorine and other disinfectants are added to water supplies.

We are told that the benefits of chlorine outweigh its risks. Chlorine kills the bacteria that used to cause epidemics of cholera, typhoid, and other illnesses. But this does not erase the fact that chlorine is also poisonous to humans. Although the risk of immediate harm is small because of the low concentration, its long-term consumption over the course of time is of great concern. Not only is chlorine itself harmful, but chlorine byproducts are recognized by the EPA as a source of contamination. Chlorine reacts chemically with organic matter that naturally occurs in water to produce carcinogenic compounds. Several long-term health studies have suggested increased cancer rates among drinkers of chlorinated water. Evidence also links chlorine to bladder and rectal cancer, heart disease, and stroke.

Exposure to chlorine is not limited just to drinking water, but also includes absorption and inhalation. Chlorine and other chemicals are absorbed through the skin while showering or bathing. In a 10-minute shower, the body can absorb the equivalent amount of chlorine contained in eight glasses of drinking water. An additional threat, particularly while showering, is inhaling chloroform gas, a toxic chlorine byproduct.

Using a well for your water needs will help you avoid chlorine, but will not prevent contamination. Bacteria is always a threat, especially in areas where there is livestock. Groundwater which feeds wells is often just as contaminated as any other water. The likelihood of contamination is greatest if the well is within a few miles of a farm (a source of pesticides, herbicides, chemical fertilizers, and animal waste), gas station, refinery, chemical plant, landfill, or military base. These sources not only contaminate our ground water but our reservoirs as well. Nowadays, no water is safe.

AIR CONTAMINATION

"Britain has run out of fresh air," reported *The Daily Telegraph*. Some 11,000 Britons die annually from car-

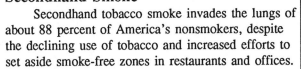

Secondhand Smoke

Secondhand tobacco smoke invades the lungs of about 88 percent of America's nonsmokers, despite the declining use of tobacco and increased efforts to set aside smoke-free zones in restaurants and offices.

Blood samples from 10,642 people, ages four and over, indicated there is almost universal exposure to tobacco smoke, even among people who do not smoke nor work or live around people who do, according to a recent study. —UPI News Service

induced air pollution. Professor Stuart Penkett, of the University of East Anglia, warned: "Motor cars are changing the chemistry of the whole of our background atmosphere." The World Health Organization says: "Around a half of all city dwellers in Europe and North America are exposed to unacceptably high levels of carbon monoxide."

The pollution of our air is one of the most serious health threats we face. Air pollution can affect us no matter how hard we try to avoid it. A factory can spew out noxious debris miles away, and the toxic elements can drift down and engulf you without warning. We all know the health hazards of smoking. Even second-hand smoke can have the same adverse effects on those who do not smoke. Pollution from factory and automobile exhaust is relatively easy to identify and sometimes smell, but there are many other air pollutants just as hazardous which we can not smell or are undetectable. Carbon monoxide is an odorless gas emitted by automobiles, home furnaces, gas stoves, and other appliances. This gas is highly poisonous.

Since we breathe polluted air all the time, we have come to regard it as just a part of life. We usually see no immediate effects resulting from the inhalation of these pollutants other than perhaps a few sniffles, occasional coughs, or headaches, and so we ignore the danger. But pollutants in the air from industry, automobiles, cigarettes, as well as household chemicals, can have a devastating effect on your health. Like chemicals in our water and food additives, the effects are not immediate, but over time can have serious consequences.

James Fraly, M.D., Medical Director of the Immuno Labs in Fort Lauderdale, Florida, recalls treating one hay fever patient who felt as though he were under attack from all sides. "He was sniffling, which he remarked was his permanent reaction to pollen, dust, cigarette smoke, and the sulfites found in many foods. His hands were covered with a fiery rash, and he was having frightening bouts of light-headedness. He'd been to several doctors already and was leery of adding even more medications to the several he was already taking."

Dr. Fraly traced the man's light-headedness to petrochemicals in the drapes and rug of his new office. He began a program of aggressive supplementation to boost his immunity and the offending drapes and rug were replaced with slatted blinds and tile.

"Eight months later, the patient's symptoms were so improved that for the first time in his life he didn't have to carry around a packet of Kleenex like a security blanket."

People don't realize how dangerous some household products are until a serious incident occurs. One morning Al and Gail Bustaque noticed as they were getting up that the van which belonged to their 16-year old son, Freddy, was still parked in the driveway. Freddy, a bright, articulate, computer whiz, normally left in the morning for his summer job before his parents awoke. Thinking Freddy overslept, Al went to Freddy's room.

Al called his son's name as he knocked on the door. There was no reply. He called again as he opened the door. Sprawled across the bed Freddy lay face up, still dressed in the clothes he'd worn the night before. Freddy's body was cold and lifeless.

During the tragic ordeal, Al noticed a spray can of air freshener nearby on his son's bed. Later, an autopsy revealed that Freddy died from inhaling fumes from the air freshener. The toxic chemicals that formed the gas propellant for the spray had stopped his heart. A death such as Freddy's is called sudden sniffing death (SSD). Many people try to get a cheap high by inhaling, or "huffing," household products. Too much huffing as well as accidental exposure can lead to SSD.

Household, as well a industrial, chemicals can damage crucial cells in the liver and kidneys, impairing the ability of these organs to function properly. The liver and the kidneys are the body's two main organs of detoxification. If they do not work efficiently, our bodies will accumulate seriously high levels of toxins.

Damage caused by household chemicals, in some cases, is irreversible. Dr. Milton Tenenbein, a pediatrician and toxicologist at the Children's Hospital in Winnipeg, Canada, has been treating people exposed to heavy doses of household chemicals for almost 20 years. In addition to the brain damage typically associated with huffing, he's seen a variety of effects such as deafness and lung and kidney damage. He also notes that in some cases a person's arms and legs can become paralyzed because of a condition known as peripheral neuropathy—after just six months of heavy exposure. Those who are paralyzed can get better, he says, although it can take as long as two years. Those with brain damage are not so lucky. According to Tenenbein, if you are exposed to these chemicals long enough, it's not a question of *if*, but *when* you will suffer irreversible brain damage. Incidental exposure to chemicals can be just as dangerous as huffing.

Most of us are unaware that the fumes of simple household products such as air fresheners are poisonous. After all, air fresheners are supposed to "clean" the air and make it more breathable. Our homes are filled with a myriad of toxic chemicals that can be deadly. Fumes from products such as felt-tip markers, lighter fluid, glue, typewriter correction fluid, paint, paint thinners, gasoline, aerosols, cleansers, detergents, fabric softeners, bug spray, etc. as well as residual chemicals and particles in carpets, drapes, cleaners, fiberglass insulation, plastics, wallpaper, paneling, solder, and other building materials. Each by

itself generally poses little threat if exposure is brief and very small. But if you are exposed to a relatively large amount, as Freddy was, they can cause immediate illness or death. Exposure to small amounts over a long time have an accumulative effect. Eventually symptoms will surface as the body's defenses weaken. The resulting symptoms depend on the types of chemicals as well as other factors such as lifestyle and diet. For this reason, environmental illnesses caused by air pollution are usually attributed to aging, genetics, a virus, or some other factor beyond our control and, therefore, there is nothing you can do about it except to suppress the symptoms and continue living as you have been until you die, or so we are told.

If you live or work in a building made from standard construction materials and use chemical household products, you are being exposed to air contamination. Combined with the exhaust from cars and factories and cigarette smoke, we are continuously exposed to enormous levels of pollutants. Unless you live out in the country miles from any civilization and in a home made of all natural products and use no aerosols or other chemical contrivances, it is impossible to avoid air pollution.

BODY CARE AND HOUSEHOLD PRODUCTS

We are exposed to dangerous levels of toxins with common products we use everyday. Some of these products are put in our mouths; others on our skin. In either case poisons penetrate our skin or mucous membranes and enter our blood stream.

Many of our everyday body care and household products are health hazards. Baby shampoo, for example, is touted as being gentle enough that you can use it on babies without worry. Because it doesn't burn their eyes, it must be good, right? Wrong! This gives a false sense of

Risks in the Workplace
The Danish Cancer Registry states that a twenty-year study shows women who handle dry-cleaning compounds have an almost five times greater incidence of liver cancer. Nurses working the cancer wards in hospitals had an almost ten times greater risk of leukemia. This is from handling anti-cancer drugs routinely used in cancer cases. Smoking, as you would expect, however, was by far the greatest risk hazard.
—*The HealthKeepers Journal*, Vol. 16, N. 6.

security as baby shampoo is very harsh on the eyes; the reason it does not burn is because manufacturers have added anesthetics—pain killers—which attack and deaden the nerves so pain messages are not relayed to the brain. This is not unique to shampoo, but is used in many common products. Air fresheners, the type that killed Freddy, do not freshen the air or remove foul odors. All they do is mask the smell with perfume and deaden the sense of smell with anesthetics.

Another ingredient commonly found in household and toiletry products is mercury. Mercury is the most toxic inorganic heavy metal known to man. Its effects are enormously widespread and really leave no part or system of the body untouched. Exposure to mercury through its numerous industrial and commercial uses (including hair dye, mascara, and skin creams) accounts for significant accumulation in our bodies. Studies have shown that mercury affects the kidneys, brain, heart, intestines, liver, testes, ovaries, and pancreas as well as thyroid, adrenal, and pituitary glands. The entire immune system is affected, thus lowering the body's ability to maintain health.

A recent study by the Fred Hutchinson Cancer Research Center in Seattle, Washington, has linked ovarian cancer with genital products. The study compared 735 women, ages 20 to 79. The group included 313 women diagnosed with ovarian cancer and 422 randomly selected women with no history of ovarian cancer. The study found that women who use genital deodorant sprays and powders had as much as a 50 percent higher risk for developing ovarian cancer.

Only a few items have been mentioned here, but how many products do you use at home or at work that have been made with plastic, glue, paint, varnish, and other chemical compounds? Not all may be harmful, but a good many are, and their combined effect can and does cause environmental illness.

ENVIRONMENTAL HORMONES

Hormones are chemicals secreted by organs to control bodily functions and development. The secretion of too much or too little of any hormone can have serious consequences and can lead to a variety of abnormalities. For example, secretion of growth hormone controls the rate of physical growth. Too much growth hormone results in gigantism and too little in dwarfism. Production and secretion of the proper amount are vital to our health. It is almost impossible to exaggerate their importance. Hormones are the main regulators of metabolism, growth and development, reproduction, and many other body activities. They play important roles in maintaining homeostasis, or

Hysterectomy

Every year 750,000 American women undergo hysterectomies. In fact, it's the most frequently performed major surgery in the United States. If the trend continues, one out of every three women in the United States will have had a hysterectomy by the time she reaches her 60th birthday.

Complications occur in up to half of all patients following hysterectomies, and of those patients, six hundred women die each year.

equilibrium, within the body. They are important not only for the healthy survival of each one of us but also for the survival of the human species.

A great many disease conditions exist today due to the over- or undersecretion of hormones including: Graves' disease, cretinism, goiter, hypocalcemia, diabetes, Addison's disease, Cushing's syndrome, hypoglycemia, osteoporosis, infertility, mental illness, allergies, and many others too numerous to list. When the sex hormones, testosterone, estrogen, and progesterone are out of balance, numerous abnormalities can exist in the reproductive system. Imbalances in parents can also affect the health of unborn children, creating in them not only deformities and dysfunctional tissues at birth, but predisposing them to many types of disease later in life.

Why is the hormonal production in some people out of balance with nature? Conditions causing hormonal imbalances have increased dramatically over the past few decades. It is apparent that this worldwide problem is a product of modern civilization.

Pollutants in our food and environment have a pronounced effect on hormone production and secretion. Chemicals which mimic estrogen, a female hormone, are widespread in our environment. Environmental estrogens are derived, in part, from polychlorinated biphenyls (PCBs), plastics, solvents, fungicides, and pesticides. The use of these materials is found everywhere. Pesticides are dumped by the ton on farmland as well as home gardens and lawns, contaminating our land, our food, and our water supply. Plastics are found everywhere. They seem to be a component of almost everything—cars, furniture, toys, clothes, dishes, water containers, electronic equipment, plastic bags, food containers, etc. Although plastic appears to be harmless, minute particles are continually released into the air and on anything it comes in contact with. If you can smell the plastic in an object, you know that tiny particles are being released into the air or your smell sensors would not be able to register it. Fill a plastic jug full of water and let it sit for a couple of hours. When you drink it, you can taste the plastic leached from the container. Plastic finds its way into dump yards and streams, and is scattered virtually all over the countryside. These environmental toxins work their way into our food supply. The overabundance of estrogen-like compounds in the environment alone has had drastic effects on wildlife and human health.

The first indication that estrogen-like chemicals could affect men appeared in studies of wild animals. In 1947, ornithologists noticed that eagles in Florida had lost their drive to mate and nest. In the 1960s, ranch minks that were fed fish from Lake Michigan failed to reproduce. In 1977, female gulls in California were nesting with females. In the 1980s a researcher at the University of Florida discovered that pesticide runoff led to elevated estrogen levels which caused the underdevelopment of sex organs in male alligators. Other researchers reported that pesticide exposure led to larger female populations of Western gulls and sterility in males. Laboratory experiments have since confirmed that estrogen imitators encourage feminine characteristics in animals.

These effects are not limited to just wildlife. In 1992, Danish researchers announced that human sperm counts worldwide had plunged by 50 percent between 1938 and 1990. Studies of children whose mothers ate PCB-laced fish during pregnancy find IQ deficits of about four points and abnormalities such as attention deficit disorder. PCBs, which mimic thyroid hormones, have a profound effect on the developing brain.

Although some hormone-mimicking pesticides, such as DDT which has not been used agriculturally in the United States since 1972 and is also banned in many other Western countries, are widely used around the world to spray food crops, much of the produce grown with the use of DDT is imported into the United States and other Western countries, so banning its use has not protected us. DDT does not degrade quickly and even after more than 20 years it is still found as a contaminant in water and agricultural land. DDT, however, is only one of dozens of actively used man-made chemicals that have the ability to mimic powerful natural hormones.

Wildlife as well as domesticated animals raised for meat and dairy production are exposed to estrogen-like chemicals in the environment. Animals raised commercially for meat are also given estrogens in their feed to promote weight gain. Significant amounts of these chemicals, when digested by animals, are stored in their fatty tissues. When we eat animal fat in meat and milk products, we are consuming these hormone-disrupting chemicals.

Testicular cancer, while relatively rare, is the most common type of cancer among men ages 15 to 35, and its worldwide incidence has increased as much as fourfold since 1940. During this same period—since the introduction of synthetic estrogens into the environment—incidence of undescended testicles in young men has doubled and sperm counts have dropped by 50 percent. In addition to diet, researchers have also fingered environmental estrogens as a cause of prostate enlargement, prostate cancer, and other male reproductive cancers.

In women, these chemicals may cause a relative progesterone deficiency which also contributes to a rising incidence of female reproductive problems, including endometriosis, PMS, infertility, fibroids, and bleeding and difficult menopause. Exposure to estrogen-like contaminants also increases the risk of breast cancer and cancer of the reproductive system. Is it any wonder why mastectomies and hysterectomies are the most common surgeries performed on women?

Pregnant women not only run a risk for themselves, but also for the unborn baby whose development can be severely affected by these chemicals.

Synthetic estrogen is also found in some drugs. "If pollutants are acting as estrogens, their effects may parallel those of the notorious drug diethylstilbestrol (DES)," observed John Rennie in *Scientific American*. DES, given to women from 1948 to 1971 to prevent miscarriage, was banned because it increased the risk of breast cancer in the daughters of these women. It also predisposed them to reproductive problems. As it turns out, the sons of women who took DES suffer an above average incidence of reproductive disorders including undescended testicles, penile deformities, and testicular cancer.

Many synthetic chemicals polluting the environment can imitate estrogenic hormones, notes Niels E. Skakkebaek, MD, an endocrinologist at the University of Copenhagen, Denmark. One of the estrogen links comes from similarities among the sons of women treated with DES. As early as the 1970s, Skakkebaek noticed that many male patients with reproductive malformations eventually developed testicular cancer. He found that some of the abnormal, precancerous cells from children were similar to fetal cells, suggesting that something went wrong while they were still in the womb. Many people whose parents were exposed to estrogen-like chemicals may be predisposed to reproductive and developmental problems. If they too are exposed to environmental hormones or other toxins, they run the risk of developing reproductive disease as well as passing on to their children inherent weaknesses that would predispose them to a similar fate.

Dietary and environmental estrogen-like chemicals can contribute to a variety of reproductive and health problems in men, women, and unborn children. Endometriosis is one such condition that is growing more and more common among women. Endometriosis occurs when tissue similar to that which normally lines the inside of the uterus grows in parts of the body where it shouldn't. This happens most commonly in the bottommost part of the pelvis, the uterine ligaments, the outside surface of the uterus, tubes, and ovaries, the lower end of the large bowel, and on the membranes covering the bladder. It is a chronic, often painful, disease that can lead to infertility. There are usually only two avenues open to women to treat this problem, harsh expensive drugs or complicated surgery. Drugs include synthetic progesterone (provera), a synthetic male hormone known as danazol, and a new class of drugs known as hormonal drugs, such as lupron and synarel. These drugs cause certain areas in the pituitary gland to shut down. The net effect of this new class of drugs is a severe pseudo-menopause and bone loss. These drugs may

Dietary Hormones

The author of *Modern Meat*, Orville Schell, interviewed Dr. Carmen A Saenz, a physician working in Puerto Rico, regarding abnormal sexual development and disease in children:

"'For years I have been encountering periodic cases of precocious puberty,' Dr. Saenz tells me when she is finished seeing the last of that morning's young patients. 'But in 1980, when I started finding one or two children like this in my waiting room every day, I knew that something quite serious was wrong. From the symptoms they were exhibiting, I was sure that they were being contaminated with some kind of estrogen.'

"I ask Dr. Saenz to describe the symptoms. Without replying, she picks up a handful of Polaroid photos from the top of her desk and hands them to me. Each shows the small body of a naked young girl. As I slowly thumb through them, Dr. Saenz gives me a case-by-case commentary in a tone of voice that matches the expression on her face—a mixture of outrage, sadness, and determination.

"In the first photo, a four-and-a-half-year-old girl with delicate coffee-colored skin, doelike brown eyes and almost fully developed breasts lies on an examining table. She smiles with a sweet innocence at the camera, seemingly unaware of the dramatic changes that have gone on in her body.

"'She had an ovarian cyst,' says Dr. Saenz tersely.

"A twelve-year-old boy stands against a white wall looking with blank bewilderment into the camera. He wears a silver crucifix around his neck, which dangles down between two grossly swollen breasts.

"'We've had to schedule him for surgery,' says Dr. Saenz matter-of-factly. 'A one-year-old girl, whose teeth have not even completely come in, lies on the examining table with a ruler stretched across her chest to measure the diameter of her enlarged breasts. She has a pacifier in one of her hands. Dr. Saenz says nothing. She just shakes her head.

"A five-year-old girl, looking wild-eyed into the camera as if a weapon were being aimed at her, lies on the examining table. Her breasts are as large and well-developed as a fourteen-year-old's...'This one had a well-developed uterus and had begun to have some vaginal bleeding,' says Dr. Saenz. 'These are developments that we would not usually expect until eight or nine years of age at the very earliest...I have seen hundreds of children like this, and I am certain that there are thousands more going undiagnosed because this problem has become so widespread that even many doctors are no longer getting alarmed about it.'"

Dr. Saenz explained that the cause of premature sexual development was due to medications or creams containing estrogen, and the consumption of milk, poultry, and beef. Livestock are routinely given hormones to bulk them up and to stimulate milk and egg production in dairy cows and chickens. Estrogen-like chemicals from pesticides also contaminate their feed. These artificial estrogens, unlike natural estrogens, do not break down easily and collect in fatty tissues of animals and humans.

When Dr. Saenz was asked how she could be sure the children were contaminated with hormones from meat and milk rather than from some other source, she replied:

"When we take our patients off meat and fresh milk, their symptoms usually regress."

relieve pain, but they also contribute to the toxic load already in the body. They don't cure the problem and may eventually make it worse.

No one knows exactly what causes endometriosis; it is generally thought to be the result of an autoimmune disease. A newer theory is that this condition is the result of cells left behind during fetal development. Later on, certain triggers activate the disease. Those triggers could include environmental contaminants such as dioxin and other industrial chemicals, radiation, stress, diet high in meat and dairy, vitamin and mineral deficiencies, chronic yeast infections, or hormonal imbalances.

Studies performed by the Environmental Protection Agency and The Endometriosis Association have shown direct correlation between endometriosis and dioxin (a common estrogen-like industrial solvent). A notable example was a long-term study on the effects of adding dioxin to the food of monkeys. They found that 79 percent of the monkeys exposed to dioxin developed endometriosis. The disease increased in severity in direct proportion to the amount of dioxin exposure.

Many industrial chemicals cause adverse estrogen-like effects. Thus an unintended side effect of industrialization is an environment that bathes its inhabitants in a sea of pollutants that can cause hormonal imbalances and disease.

SPONTANEOUS HEALING

Rebecca consulted three gynecologists after experiencing chronic pain and bleeding from endometriosis as well as a benign ovarian tumor. Their diagnoses were unanimously in favor of a hysterectomy, the surgical removal of the uterus, fallopian tubes, and cervix, and a bilateral oophorectomy, the removal of both ovaries. The night before she was to go into the hospital, a friend handed her a book on natural health. She spent the evening reading.

"That night I made the decision to follow the program outlined in the book and see what it would do for me," says Rebecca. "It took courage to back out of the operation, but the next day I told my doctor, 'I know where your office is. If this doesn't work, I'll be back.' His response was, 'You have to live with your condition. It's your body.' And I said, 'That's it exactly. It's my body.'"

The program Rebecca followed stressed detoxifying the body, removing harmful poisons, and preventing additional ones from entering her system. Central to this program was her diet. She eliminated most meat, dairy, and sugar products and concentrated on preparing low-fat meals centered around foods rich in complex carbohydrates.

"I'll never forget my first meal," she says. "I cooked brown rice, butternut soup, and daikon radishes. I didn't really believe it would work, but I figured, what do I have to lose? The amazing thing is, I started feeling better within 24 hours, and that gave me the motivation to stick with it."

Three months later, she was examined by her doctor. "He said, 'Frankly, I'm amazed. Endometriosis doesn't reverse itself; however, I can't find any of the nodules from when I examined you last time.'"

Rebecca continued with her detoxification program which, besides diet, included hot mineral baths, exercise, and mental visualization among other things. "I put all these positive things together, and it worked," says Rebecca. "I healed myself, I lost weight and was happier. It was a turning point in my life."

Eating nutritious foods and living a healthy lifestyle saved Rebecca from the pain of undergoing surgery, the $40,000-plus hospital expenses, and being dependent on costly hormone supplements for the rest of her life. It sounds too easy, but it's true.

The stories of Carrie, Neva, Rick, and Doris mentioned at the beginning of this chapter are typical examples of people struck with degenerative disease and the agony it caused them and their families. Cancer, heart disease, diabetes, and other degenerative conditions can affect anyone at any age. Most people live out their lives relying on medications and surgery to keep them alive. As a consequence, they suffer great pain and financial loss with medical care until the day they die. For many people who are incapacitated or in pain, death is a welcome relief.

We should not have to suffer degenerative diseases and pain and agony until we die. We should live life with energy, relatively symptom free, and happy.

Some people do live long, active, healthy lives without suffering any debilitating degenerative condition. Others, like Rebecca, recover from serious degenerative diseases and live symptom free for the rest of their lives—without surgery, pain, or medications. Rebecca's case is not unusual, it happens all the time. Doctors call it spontaneous healing. Spontaneous healings are what modern medicine refers to when incurable cancer suddenly goes away, or a cyst inexplicably disappears, or a lifelong symptom mysteriously vanishes. Because doctors can't explain why these so-called miracle recoveries happen—or duplicate the results at will—such incidents are ignored.

> Modern Americans and Britons have 1,000 times more lead in their bones than did preindustrial peoples who lived a millennium ago. —*Science News*

Why can some people spontaneously recover without any medical treatment, while others, with similar conditions, get the best medical care available, suffer, and die?

DETOXIFICATION IS THE ANSWER

We will never be able to clean our environment from the mess we have made of it. We may be able to make it better, but toxic chemicals are everywhere. Even if there was suddenly a worldwide ban on all toxic chemicals, residue would remain for decades, perhaps even centuries. Since we cannot completely remove toxins from our environment, nor can we completely avoid them in our everyday life, we must learn to deal with them the best we can. We can do this by making sensible lifestyle choices and using periodic detoxification methods. Detoxification will purge harmful substances from your body, including poisons that may have been accumulating for decades.

The body has an amazing capacity to heal itself. We get a cut, break a bone, tear a muscle, or get a bacterial infection, and the body immediately goes to work to repair the damage. We develop symptoms (mucus discharge, fever, coughing, vomiting, diarrhea, fatigue, etc.) to fight and remove harmful substances. The body knows what to do in every case—no matter how old it is. The only time the body makes mistakes (such as in autoimmune diseases) is when it is over-encumbered with toxins, or functionally damaged by injury or other negative factors which alter the body's normal processes. If the body is healthy, it can quickly heal injury and ward off countless diseases without suffering symptoms of sickness. When our bodies are weakened by toxic accumulation and stress, and lack essential nutrients, our resistance to infection is decreased, sickness is more severe and more frequent, and recovery is slow.

Given the chance, the body will eliminate harmful toxins that weaken our immune system and cause degenerative conditions to develop. The body will heal, replacing damaged, diseased tissues with new healthy cells. But as long as irritating contaminants remain in the tissues and new toxins are continually added, recovery is impossible. Surgically removing a cancerous growth, for example, from one part of the body may relieve pain, but will not eliminate the cause of the cancer. The disease-causing factors remain, irritating other tissues, and eventually the cancer returns. Removing the symptoms of disease does not cure the disease. The only way to remove the cause of degenerative disease is to allow the body to cleanse itself. Surgery won't do this, drugs won't do this, radiation won't do this. It has to be done internally.

A poor diet is a major cause of illness and physical and mental deterioration. By making proper dietary choices, you will get stronger and healthier. For some people, a simple dietary change may be all they need to overcome annoying health problems. But for others, diet alone may not be enough. If toxic accumulation has been going on in the body for many years, degeneration has progressed to such a state that dietary changes alone may be too slow and even ineffective. This is especially true for serious degenerative conditions that are routinely treated today by prescription drugs or surgery.

Using a variety of drugless natural detoxification methods, harmful poisons can be extracted from the body and eliminated. The body then can repair and rebuild itself with healthy tissues, thus overcoming deteriorating conditions.

How do you know if you need to detoxify your body? If you have any serious degenerative condition like those mentioned in this chapter, you have a toxic accumulation problem. But most people have not experienced any "serious" or life-threatening health problems; does that mean they are in good health? No! If you eat a diet composed of typical grocery store and restaurant foods, chances are you are in serious need of detoxification. If you have any degenerative health problems, no matter how minor they may seem, you have excess toxins stored in your body. Some of the symptoms of toxic overload include: constipation, fatigue, skin problems (acne, psoriasis, eczema), back pain, body odor, bad breath, poor digestion, gas, excess body weight, poor memory, depression, allergies, frequent illnesses (ear infections, colds, etc.), irritability, restlessness, quarrelsomeness, lack of endurance, reproductive problems, and any other annoying condition that a "healthy" body should not have. Through detoxification you can rid yourself of these dis-ease conditions and enjoy symptom-free health for life.

The detoxification methods discussed in this book have been used successfully for years, some for centuries, to overcome health problems. Detoxification can help those with chronic fatigue, ulcers, fibrocystic breast disease, chronic headaches, hypertension, heart disease, diabetes, yeast infections, premenstrual problems, hyperactivity, multiple sclerosis, atherosclerosis, skin rashes, allergies, respiratory problems, leg aches, hearing loss, senility, vertigo, arthritis, gout, kidney stones, osteoporosis, acne, constipation, numerous forms of cancer, and other degenerative conditions.

The methods described in this book are all harmless, yet effective, means of internal cleansing that can be self-administered. Not only will they stop or reverse deterioration, but they will strengthen your immune system, allowing it to fight off infectious diseases, thus reducing your chance of getting colds, flu, and other infectious illnesses. Body chemistry, too, will return to normal, allowing for the production of enzymes, hormones, antibodies, and other substances in the proper amounts and at the proper times. The entire body will work and function as it was designed to do. You will look younger, feel better, have more energy and more vitality, and think clearer than you have for years.

In the following chapters, you will learn what foods cause health problems and contribute to degeneration. You will see how and why toxins build up in the body. You will learn which foods reverse degeneration, and the methods of detoxifying and purging the body of harmful substances. You will also learn about the "healing crisis" which is greatly misunderstood by conventional medical practitioners who see it only as symptoms of disease that must be suppressed with drugs. You will learn how to initiate a healing crisis and how to recognize it. Most of all, you will learn the process by which the body heals itself.

Please keep in mind that the detoxification programs described in this book are not offered as *cures* for disease. They are designed to support and encourage the body's own inherent healing power to accomplish this task. There is no procedure, no vitamin, no herb, or drug that can cure disease. Cure comes only through the body's natural healing processes. The programs suggested in this book are aimed at assisting in these processes by eliminating the causes of disease and creating conditions that encourage the body's own healing forces to bring about healing.

The purpose of this book is not meant to replace sound medical care but is provided as a means of helping you take control of your health and give you new hope for a better life and better future. Modern medicine has an amazing capacity to deal with trauma and emergency situations, including dangerously advanced degenerative disease for which natural treatment might be too slow to resolve. Serious medical problems should not be self-diagnosed, but brought to the attention of a competent medical practitioner.

 ## ADDITIONAL RESOURCES

Body/Mind Purification Program. Chaitow, Leon, N.D., D.O. New York: Simon & Schuster, 1990.

How to Survive in America the Poisoned. Regenstein, Lewis. Herndon, VA: Acropolis Books, 1982.

Our Stolen Future. Colborn, Theo; Dumanoski, Dianne; Myers, John Peterson. New York: Dutton, 1996.

Silent Spring. Carson, Rachel. Boston: Houghton Mifflin, 1962.

Pesticides and the Living Landscape. Rudd, Robert. Madison, Wisconsin: University of Wisconsin Press, 1968.

The Withering Rain. Whiteside, Thomas. New York: E.P. Dutton, 1971.

Chapter 2

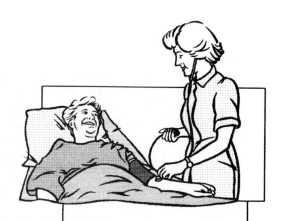

THE GENESIS OF DISEASE

MECHANISMS FOR DISEASE

According to standard medical philosophy, the mechanisms that cause all disease are: biologic organisms, genetics, degeneration, autoimmunity, abnormal growths, inflammation, physical and chemical agents, and malnutrition.

The mechanism that is credited with causing the most disease and upon which most treatments focus is biologic organisms. Biologic organisms include viruses, bacteria, fungi, protozoa, and pathologic animals such as parasites. Since the discovery of the "germ" by Louis Pasteur in the mid-nineteenth century, microorganisms have been blamed for nearly every ill of mankind. The concept of pathologic organisms causing disease became so prevalent that it even overcame common sense. A century ago almost all disease was considered caused by these creatures. Antibiotics and other germ-fighting medicines quickly became popular. Allopathic medicine achieved great success fighting tuberculosis, cholera, pneumonia, and a host other diseases by using these drugs. The great success drugs achieved in halting biologically-caused disease was phenomenal. At first, much good was accomplished. But the medical profession focused too much on germs as the cause of disease, and other forms of medical treatment (herbology, homeopathy, etc.) were ignored.

In the late 19th century, the practice of polishing rice became widely popular. Polishing rice removed the vitamin-rich outer layers of the grains and made them whiter and more pleasing to people. As this practice became widespread, a rare disease called beriberi spread like a plague throughout the Far East. Beriberi is characterized by swelling, tissue degeneration, pain, loss of strength, involuntary nervous twitching, mental confusion, paralysis, and heart failure. Rice comprised the staple diet for most people in these countries. The poor who subsisted primarily on polished rice and fish were the most affected. No one knew the cause of the disease.

Because it was believed that germs were responsible for most all illness, beriberi was first believed to be the result of some pathogenic microorganism. Medical researchers wasted much time and energy seeking a microbial cause before they realized that the problem was not a germ, but a lack of nutrients, specifically thiamin (vitamin B_1). Hundreds of thousands of people died from thiamin deficiency as a result of eating processed grains deficient of vital nutrients. Until this time, no one suspected that a lack of something in the diet could be the cause of disease. Thiamin as well as other vitamins are found in abundance in the hulls of the rice kernel, and people ate brown rice as a staple for centuries without suffering any nutritional diseases.

The ultimate cause of human disease is the consequence of our transgression of the universal laws of life.
— Paracelsus (1493-1541)

He's the best physician who know the worthlessness of most medicines.
— Benjamin Franklin

Age is no excuse for disease.
— Dr. M. Ted Morter, Jr.

Similar occurrences happened with wheat when the use of white flour became common. One notable case occurred among the Eskimos. A ship was wrecked in the Arctic, and upon salvaging the white flour, the Eskimos lived on this almost exclusively and soon developed beriberi. After returning to their normal diet, the disease disappeared. Because of the increasing incidence of beriberi and other nutritional diseases, instead of going back to the use of whole grains, manufacturers started adding synthetic vitamins to processed flours. That is why we have bread that is "fortified" with vitamins and minerals. Removing the bran of the wheat takes away some 20 nutrients, only four are added back, but the bread is labeled as "vitamin enriched." This so-called enriched bread lacks at least 16 nutrients as well as the fiber necessary for proper digestion.

The lack of Vitamin C has also caused widespread deficiencies. This was most common with sailors who subsisted on diets devoid of fruit and vegetables. Produce was used up in the early part of the journey, and for the rest of the time the diet consisted of biscuits and salted meat. Lack of vitamin C resulted in scurvy. Scurvy is characterized by bleeding gums, loosened teeth, muscle degeneration, pain, depression, bone fragility, and joint pain, and can lead to death. It was noted even before the discovery of vitamins that fresh produce would prevent and cure scurvy. Because of the many deficiency diseases caused by a lack of nutrients, nutrition has been recognized as an important factor in health and disease. Doctors, in general, have been reluctant in accepting diet as a major factor in health. They prefer to prescribe pills rather than wholesome foods.

From research over the past 150 years, it has become evident that germs are not the only cause for disease. Some conditions are clearly not caused by pathogenic organisms.

Babies born with problems provided evidence that some physical conditions are inherited. Another cause that has become popular with medical science is genetics. As more and more disease conditions occur that are not related to biologic origin, the answer is conveniently labeled as "genetic." The person was born this way, or was born with a predisposition to develop a certain condition. These so-called genetic diseases, rare a century ago, are running rampant today. In fact, it is estimated that most people have some genetic predisposition to disease or other inherent weakness. This makes a convenient excuse for the occurrence of diseases that have an otherwise unknown cause and no medical cure.

People who don't get sick or live long are explained away as having strong genes. Those who get sick often, die early, or acquire degenerative diseases are labeled inherently weak. The concept basically takes responsibility of health away from the individual and puts it in the hands of fate.

Only through drugs and surgery can these poor victims be saved from their misery. Drugs, however, only suppress the symptoms. The cause for the condition is not taken care of. Like the germ theory in which microbes can attack anyone at any time, genetic diseases can occur in anyone regardless of lifestyle.

Another mechanism of disease is attributed to degeneration. By some unknown means tissues begin to degenerate and fall apart. Degenerative disease is considered a normal consequence of aging. However, degeneration of organs and tissues, resulting in disease, can occur at any time in a person's life. The number of degenerative diseases has been skyrocketing over the past century. It is estimated that almost everyone will be affected by some type of degenerative disease in their lifetime. It is not limited to the elderly. Even children are becoming affected. It has become a major threat to health in industrialized countries. Interestingly, degenerative diseases are relatively rare in Third World countries.

Abnormal growths such as tumors and cancer are classified as a degenerative condition. Some medical experts attribute them to genetic causes, although more and more evidence has accumulated pointing to carcinogenic

Diabetes

The number of Americans developing diabetes has surged over the past decade, according to statistics released by the American Medical Association and the American Diabetes Association. The numbers have increased from 11 million during the early 1980s to 16 million today.

This growth in the incidence of diabetes is due, in part, to an increase in obesity, which increases risk. Many people are prediabetic or in the early stages of diabetes without even realizing it. The condition can often be controlled with diet and exercise. If not, daily oral medication or insulin injections may be necessary.

The conditions that cause diabetes often lead to many other complications. People with diabetes are 2.5 times more likely to have strokes than are those without diabetes—and they're two to four times more likely to develop cardiovascular disease; 60 to 65 percent of people with diabetes have high blood pressure; diabetes is the leading cause of new cases of blindness in adults 20 to 74 years old; it's also the leading cause of end-stage kidney disease; and 60 to 70 percent of diabetics have mild to severe forms of nerve disease.

—American Medical Association

or toxic chemicals in food and environment as the cause. The treatment is to remove the *symptoms* with drugs, surgery, and radiation and hope the cause goes away.

Another mechanism for disease is autoimmunity. Some diseases result from the immune system attacking the body or from mistakes or overreactions of the immune response. Allergies are the most common autoimmune disease. In other words, the body doesn't know what it is doing and makes mistakes.

A mechanism closely related to autoimmunity is inflammation. The inflammatory response is a normal mechanism that usually speeds recovery from an infection or injury. However, when the inflammatory response occurs at inappropriate times or is abnormally prolonged or severe, normal tissues may become damaged. Thus, some disease symptoms are caused by an inappropriate inflammatory response. The body is malfunctioning when this happens.

Physical and chemical agents are also recognized as a cause for disease. Agents, such as toxins or destructive chemicals, extreme heat or cold, mechanical injury, and radiation, can affect the normal functions of the body. It is interesting to note that all medical treatments involve methods which fit into this category. All drugs are foreign chemicals to the body and as such are toxic. All drugs have adverse side effects. But these effects are ignored because the philosophy is that the drug will do more good than harm. This, however, is not always true. Mechanical injury is caused by doctors during surgery. The skin and tissues are cut, organs are dissected and removed. Some of the organs are vital to health. The thyroid, for example, excretes hormones necessary for proper bodily functions; when it is removed, the hormones must be supplied by synthetic hormonal supplements which must be taken for the rest of the person's life. Similarly, other organs in the body that are removed cause deficiencies in normal body function. We all know that radiation is dangerous, but it is also used to treat patients. The philosophy is that radiation will kill mutating cancerous tissues, but if it kills these rapidly growing cells, what is it going to do with the healthy cells around it?

There is no denying the fact that toxins, mechanical injury, and radiation cause disease, but because these are the very methods by which doctors treat symptoms, little emphasis is put on them. The blame for the vast majority of disease is given to microorganisms, genetics, abnormal growths, degeneration, autoimmunity, and inflammation. The two primary causes for disease, malnutrition and chemical agents, are largely ignored.

Another cause is entirely overlooked by many, and that is excessive stress (physical and mental). Stress can cause physical injury (e.g., pulled muscles, broken bones, bruising, etc.), chemical imbalances (such as increasing acidity of body fluids), breakdown of the immune system, overworked organs, or it can drain vital nutrients from the body, as well as cause mental and emotional fatigue. Emotional trauma can have a drastic effect on physical health as well as mental health.

The underlying cause for all disease is malnutrition, toxic accumulation, and excess stress. The other mechanisms clung to by the medical establishment all play a part, but usually only as secondary factors. The real cause for disease, and consequently the solution, involves diet, detoxification, and stress reduction. The accumulation of toxins in the body and/or inadequate consumption of nutrients (vitamins, minerals, proteins, fats, carbohydrates, water, and phytochemicals) will cause the body to degenerate, leading to degenerative diseases, abnormal growths, autoimmunity dysfunction, inappropriate inflammatory response, and infections. These conditions are NOT the cause of disease, but a consequence of it! They are symptoms caused for the most part by malnutrition, excessive stress, or toxic accumulation in the body. By removing the toxins, reducing stress, and supplying essential nutrients, your body will heal itself from all of the conditions attributed to these other causes.

Cataracts

An estimated 46 percent of all people aged 75 to 85 have cataracts, and, as a result, cataract surgery has become the most common surgical procedure among people who are 65 years of age or older.

In fact, over 40,000 Americans will become blind in 1996 due to cataracts, the formation of many of which could have been prevented through proper nutrition.

A cataract is any yellowish fogging over the lens of the eye. Normally, the lens, situated behind the pupil, focuses light on the retina at the back of the eye to produce a sharp image. When a cataract forms, the lens becomes so opaque that light cannot be transmitted easily to the retina.

According to Anita M. Van Der Hagen, and colleagues, in an article which appeared in the *Journal of the American Optometric Association* (1993), "It is possible that the damage could be prevented or moderated by supplementing the diet with specific antioxidant vitamins and minerals that enhance the body's natural defenses against free radicals."

THE GENETIC CONNECTION

Many people are brainwashed into believing that genetics has control over their life. One of their parents had cancer, so they will have it too. This is a form of self-fulfilling prophecy. They program themselves to get cancer, or diabetes, arthritis, or any other disease, because they believe it is genetic and there is nothing they can do about it. This is a lie. Disease is not genetic, although we may have weaknesses that predispose certain target organs, they don't have to break down, but can do their job adequately for a lifetime if toxic thoughts are not allowed to interfere and the body is kept unpolluted.

Genetics is not the problem it is claimed to be. So-called genetic conditions are responding to dietary and detoxification treatments. Many doctors refuse to accept it, but it is happening.

This is not to say that genetics plays no role in our health, for it does. Some people are genetically stronger than others. A person with a strong constitution will have fewer illnesses and live longer than one who was born with a weaker genetic makeup. But if the stronger abuses himself with poor dietary choices and lifestyle habits, and the weaker person does not, then the genetically weaker person will be healthier and live longer.

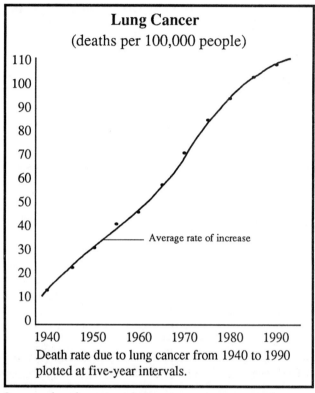

Death rate due to lung cancer from 1940 to 1990 plotted at five-year intervals.

Lung, colon, breast, and prostate cancer account for more than half of all cancer deaths. The rate at which cancer occurs is steadily increasing in industrialized nations.

We are all born with inherent strengths and weaknesses. Generally, we are as healthy as the weakest organ in our body. For if that organ malfunctions, the entire body suffers. If the weak organ, for example, happens to be the pancreas, its dysfunction could result in the development of diabetes. Diabetes affects the entire digestive system, as well as the blood, liver, eyes and many other organs. Dysfunction of the pancreas causes a disruption in the function of many other organs and disease-like symptoms occur.

Most of us are born with completely functional organs that, although they may be inherently weak, will function adequately if supplied with adequate nutrients and kept toxin-free. But when toxins invade the body and enter the bloodstream, they circulate throughout the body. Most toxins are neutralized by the liver or immune system and removed through one of the body's channels of elimination—lungs, kidneys, colon, and skin. But not all toxins are removed. These toxins accumulate in areas of the body which are weakest or where circulation is slowest. These usually are the inherently weakest parts of the body. These organs become encumbered with toxins and slowly deteriorate, becoming dysfunctional. If the

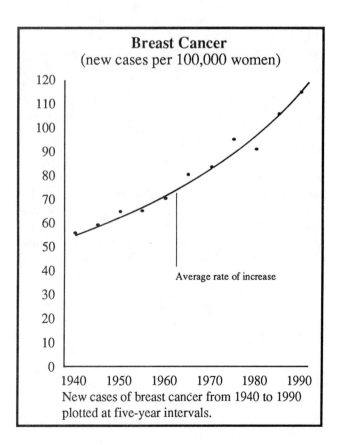

New cases of breast cancer from 1940 to 1990 plotted at five-year intervals.

organ secretes hormones, hormonal secretions can be either elevated or suppressed, causing abnormal chemical reactions leading to numerous symptoms.

Many conditions, which are incurable by standard medical practices, are attributed to genetics. Mental retardation, autism, hyperactivity, cancer, and a host of others have all been blamed on genetics. There is nothing, so we are told, that we can do about it but submit to drugs and surgery and a lifelong commitment to medical care.

Most of these so-called genetic conditions can and have been cured, or at least helped, by diet and detoxification therapies. Endometriosis, which has been considered a genetic condition, as we have seen in the previous chapter, can be cured by natural means, demonstrates that many of the conditions attributed to genetics are really a nutritional or toxic accumulation problem. Some conditions are without question inherent—people are born with them—but they are not genetic. Faulty genes are not the cause of many, if not most, inherent diseases. Inherent diseases are defined as those which a person is born with, but not necessarily genetically induced. For example, a pregnant

Caffeine and Pregnancy

Foods and beverages containing caffeine which are consumed before and during pregnancy can seriously affect the health of newborn babies and even lead to fetal loss.

This is the conclusion from a recent study that featured 331 women who experienced fetal loss and 993 controls who had a normal pregnancy. The study confirms that caffeine is rapidly absorbed and even crosses the placenta. The researchers agree with the Food and Drug Administration's 1980 recommendations that caffeine should be considered potentially hazardous to the unborn child. In addition to causing fetal loss, caffeine is believed to inhibit fetal growth and cause chromosomal problems.

Caffeine has also been shown to be addictive and can induce headaches, insomnia, and anxiety. Four or more cups of coffee per day (decaf or not) increases the risk of heart disease by 60 percent in women. Coffee can also aggravate ulcers and heartburn. Beverages, besides coffee, which contain caffeine, such as black tea and soft drinks, have the same effect.

—*Journal of the American Medical Association*, Vol. 270, No. 24.

woman who contracts the rubella (German measles) virus, may give birth to a baby which is deformed or has some physical dysfunction. The birth defect was not caused by faulty genes from the parents, but by toxins (rubella virus).

A woman's diet prior to and throughout pregnancy is crucial to her health and the growth, development, and health of the infant she carries. The consumption of alcohol during pregnancy, for instance, can have tragic effects on a fetus. Even very limited consumption of alcohol during pregnancy poses significant hazards to the developing baby because alcohol can easily cross the placental barrier and enter the fetal bloodsteam. When alcohol enters the fetal blood, the potential result, called fetal alcohol syndrome (FAS), can cause tragic congenital abnormalities such as a "small head" or low birth weight, developmental disabilities such as mental retardation, and even death.

Pregnant women who smoke are 50 percent more likely to have mentally retarded children. Smoking during pregnancy is linked to low birth weight, infant mortality, and lower intelligence in children. Even secondhand smoke can place unborn children at risk. Lack of nutrients and the exposure to toxins (viruses, alcohol, tobacco, or any other chemical, drug, or biological contaminants) unquestionably cause problems to unborn children. Environmental and dietary chemicals including drugs (both pharmaceutical and recreational) are all toxins! They collect in the body to aggravate tissues, disrupt hormonal balance, and weaken immunity.

Most inherent diseases, which are attributed to genetics and therefore assumed to be unavoidable, *are* preventable. This can be illustrated with an understanding of the critical period of development in unborn babies. The growth of each organ and tissue type in the developing baby has its own characteristic pattern and timing. Each organ is most dependent on an adequate supply of nutrients during its own intensive growth period. In the fetus, for example, the heart and brain are well developed at 14 weeks, but the lungs are still not functional for at least 10 more weeks. Therefore, early malnutrition affects the heart and brain; malnutrition later in the child's development affects its lungs.

The initial development during a critical period occurs at only that time, and at no other. Necessary nutrients must be supplied during this period if the organ is to reach its full potential. If the development of an organ is hampered by lack of essential nutrients or contamination from toxins during a critical developmental period, recovery is impossible. Thus, early malnutrition can have irreversible effects, although they may not become fully apparent until maturity. The effects of malnutrition during critical periods

Antibiotics and Developmental Delays in Children

A recent survey of 700 children ages 1 to 12 years has demonstrated a possible link between the overuse of antibiotics and developmental disorders in children.

The survey, conducted by the Developmental Delay Registry in Silver Spring, Maryland, found that children who have taken more than 20 cycles of antibiotics in their lifetime are 50 percent more likely to experience developmental delays than children who haven't. Additionally, developmentally delayed children were 37 percent more likely to have had three or more ear infections than unaffected children.

Studies have also shown that antibiotics are essentially worthless for the treatment of ear infections. Those children who are not treated heal just as quickly as, and have fewer reoccurrences than those who use antibiotics.

The Developmental Delay Registry warned "Parents should be put on notice that utilizing antibiotics prophylactically could jeopardize their children's development. We believe alternative approaches to treating ear infections should be considered."

—Adapted from a report by the Developmental Delay Registry

is readily seen in the poor dental health of children whose mothers were malnourished during pregnancy.

Problems in development during critical periods often surface later in life as a predisposition or susceptibility to disease. A person whose pancreas development was hampered by inadequate nutrition or toxic exposure may develop hypoglycemia or diabetes as a result of the overconsumption of sugary foods and/or the accumulation of environmental toxins in that organ. Organs which are susceptible to disease due to developmental problems can function adequately for a lifetime without giving any trouble if they are taken care of. You have no way of knowing which organs may be predisposed to give you trouble until something begins to go wrong. By keeping toxins out of the body and providing yourself adequate nourishment, these organs will, for the most part, hold up your entire life without giving you problems.

It is especially important that women during their childbearing years take special care to eat healthfully and avoid unnecessary exposure to toxins. The first organs to

develop in the embryo are the brain and spinal cord. These organs begin their critical period of development before a woman is even aware that she is pregnant. A woman who protects herself from exposure to toxins and eats a variety of nutrient-dense foods prior to pregnancy establishes habits that will nourish herself and the growing fetus.

An infant's birthweight is the most important indicator of an infant's future health. A low-birthweight baby, defined as one who weighs less than 5½ pounds, has a statistically greater chance than a normal-weight baby of contracting disease and of dying early in life. About 1 in every 15 infants born in the United States is a low-birthweight infant, and about one-fourth of these die within the first month of life.

Another reason why a mother's prepregnancy nutrition is important is that it determines whether she will be able to grow a healthy placenta during the first month of gestation. The only way nutrients can reach the developing fetus in the uterus is through the placenta. In the placenta, nutrients and waste materials are exchanged between the mother's and baby's blood vessels.

If placental development was affected by a lack of adequate nutrition or the overexposure to toxins, then no matter how well the mother eats later on during pregnancy, the fetus will not receive optimum nourishment. The result will be a low-birthweight baby, with all of the potential health consequences. This can affect not only the unborn child but also grandchildren. If the infant is a female, her ability to store nutrients as a young adult may be affected. She may also be unable to grow an adequate placenta. In turn, she may bear an infant who is unable to reach full developmental potential.

Women considering having children need to prepare themselves *before* they become pregnant. Avoiding toxins and eating wisely will help to ensure the health of future generations. If this were done, many of the so-called genetic diseases could be conquered.

AGING AND DISEASE

Most degenerative diseases and frequent infections, we are told, are a normal part of aging and we must expect them. Growing older is blamed for many degenerative conditions which standard medical treatments fail to correct. Aging, however, is not the cause of disease. There are many seniors who lead active healthy lives without experiencing any of the degenerative diseases attributed to aging. If you look at people in less developed countries where degenerative disease is rare, some live to be 90, 100, and more without experiencing the so-called age-related diseases. Many of these people continue to work, which is usually physically demanding, until the day they die. They aren't incapacitated by old age. Degenerative disease is clearly not a condition of aging.

Some of the major conditions which have been attributed to aging include:

- Development of bone spurs
- Bones become porous and fracture easily (osteoporosis)
- Degeneration of joints (osteoarthritis)
- Calcification of cartilage
- Dry, wrinkled, discolored skin
- Loss of urinary function and inability to void completely
- Wasting of respiratory muscles decreasing respiratory efficiency
- Degenerative heart and blood vessels
- Hardening of the arteries (arteriosclerosis)

Prostate Cancer

For years, prostate cancer was considered a disease of elderly men, most of whom died of other causes without ever having any symptoms of prostate cancer. Prostate cancers generally grow slowly and when the disease occurs later in life, other conditions often cause death first.

The incidence of prostate cancer has been increasing among men in their 40s and 50s in many Western countries. Unlike most prostate cancers, invasive cancer rapidly engulfs the organ and spreads throughout the body. This type of cancer killed actor Bill Bixby and musician Frank Zappa.

Animal protein found in meat and dairy products may be a contributing factor in the development of prostate cancer reports the *Journal of the National Cancer Institute*.

In an analysis of several hundred cases of prostate cancer among 51,000 men, Edward Giovannucci, M.D., of the Harvard Medical School in Cambridge Mass., found that men eating large amounts of meat were *80 percent* more likely to die from prostate cancer than those who ate meat sparingly.

Men consuming meat five times a week were two to three times more likely to develop invasive prostate cancer than those who ate meat one a week.

Meat consumption has steadily increased over the past several decades. Along with the increase in meat consumption has been an increase in prostate cancer.

- High blood pressure (hypertension)
- Decrease in near vision (presbyopia)
- Pressure in eye which can lead to blindness (glaucoma)
- Loss of transparency of lens or cornea of the eye (cataract)
- Loss of hearing, smell, and taste
- Loss of memory, senility (Alzheimer's disease)

We are told that when we get older (usually after age 40), expect to get one or more of these conditions. A few decades ago the effects of aging were expected when people reached 60 or 70 years of age. In time, the age in which these conditions were becoming evident dropped to 50, then to 40. Now we see "old age" diseases in people who are only in their 30s and 20s and even in teenagers! These are not natural conditions and they don't develop in healthy bodies—regardless of age!

In Third World countries, degenerative diseases have been relatively rare. In countries where people become more affluent, they begin to take on lifestyle habits of Western societies, eating rich, toxic-laden foods and, consequently, developing the same degenerative diseases, while their poorer countryfolk remain free of these conditions. Data from international epidemiological comparisons clearly shows that immigrants from Third World countries which have a low incidence of degenerative disease, yet take on the lifestyle habits of Western societies, rapidly acquire the disease rates of their adopted countries. Thus environmental factors, including diet, are more important in the genesis of degenerative diseases. The Eskimos of Alaska, for example, had much fewer diseases than the white folks living around them when they remained on their traditional diets, but when they started to eat packaged and processed foods, their disease rate soared. These statistics clearly indicate diet as a major factor in degenerative conditions—not heredity and not age. Disease does not come by chance and is not normal.

Ill health can be reversed by changing factors that contribute to disease. Diet is one of these factors. By eating a more "primitive" diet, we avoid foods which are nutrient poor and laden with toxins. The reversal of the damaging effects of modern foods was clearly demonstrated during the Biosphere 2 experiment which began in September 1991 and ended two years later. In the experiment, eight men and women lived the entire time in an environmentally sealed enclosure. Their food consisted entirely of what they raised themselves without chemicals and without modern processing methods. Their food retained all its naturally occurring nutrients and fiber. No chemicals were added. What they ate was limited to what they could grow, which also limited the quantity they could eat. Risk factors associated with heart disease, cancer and other degenerative conditions, such as high blood pressure, and body weight, fell to optimal levels.

Within only six months, average weight decreased by 26 pounds in the men, 15 pounds in the women. Blood pressure levels dropped from an average of 110/75 to 90/58; memory, mood, and energy levels also improved. In short, the functional age of the participants decreased. Essentially, they became physically and mentally younger and healthier.

LIFE EXPECTANCY

Life expectancy in the United States for women is 78.8 years and for men 71.8 years, or 75.4 years on average for both men and women. The life expectancy for all industrialized countries varies by only a couple of years. Japan has the highest life expectancy at 79 years on average for both men and women.

Life expectancy is often cited as proof of the effectiveness of modern medicine and the reason for the prevalence of degenerative diseases now. In 1900 the life expectancy was only 45 years. It is now nearly twice that, thanks to modern medicine, or so they say. Since people are living longer, according to their theory, more people are experiencing degeneration or aging diseases. It is just a consequence of the long life span of people now.

This argument, however, is false. The statement that life expectancy was 45 years in the past is misconstrued as indicating that everyone at that time would only live to about 45 years when they die of old age. This is not true. Life expectancy is defined as the length of time, *on average*, a person can expect to live. It is *not* an indicator of life span, which is how long a person can live. Scientists estimate that the maximum life span for humans is around 120 years. But on average we can expect to live to about 75 years. With the exclusion of deaths caused by accidents, violence, and plagues, all of which bring premature death, the "true" life expectancy* for humans has not changed for at least 3,000 years. In the Bible the average life for man after the great flood is given as between 70 and 80 years (Psalms 90:10)—which it still is today. Life expectancy, as it is calculated today, figures in infant mortality and deaths from all causes. In years past when sanitation practices were unheard of, many people died prematurely from

---

*"True" life expectancy is defined here as the average length of time we can expect to live if not shortened by accident, violence, plague or other fate which attacks people of any age.

infectious disease. Thus the life expectancy, on average, was very low. But people, who survived plagues, wars, and other life-threatening situations, lived just as long then as they do now.

Before the 20th century, infant mortality was extremely high, as was death from infectious diseases, especially in large overcrowded cities where sanitation was poor and disease-causing microorganisms, insects, and rodents lived alongside man. Bubonic plague has struck many times throughout history. Known as the Black Plague, it devastated Europe several times during the middle ages and again later in the 17th century. It was intensified and perpetuated by filthy living conditions. It was carried by infected rats and transmitted by fleas to man. The disease was controlled in London after fires destroyed much of the city, and rodents and filthy living conditions were eliminated.

Sanitary conditions, in general, were appalling before the 20th century. Hospitals were often breeding grounds for disease. It was not uncommon, when they were overcrowded, for patients to be stacked like sardines. Even operating tables were simply doused with a bucket of water to "clean" them for the next patient. Childbed fever, a mysterious disease, which killed women and their newborn infants, rose to epidemic proportions, claiming the lives of up to 50 percent of the women in certain hospitals. Its cause was finally shown to be a result of physicians not washing their hands between patients. Such unsanitary conditions resulted in an unnecessarily high death rate from infection and contagious disease.

With the discovery of microorganisms and the subsequent conscious effort to maintain sanitary conditions, the death rate has been drastically reduced. In 1900 the average life of a person was only 45, not because people did not live to 70, 80, 90 years or more, but because so many died prematurely. This figure represents an average for all people, including those who died in infancy. Since the infant death rate was enormously high, as was death from infectious diseases, the figure derived for life expectancy is misleading.

It wasn't drugs and it wasn't technology that improved life expectancy, although modern medical technology has prolonged the life of many and has been valuable in accident cases. The real factor has been improved sanitation. Deaths from infectious diseases as well as infant mortality have been drastically reduced, primarily because sanitation is better.

Many Third World countries, without the benefit of modern medicine, have people who live much longer than average. The Hunzas of Pakistan, for example, have more centurions per capita than any other people on earth. In fact, those societies who live the longest and are the most disease-free, do not have the modern technology, nor the pollution, we have.

Some people claim that because of the advances in modern medicine we live longer now than people did in the past. They disregard the threat toxins have in the environment, feeling medical science has all the answers and that we are really better off now than at any time in history. They often cite life expectancy over the years ranging from the 20s in ancient times to the 70s of today. To test this theory, a *random* selection of notable people were selected who lived during the 18th century. This period of time was chosen to narrow down the possible choices. At this time, the life expectancy is estimated to be about 40 years of age. The people chosen for this informal survey were taken straight from standard historical references. Each person in the survey was selected at random. The only criteria was that all of them, as far as could be determined, died of "natural causes" rather than acts of war, crime, accident, starvation, etc. This informal survey is by no means a detailed or complete analysis. But it does give an idea of the length of a person's life two centuries ago when people were not suppose to live as long as they do now.

A total of 50 subjects (all men because age data was easier to acquire) were chosen from scattered geographic locations. Of these subjects, the oldest, the famed violin maker Antonio Stradivari, died at the age of 93. The average age at death was 76 years. Compare this with the life expectancy of 72 for men now. This is a far cry from the so-called 40-year life expectancy we are led to believe. The 40-year life expectancy is correct when you factor in deaths occurring from infant mortality, wars, accidents, plagues, etc. that shorten the normal or expected life span. So you see, not only was the "true" life expectancy of people 200 years ago no less than ours today, but in fact, longer. They had a four-year edge over us. We have actually *lost* four years in "true" life expectancy over the past two hundred years. This is even more significant when you consider that people are kept alive longer than they normally would with the use of modern drugs, surgery, radiation, iron lungs, dialysis machines, etc. If it were not for these modern medical wonders, our life expectancy would be many years less than those of previous generations when only herbs and good foods were the medicines of choice.

Another big difference between life now and previous generations is that they did not suffer with decades of degenerative disease slowly eating away on their bodies. Many died of infectious illnesses that affected an aged body or their bodies just simply gave up the ghost. In other

Lifespan of Notable 18th Century Figures

Person	Years Lived	Age
Benjaman Franklin	1706-1790	84
George Washington	1732-1799	67
Samual Johnson	1709-1784	75
Thomas Jefferson	1743-1826	83
Henry Grattan	1746-1820	74
John Adams	1735-1826	91
Jacques Germain Soufflot	1713-1780	67
Thomas Paine	1735-1809	74
Authur Wellesley	1769-1852	83
Antonio Stradivari	1644-1737	93
Andre Ampere	1775-1836	61
King George III	1738-1820	82
Thomas Augustine Arne	1710-1778	68
Bishop A. G. Spengenberg	1704-1792	88
Albert von Haller	1708-1777	69
Edmund Halley	1656-1742	86
Yokai Yagu	1702-1783	81
Johann Wolfgang Goethe	1749-1832	83
John Fothergill	1712-1780	68
John Quincy Adams	1767-1848	81
James Madison	1751-1836	85
F. A. Mesmer	1733-1815	82
Giovanni Viotti	1753-1824	71
James Monroe	1758-1831	73
George Frederick Handel	1685-1759	74
James Watt	1736-1819	83
Henry Cavendish	1731-1810	79
Samuel F. B. Morse	1791-1872	81
David Mendoza	1763-1836	73
Charles Bonnet	1720-1793	73
Francesco Guardi	1712-1793	81
Ferdinand Waldmuller	1793-1865	72
Rossini	1792-1868	76
Joseph Priestly	1733-1804	71
N. I. Lobachevsky	1793-1856	63
John Trumbull	1756-1843	87
Heinrich Marschner	1795-1861	66
Karl Loewe	1796-1869	73
Edward Jenner	1749-1823	74
Richard Colley Wellesley	1760-1842	82
Willibald Alexis	1798-1871	73
Adolphe Thiers	1797-1877	80
Pope Pius VI	1717-1799	82
Ando Hiroshige	1797-1858	61
Charles Bonnet	1720-1793	73
John Wesley	1703-1791	88
William Cowper	1731-1800	69
Friedrich Ruckert	1788-1866	78
Gottfried Treviranus	1776-1837	61
Louis I	1786-1868	82

words, these people died of "old age" rather than debilitating degenerative disease so common today. And they did not suffer the "torture" of medical treatments that people are subjected to today in a, too often, vain attempt to keep people alive despite terminal illnesses. Many such treatments only quicken death or make illnesses more unbearable.

According to *Confessions of a Medical Heretic*, written by Dr. Robert S. Mendelsohn, modern medical treatment can actually shorten life. Dr. Mendelsohn gives several examples. As a protest to soaring rates for malpractice insurance, doctors in Los Angeles went on strike in 1976. As a result, the death rate dropped by 18 percent. That same year, doctors in Bogota, Colombia, refused to provide any services except for emergency care. This resulted in a 35 percent drop in the death rate. When Israeli doctors drastically reduced their daily patient contact in 1973, the Jerusalem Burial Society reported that the death rate was cut in half.

It is of interest to note that according to Dr. Joel Wallach* the average life span for a medical doctor is only 58 years! Doctors who are trained in the most modern methods of health care using the latest scientific equipment and drug therapies, and who have easy access to these methods for themselves have only accomplished in shortening their own lives. All the medical advances in the world have done little for them. The people who lived during the 18th century using herbs, simple remedies, natural foods, and living in a relatively unpolluted environment, outlived today's medical experts by an average of 18 years!

It has been estimated that if given healthy clean foods, avoiding excess, getting daily exercise, in a toxin-free environment, humans could live to be 120 years of age without suffering debilitating or crippling degenerative disease. This estimate is based on animal studies where life span has doubled when these conditions exist. Further proof comes from people and cultures around the world who actually live this long.

Most every country in the world has citizens who live past the age of 100 years. Some countries or areas of the world have more than others. There are a few places on earth where the life span of man is extraordinarily long compared to modern standards. Interestingly enough the places where the people live the longest and are the healthiest are in remote areas separated from industrialization, free from environmental toxins, and contaminated food and water. These people raise their own food, work with their hands, till their own fields, and

---

Rare Earths: Forbidden Cures by Joel Wallach, DVM, ND and Ma Lan, MD

Aging and Degenerative Disease

Chronic condition among persons aged 65 and over

Disease	Persons with conditon(%)
Arthritis	46.5
Hypertensive disease	37.9
Hearing impairments	28.4
Heart conditions	27.7
Chronic sinusitis	18.4
Visual impairments	13.7
Orthopedic impairments	12.8
Arteriosclerosis	9.7
Diabetes	8.3
Varicose veins	8.3
Hemorrhoids	6.6
Urinary system disease	5.6

If disease were a "natural" consequence of aging, we would all develop essentially the same conditions at about the same times of life. After all, we all follow the same general pattern of progress in our development: we teethe, learn to walk and talk, go through puberty, etc. at approximately the same ages. Although there are minor variations in the timing of the onset for each of us, the pattern is consistent. The development of disease, however, is not consistent. Degenerative disease can strike at any age. Furthermore, not all people develop degenerative disease even in old age. If degenerative disease were a part of the aging process, we should all expect to develop these conditions as a consequence of aging. As shown in the list above, degenerative disease doesn't affect everyone. Although as we age the body as a whole degenerates, or loses some degree of efficiency, it does not have to develop degenerative disease.

harvest their own fresh produce. Their environment and food is relatively clean. They work with their hands and even in old age they remain physically active, contributing to the society as a whole. In these places degenerative diseases are almost unknown. It is not uncommon for people to live to be 100 or more.

Some of the most notable societies include the people of Tibet, Southern Russia (Georgia, Abkhazian, Azerbaijan, and Armenia), Vilcabamba (Peru), and Hunza (Pakistan). Newspaper articles frequently appear describing the birthdays or deaths of people from these areas who have reportably lived to be 120 or more. One news story that appeared a few years ago told of the 168th birthday of Shirali Mislimov, a resident of Azerbaijan, in Russia, then believed to be the oldest living person. Mislimov celebrated his birthday by working in his garden and taking his daily half-mile walk. The article stated that Mislimov, who lives with his 107-year-old wife, was as fit as a fiddle. He had recently recovered from a winter bout with pneumonia, the first time in his life he had been sick, according to the Russian news sources.

Mislimov says he tried smoking cigarettes once about 150 years ago, but got sick after three of four puffs and has not smoked since. The only time he ever tried whiskey was in 1831. "I thought I was burning inside," Mislimov said.

In the region between the Black Sea and the Caucasus Mountains in southern Russia where Mislimov is from, live some of the oldest people in the world. It is reported that this region is inhabited by over 500,000 people, approximately 5,000 of which are over 100 years old. In other words, nearly 1 out of every hundred people living in this region is over a century old. The people in the Lhasa Valley of Tibet, Vilcabamba in Peru, and the Hunzas of northern Pakistan all show similar percentages of centurions. In comparison, the United States (which is similar to other industrialized countries in life expectancy) has a ratio of only three centurions for every 100,000 people.

The people in these areas do not die from heart disease, cancer, diabetes, and other degenerative diseases that plague western cultures. They do not spend their last days, months, or years suffering with a body that is slowly deteriorating, banished to nursing homes and hospitals or hooked up to tubes and fed a constant stream of medications. When they die, it is relatively sudden and painless—the way it should be for all of us. Their bodies age, of course, and functions do slow down, as you would expect, but the pain and disability common with us is not the norm with them.*

The dietary habits of these long-lived people are rather varied. They eat a mixture of foods, primarily grains, vegetables, fruits, and nuts, with some meat and milk. The one similarity they have which contrasts with

---

* Critics may argue by saying aging is a degenerative process, so even people in long-lived societies degenerate just like those in industrialized nations. Although it is true that aging involves some degree of degeneration, aging does not necessarily mean the development of degenerative disease. Our bodies can degenerate with age without acquiring degenerative diseases. Degenerative disease can occur at any age. It is seen more in the older population because they have been exposed longer to environmental toxins and other negative factors.

> With the thousands of cases that have been observed during the practice of environmental medicine, we have seen one astounding fact: the body can heal just about anything, if given the opportunity.
> —Sherry A. Rogers, M.D.

most Western cultures is the absence of toxins in their environment and their foods. All food is grown locally in pesticide-free farmland which is organically fertilized. Little or no man-made chemicals are used in their environment, so their water is clean and rich in natural minerals. Their air is fresh. Their food, including the little meat and milk they eat, is free from toxic contamination. They also get plenty of exercise, as they rely on physical labor for most of their work. Even the elders remain physically active.

INFECTIOUS DISEASE

Toxins, malnutrition, and excessive stress are the culprits for most of our health problems today, not genetics, not aging, and not germs. Disease-causing microorganisms have troubled mankind since the beginning of time. We all live in a sea of germs. They are in the air, on our food, on our skin, and even inside our bodies. We will never be free from germs. Some of these microorganisms are beneficial to us, others cause disease. Before the days of antibiotics, harmful bacteria caused sicknesses in populations where conditions were unsanitary or people were malnourished—two very common conditions in ages past. Although antibiotics have been credited with conquering illnesses caused by bacteria, antibiotics did not remove the major cause of infectious disease like cholera, typhoid, and typhus; better nutrition, pure water, and sanitation did it. Childbed fever and other postsurgical infections declined simply when doctors began washing their hands between patients and not because they were given antibiotics.

Infectious diseases are still the most common health problem we face. Hardly a year goes by without most people suffering from bouts with colds or flu. These infectious illnesses, however, are primarily a result of toxic accumulation, malnutrition, or excess stress. If stress or toxins build up in the body, the immune system becomes overworked; this is especially true if nutrition is inadequate. With a suppressed immune system, microorganisms—the type that surround us every day—are more easily able to gain a foothold and multiply, causing illness.

A person who is relatively stress- and toxin-free and

Influenza

Influenza, or the flu, is caused by a virus—a cousin to the common cold. And unlike bacteria infections which are treated with antibiotics, there are no anti-viral medicines. Once a person becomes infected, the disease must run its course. Your only defense is your immune system. The strength of that system profoundly influences the outcome, whether the symptoms will be mild or severe and whether it will end in life or death.

The secret to the flu virus's endurance is its versatility. The virus changes its molecular form with each new outbreak. It is never dormant, has no geographic limitation, and quickly sidesteps the immunity conferred by vaccination by changing itself into something else. Flu can penetrate the tightest quarantines and, once contracted, cannot be kept from running its course.

Flu epidemics have been recorded throughout history, some more devastating than others. Flu viruses are always present to some degree and, generally, are not much more threatening than a bad cold. Even so, only the Black Death, which decimated Europe in the Middle Ages, was more deadly than the great influenza epidemic of 1918 and 1919. During this epidemic some 20 million people worldwide died.

The 1918-1919 pandemic came to be known as the Spanish Flu. In the spring of 1919, the Spanish Flu virus vanished as suddenly as it had appeared. Researchers have never been able to identify the lethal strain, and no one knows if it still exists or if it will strike again.

In recent years tissues taken at autopsy in 1918 and preserved in formaldehyde and wax have been studied. Genetic analysis of the virus does not match any virus that has been found since, but appears to be related to the swine flu. Two other flu viruses spread all over the world since 1918—Asian flu in 1957 and the Hong Kong flu in 1968—and it is believed that both mutated in pigs.

Most experts believe that flu viruses reside harmlessly in birds, where they are genetically stable. Occasionally, a virus from birds will infect pigs. The swine immune system attacks the virus, forcing it to change genetically to survive. The result is a new virus, which when spread to humans, can be devastating.

Over the past century it has been noted that flu mortality has increased among the older age group, from 25 percent in the 1918 epidemic to 88 percent in 1951 to the upper nineties in more recent outbreaks. This increase in mortality has been attributed to underlying chronic degenerative diseases in older people, which were not as prevalent in past generations. Vaccines, which have only moderate success and are only effective for a few months or a year, are now routinely recommended for the old and very young who are the most susceptible.

---

is well nourished will have resistance to pathogenic disease. This person will have few, if any, colds and other seasonal illnesses. The microbes just can't penetrate this person's immune defenses.

Infectious diseases are on the rise. One reason is because people's resistance to disease is becoming weaker. You hear in the news outbreaks of viruses or bacteria that affect or kill dozens of people. What you don't realize is that a far greater number of people have been exposed to the same pathogenic microbes, yet have relatively mild symptoms or have no adverse effects at all. It is only those people who are either toxic laden, malnourished, or under undue stress that get deathly ill. A truly healthy person can resist almost any infectious disease.* We are born with the ability in our immune system to handle any type of disease causing microbe. Only if the body is weakened will the microbes overpower us.

Good nutrition plays an important part in the health of our immune system. Even though food is relatively abundant in Western countries, many people are marginally malnourished because they live almost entirely on processed refined foods low in vital nutrients.

When we hear the word "malnutrition," we think of disease conditions such as beriberi or starvation. Malnutrition can manifest itself in many ways, disease conditions as drastic as those mentioned or in lesser symptoms such as anemia, fatigue, frequent infections, headaches, etc. In order for the symptoms of nutritional deficiencies to be clearly identifiable, malnutrition must be chronic over a long period of time. The recognition and diagnosis of a deficiency disease is seldom made until the disease is far advanced and gross pathological symptoms are present.

---

*Although aging is not an excuse for the development of disease conditions, as we age and our immune system weakens we become more susceptable to infection. Death in the elderly is often due to infection even when degenerative disease is absent. We all have to die sometime.

Few good clinical tests exist for the determination of subclinical deficiency states. In Western countries where food is readily available, full-blown malnutrition is relatively rare. However, the use of processed and convenience foods where nutrients have been destroyed or removed has led to widespread subclinical malnutrition. Subclinical malnutrition, in a sense, is worse than full-blown malnutrition because it goes unrecognized and the body slowly deteriorates. Aches and pains come and go. Infections become more frequent and last longer. Aging—wrinkles, gray hair, decreased energy—comes prematurely. Teenagers are particularly vulnerable because they live on diets of convenience and snack foods devoid of essential nutrients. It is no wonder they develop degenerative diseases later in life.

YOU HAVE CONTROL OVER YOUR HEALTH

We have control over our health, for the most part. How we live, eat, act, and react determines our level of health. We are not subject to random chance of disease. We create disease in ourselves though our lifestyle and our habits. We have the power to make ourselves sick or to make ourselves healthy; we only need to make the choice.

Our bodies have miraculous God-given power of rejuvenation. It is inherent in all of us. Our cells, if nourished properly and kept free from toxins and stress, could live indefinitely. Cell cultures in scientific laboratories have been kept alive in such environments for many decades without disease or death. These cells will continue to thrive so long as they are properly nourished and harmful toxins are shut out. Our bodies, likewise, will live to their full capacity so long as we nourish them and keep them toxin-free.

Through a series of detoxification methods, you can cleanse your body from the toxins that bind it to sickness and poor health. You can overcome addictions to over-eating, sugar, fatty meats, caffeine, alcohol, tobacco, drugs, laziness, and other health destroying factors. All you have to do is put forth the effort. You cannot sit back and do nothing and expect your health to improve. That is the concept of the pill. You take a magic pill and your symptoms go away. Little effort is required on your part and you continue with your health destroying lifestyle. As you do, your body ages, degenerates, decomposes, and dies. It's an easy life down the road to ill health.

Achieving good health requires effort, but the rewards are great: freedom from pain, discomfort, fatigue, irritability, and a host of other negative symptoms. You have control over your health even if you

Worldwide Deaths from Disease

Disease	Est. Annual Deaths	Primary Cause
Cardiovascular disease[1]	12 million	Lifestyle & environmental factors
Diarrheal disease[2]	5 million	Protozoa & bacteria
Cancer[1]	4.8 million	Lifestyle & environmental factors
Pheumonia[2]	4.8 million	Bacteria
Tuberculosis[2]	3 million	Bacteria
Obstructive lung diseases[1]	2.7 million	Lifestyle & environmental factors
Measles	1.5 million	Virus
Malaria[2]	1-2 million	Protozoa
Hepatitis B	1-2 million	Virus
Tetanus[2] (neonatal)	775 thousand	Bacteria
Maternal mortality[2]	500 thousand	Various causes
AIDS	200 thousand	Virus
Schistosomiasis[2]	200 thousand	Parasite
Amebiasis[2]	40-110 thousand	Protozoa
Hookworm[2]	50-60 thousand	Parasite
Rabies	35 thousand	Virus
Typhoid[2]	25 thousand	Bacteria
Yellow fever	25 thousand	Virus
African trypanosomiasis[2]	20 thousand	Protozoa
Ascariasis[2]	20 thousand	Parasite

Of the ten top killer diseases in the United States and most other industralized nations, seven are of a degenerative nature: heart disease, cancer, stroke, diabetes, lung diseases, liver disease, and atherosclerosis (the other three causes of death are accidents, suicide, and pneumonia/influenza).

1. Primarily a degenerative disease and a major cause of death in industralized nations.
2. Caused primarily by bacteria or parasite infestation. Can be avoided to a great extent with proper sanitary practices. Most common among Third World Countries.

Source: World Health Organization and National Center for Health Statistics

The Age of Supergerms

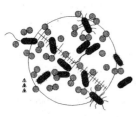

Time was running out for the 57-year-old kidney patient. For nine months Dr. Cynthia Gibert desperately tried one antibiotic after another on him, but nothing worked. The man's blood was still flooded with enterococcus bacteria which were slowly poisoning his body. "We tried six or seven different medications. Some we didn't think would work. But we had nothing else to try." says Gibert, an infectious-disease specialist at the Veterans Affairs Medical Center in Washington. Even experimental drugs proved useless. Sometimes the man's blood tested clean, but within days the infection came roaring back. One strain of bacteria would die but a few antibiotic resistant bacteria—would take the place of their more vulnerable cousins. Then they multiplied by the billions. The patient sensed his doctor's frustration. "I guess you're coming to tell me I'm dying," he said. Nothing had worked, she explained; they had run out of options. Antibiotics, the miracle drugs of the 20th century, had been useless against this new strain of bacteria. Several days later the man died of a massive bacterial infection of the blood and heart.

Today people are suffering and dying from illnesses that 40 years ago science predicted would be wiped off the face of the earth. Infectious disease like tuberculosis, pneumonia, and others considered conquered through the use of antibiotics are making a frightening comeback. Infectious diseases are now the third leading killer of Americans, behind cancer and heart disease, and are becoming a global threat. The world's population has never been more vulnerable to emerging and re-emerging infections, wrote Dr. Joshua Lederberg, a Nobel prize winner for research in the genetic structure of microbes, in an editorial in *Journal of the American Medical Association*.

Experts say our overuse of antibiotics is largely to blame: antibiotics encourage proliferation of drug-resistant bacteria. The Centers for Disease Control and Prevention (CDC) examined death records nationwide and found 65 deaths among every 100,000 people were caused by infectious disease, up from 41 of every 100,000 death twelve years before.

Staphylococcus aureus, the bacterium responsible for some pneumonias and, most worrisome, for blood poisoning in surgical wounds, is becoming a major threat. Some 40 percent of staph in hospitals are resistant to every antibiotic but one, vancomycin. "We know at some point vancomycin will succumb and the bacteria will grow and proliferate unrestrained," worries Dr. Thomas Beam of the Buffalo, N.Y., VA Medical Center. "It will be like the 1950s and 1960s, when we had nothing to treat this infection, and the mortality rates were as high as 80 percent." In those decades, thousands of people died each year of staph infections.

In 1946, just five years after penicillin came into wide use, doctors discovered a staphylococcus that was invulnerable to the drug. Pharmacologists developed new antibiotics. But new drug-resistant bacteria appeared. As new drugs were developed, new strains of bacteria arose. Pharmacologists, for the most part, were able to stay ahead, developing new drugs to combat the new strains of bacteria. Slowly, scourges such as tuberculosis, bacterial pneumonia, septicemia (blood poisoning), syphilis, gonorrhea, and other bacterial infections were vanquished, or so it seemed. People still died from these ills, but not so many. The perception in the 1980s was that we had conquered almost every infectious disease. Science was sure the real challenges would lie in the conquest of cancer, heart disease, and other chronic diseases. Funding and research in antibiotic development declined. Medicine's presumed triumph over infectious disease was an illusion.

Today every disease-causing bacterium has versions that resist at least one of medicine's 100-plus antibiotics. Some of these "supergerms" resist almost all known antibiotics. Drug-resistant tuberculosis now accounts for one in seven new cases; 5 percent of those patients are dying. Several resistant strains of pneumococcus, the microbe responsible for infected surgical wounds and some children's ear infections and meningitis, appeared in South Africa in the 1970s, spread to Europe and now are turning up in the United States. Recently, 13,300 hospital patients died of bacterial infections that resisted the antibiotics doctors fired at them. It was not that they had infections immune to every single drug but rather that, by the time doctors found an antibiotic that worked, the rampaging bacteria had poisoned the patient's blood, scarred the lungs, or crippled some other vital organ.

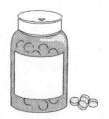

The secret to the new supergerms is the ability of the bacteria to adapt to their environment. When a colony of bacteria is dosed with, say, penicillin, most die. But a few lucky microbes, by chance, harbor genes that make them immune to the drug. They survive. The survivors pass on their resistance to their progeny—one bacterium can leave nearly 17 million offspring within 24 hours. Even more insidious, the resistant strains can share their genes with unrelated bacteria. For example, a microbe releases a chemical, attracting another bacterium; when the two touch, they open pores and exchange a loop of DNA. Through this sort of action, cholera bacteria picked up resistance to tetracycline from plain old E. coli in the human intestine.

This global threat from supergerms sounds like a plot for a horror movie. The sad thing about this is that we brought it upon ourselves. The rise of these supergerms is due to our overuse and abuse of antibiotics. Doctors routinely dispense antibiotics without knowing whether their patient's illnesses are caused by bacteria. Doctors feel they do no great harm so prescribe drugs for conditions like viral infections (e.g., colds, flus, etc.), for which antibiotics have no effect.

Eighty percent of the conditions that people see doctors for are self-limited, that is, will correct themselves without any medical care. Doctors, however in an attempt to do something for the patient, give them antibiotics. That way if the illness just happens to be caused by a bacterial infestation, then the antibiotic *may* help (although even then it usually isn't necessary). And if the illness is not caused by bacteria, antibiotics serve to placate the patient and justify the time and expense of coming to the doctor. If doctors simply told patients that their illnesses aren't serious and sent them away without medication, they feel their patients will go to other doctors who will prescribe antibiotics. For these reasons, antibiotics have been grossly overprescribed.

Another problem is that harmless bacteria that live in the intestines and keep disease-causing bacteria in check, are destroyed. Without competition, harmful bacteria, especially pathogenic supergerms, can proliferate. The result is infectious diseases that can't be controlled by the usual antibiotics.

Medical use of antibiotics is not the only problem. Farm animals receive 30 times more antibiotics than people. The drugs treat and prevent infections. But the main reason farmers like them is that they also make cows, hogs, and chickens grow faster from each pound of feed. Resistant strains emerge just as they do in humans taking antibiotics—and remain in the animal's flesh even after it winds up on our dinner table. Many salmonella strains in turkey, for instance, are resistant to several common antibiotics. Although cooking kills them, the supergerms spread from animals to people through raw or undercooked meat. At least 500 people in the United States alone die annually from microbes present in meat and poultry. An additional 6.5 million people fall ill.

Meat isn't the only problem. Milk is allowed to contain a certain concentration of 80 different antibiotics—all used on dairy cows to prevent udder infections. With every glassful, a small amount of several antibiotics is consumed, which could produce resistant germs in milk drinkers.

Pharmaceutical companies are scrambling to catch up in the race with supergerms, which have sprinted years ahead of our ability to control them. Before science catches up with the microbes, many more people will die.

Ironically, the cure for all pathogenic bacterial infections, even those caused by drug-resistant supergerms, has been with us all along and is readily available. That cure is our own immune system. Our immune systems were designed to combat and control any bacterial infection.

We will never win the race against the supergerms. The only real cure for bacterial infections is within our own bodies. If we have a healthy immune system, it can handle any bacteria nature can throw at us. It is only when the immune system is weakened that infections become dangerous. And how do they become weakened? Exposure to environmental toxins and lifestyle habits are the biggest contributing factors.

As supergerms become more prominent, the mortality rate will soar. These new supergerms will become a major threat to health because people's ability to resist infection has greatly declined with the chronic overexposure to immune-suppressing toxins.

If your immune system is healthy, you have little to fear from the emerging supergerms. A healthy immune system easily repels most bacterial invaders, regardless if they are supergerms or not. But when resistant bacteria take hold among the weak, they're hellishly hard to control.

We cannot depend on new antibiotics to be developed. Our only sure defense against the supergerm is to strengthen our immune systems through diet and periodic detoxification methods.

—Adapted from "The End of Antibiotics," by Sharon Begley, *Newsweek March 28 1994* are predisposed to certain illnesses because of inherent conditions. We all have our own unique weaknesses, but they don't have to be the cause of sickness or death, not if we treat ourselves right. If you want to continue as you are now—do nothing. If you want to reclaim your health, you must detoxify your body and begin living a healthy lifestyle. You have the power to change; the choice is up to you.

HEALTH ASSESSMENT PROFILE

As you begin the cleansing programs described in this book, you will be building a new body. You will lose unwanted fat and eliminate encrusted wastes and toxins. Your eliminative channels will improve and become more effective. Your immune system will become stronger. Your digestive system will work better and you will be capable of assimilating needed nutrients as you should. Your body and your mind will function better. You will think clearer, have a better memory, be more emotionally stable, be capable of handling stress, feel stronger, tire less easily, and enjoy life more. You will, in effect, turn back the clock and regain the health and vitality you had in years past. And you will maintain it longer throughout life.

Although we all age chronologically, we do not age at the same rate. A healthy 60-year-old can be "functionally" as young as a 45-year-old while a sickly 40-year-old could have a body comparable to a 70-year-old. The average human life span is about 75 years. Some people live much longer, and those who do are generally free of debilitating disease for most of their lives. They are functionally younger than those people whose bodies degenerate and die before their time. Toxins, malnutrition, and excessive stress accelerate functional age, increase disease susceptibility, and shorten life.

Dr. Roy L Walford, a professor of pathology at the UCLA School of Medicine and author of *The 120-Year Diet*, has identified several "biomarkers" which give us a way of measuring functional age. By measuring a person's biomarkers, functional age can be determined. By following the detoxification methods described in this book, you will become healthier and, consequently, functionally younger.

There are many types of biomarkers, some involving equipment and measurements that require medical supervision. Some you can do yourself in your own home. They are described here and are adapted from Dr. Walford's text. There is wide variation on these tests and they shouldn't be taken as absolute evaluations of health status. Some people, for example, may have youthful skin, but poor eyesight. So the following tests should all be considered together to provide you with your approximate functional age.

Skin Elasticity Test

As we age, our skin loses its elasticity and wrinkles develop. Significant changes usually occur at about the age of 45. It is a good marker for how the skin changes after age 45. At younger ages there is only slight change.

For this test, pinch the skin on the back of your hand between the thumb and forefinger for five seconds. Let go and time how long it takes for the skin to completely flatten back out. The shorter the time, the younger the functional age of the skin. Compare your results to the table below.

Time (sec.)	Functional Age (years)
1-4	44 or younger
5	45-50
10-15	60
35-55	70
56 or more	over 70

Falling-Ruler Test

This test measures your reaction time. You need a flat 18-inch wooden measuring stick. Have someone hold the ruler vertically at the top, by the 1-inch mark. Hold the thumb and middle finger of your right hand 3½ inches apart, equidistant from the 18-inch mark near the bottom of the ruler. Without warning, your assistant will drop the ruler. As soon as you see it fall, catch it between your two fingers.

Write down the inch mark on the ruler where your fingers caught it. Repeat this two more times. Take an average of all three. So, if you caught it at 10, 12, and 8-inch marks the average would be 10+12+8/3=10. Compare your average score with the table below.

Measurement (inches)	Functional Age (years)
11 or less	20
9	30
8	40
7	50
6	60
5-0	70 and older

Static Balance Test

This test is considered the best biomarker among the do-it-yourself measurements. There is a full 100 percent decline with age.

The static balance test measures how long you can stand on one leg with your eyes closed before falling over.

For this test you must be either barefoot or wearing low-heeled shoes. Stand on a hard surface with both feet together, close your eyes, and lift your foot about six inches off the ground. If you are right-handed lift the left leg and if you are left-handed lift the right leg. The raised knee should be bent at about a 45-degree angle. Don't move, just stand on one foot with your eyes closed. Have someone time you. When you fall or touch the ground with the other foot, record the time. Do the test three times and take an average. Check your results with the table below.

Time (sec)	Functional Age (years)
30 or more	20
25	30
16	40
10	50
7	60
5	70

Visual Accommodation Test

This test provides a general evaluation on visual health. If you wear glasses you can do this test with or without them, but do not use reading glasses. This test is based on the premise that as the eyes age, they lose their ability to focus up close. Here you will determine how close you can bring an object up to your eyes before it begins to blur.

Hold a newspaper at arm's length and slowly bring it toward your nose. Bring it as close to your face as you can until the regular-sized print starts blurring. Record this distance.

Distance (inches)	Functional Age (years)
4 or less	21
5.5	30
9	40
15	50
39	60

It is suggested that you measure each biomarker before you begin any of the programs in this book. Then, periodically compare your progress as you detoxify. Keep in mind that detoxification and rebuilding is a slow process. Make your second measurement after you have been detoxing for about six months and again after a year, and at yearly intervals thereafter as you desire. The primary purpose of the health assessment profile is to give you a marker upon which you can gauge your progress. Dr. Walford says that the initial tests should not be taken too seriously. You should be more interested in the rate of change thereafter. In other words, you can best use the results to monitor the rate at which you age. If you follow the recommendations in this book you should notice over time a significant decrease in the rate at which you age as judged by these biomarkers.

For the most part, this test is really just for fun. It isn't an absolute measure of disease susceptibility or aging by any means. While it does provide clues to health status, the real test is the way you feel. As you follow the programs outlined in this book, symptoms of dis-ease or aging will decrease. You will reclaim your health and maintain it as long as you follow a healthy lifestyle.

 ADDITIONAL RESOURCES

An Alternative Approach to Allergies. Randolph, Theron G., M.D. and Moss, R.W., Ph.D. New York: Bantam Books, 1987.

Anatomy of An Illness. Cousins, Norman. New York: W.W. Norton & Co., 1979.

The Betrayal of Health. Beasley, Joseph, M.D. New York: Times Books, 1991.

Beyond Antibiotics: Healthier Options for Families. Schmidt, Michael, D.C. Berkeley, CA: North Atlantic Books, 1992.

Cancer Battle Plan. Frahm, Anne E. and Frahm, David J. Colorado Springs, CO: Pinon Press.

The New Our Bodies, Ourselves. The Boston Women's Health Collective. New York: Simon & Schuster, 1992.

Vaccination and Immunization: Dangers, Delusions, and Alternatives. Chaitow, Leon. UK: Saffron Walden, 1987.

Vaccines: Are They Really Safe and Effective. Miller, Neil Z. Santa Fe, NM: New Atlantean Press, 1992.

Women's Health Alert. Wolfe, Sidney M., M.D. and the Public Citizen Health Research Group. Reading, MA: Addison-Wesley Publishing, 1991.

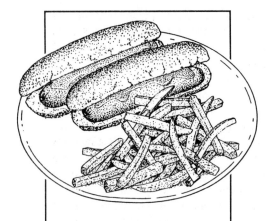

Chapter 3

EATING MAY BE HAZARDOUS TO YOUR HEALTH

*Everything in excess is
opposed by Nature.*
        —*Hippocrates*

*Last year each of us, on
average, swallowed three
pounds of flavorings, coloring,
preservatives, glazes,
antispattering agents,
emulsifiers, bleaches, and
other additives with our food.*
        —*Joan Morgan, M.D.*

Warning labels should be placed on all junk foods, "Eating this product may be hazardous to your health." Junk foods being defined as all processed connivance foods: white bread, crackers, chips, cookies, lunch meats, frozen dinners, canned vegetables, soups, stews, beans, and any other heat-and-serve type food that has been denatured and pumped up with preservatives and chemical additives. Eating such foods puts a tremendous burden on our bodies. Poisons from these foods accumulate in and around cells, agitating tissues, and causing cells to degenerate, which leads to dis-ease conditions.

Most people don't know such foods are bad for their health. They grew up eating these types of foods. Their parents fed these foods to their children believing them to be nutritious, and their children continue to feed them to their own kids. That is why the health of Western nations has been declining year after year.

Eating poor-quality foods is a habit we have become woefully addicted to. Some people, unwilling to give up their food cravings and poor dietary habits, argue that these poor-quality foods provide them with all the nutrition they need, especially since some of it is "fortified" with vitamins. When you question them about the chemical additives, they say all food is safe to eat, the government wouldn't allow toxic amounts of chemicals and contaminants into the food. Because some people sincerely believe this, they continue to eat poor-quality foods. Their actions are not controlled by their brains, but rather by their tastebuds. Sugar, as well as meat and salt and other foods, is addictive just as tobacco, caffeinated drinks, and drugs are.

Eating junk food drains the body of its vital energy. The body channels its healing forces to clean up the toxins which are continually being pumped into it. As a result, it becomes weakened and less able to fight off infection, prevent degenerative conditions from occurring, and rebuild with new healthy tissue.

One of America's foremost fasting and nutrition experts, Paul Bragg, Ph.D., demonstrated how a diet consisting of junk foods weakens the body. He challenged 10 college athletes to a test of endurance by walking across the tortuously hot Death Valley dessert during mid-summer. Death Valley, located in southern California, is the hottest spot in North America. Summer temperatures can reach 130 degrees. The challenge was to hike across 30 miles of desert in one day. A truck would accompany them carrying an assortment of refreshments and foods—white bread, buns, crackers, cheese, lunch meats, hot dogs, soda—all junk foods and all typical of the foods people, including the students, live on every day.

The young men were allowed to eat and drink as much as they wanted during the trek. Bragg, a great-grandfather at the time, would go fasting, drinking only water.

A 30-mile hike in the hot sun may seem possible for a group of healthy young college students. But for an "old" man who wasn't even going to be eating, to keep up his strength, it seemed impossible. When they started the hike in the morning, it was already 105 degrees. Temperatures got progressively hotter throughout the day. The college boys gobbled the sandwiches, drank quarts of cool water and cola drinks. Bragg drank his water and ate nothing.

Soon after stopping for lunch three of the husky college boys became violently ill and threw up all they ate for lunch. They got dizzy and turned deathly pale. They quit the hike and were driven back to Furnace Creek Ranch from which they started. The hike went on with seven college athletes continuing. As they hiked, the kids continued to drink and snack on the food. Five more eventually developed stomach cramps and become too ill to continue and had to be taken back to the ranch.

Bragg continued the hike with the two remaining students. At about 4 p.m., as the merciless sun beat down on them, the last two athletes collapsed in the hot burning sun and had to be returned to the ranch. Alone, Bragg continued the trip. "I felt as fresh as a daisy!" he said, "I was not full of food because I was on a complete fast. I drank only the warm water I needed." He finished the 30-mile hike in around 10 and a half hours and had no ill effects whatsoever. He camped out for the night and next day arose and hiked another 30 miles back to the ranch, again without any food.

The athletes, eating poor-quality foods, had less strength and endurance than the elderly Bragg, who ate nothing. Bragg even doubled the distance by walking back to the starting point. The boys ate foods that required energy to digest, foods which lacked nutritional value and contained chemical additives. Much of their internal energy was diverted to remove the toxins in the food they ate. As a result, they weren't able to finish the hike. Many people eat like this every day. Their bodies are struggling to keep up the pace of life, but it's an uphill battle that eventually leads to sickness. Bragg took no nourishment during the trek (so his performance was not attributed to eating superior food), yet he had ample energy and endurance. Surely this old man did not have youth in his favor, nor did he have exceptional strength compared to the college athletes he challenged. What he had was a lack of toxic poisons going into his body, poisons which drain the body of vital energy. The students' bodies were battling the heat and stress of the hike as well as the toxins ingested in their food. Their energy was quickly used up and they collapsed in exhaustion.

This happens to us too when we eat nutritionless toxin-laden foods. Our digestive and immune systems work at full speed, so during a busy day, we run out of energy by mid-afternoon. The effectiveness of the body to remove toxins and fight off infectious organisms is hampered because we are exhausted. Toxins build up, piling up day after day. It is no wonder degenerative disease has spread over civilized countries like a plague.

Overeating compounds the problem. Overeating puts a tremendous strain on the gastrointestinal tract and consumes huge amounts of our vital energy. This may be one reason why overweight people do not like to exercise. They are chronically tired and rundown by the loss of energy their bodies must spend processing food. The more one eats, the more energy is needed to digest what is eaten, and the more toxins are piled into the body. As a consequence, the body spends most of its energy trying to process food. Toxins rapidly accumulate in fatty tissue, weak organs, and other metabolically slow tissues. It's no wonder overweight people are plagued with contagious infections like colds and flus as well as degenerative diseases. The overconsumption of poor-quality foods is one of the worst things you can do for your health. Even eating too much healthy food is not good, as energy is spent processing this material rather than cleaning and healing.

Most of the food available in the grocery store and in restaurants is of poor-quality. It is designed for convenience, appearance, and flavor—not nutrition. Eating such foods is hazardous to your health.

QUALITY OF THE FOODS WE EAT

"Ted came to me quite sure he had a serious illness," reports Dr. William Manahan, author of *Eat For Health*. "For four to six months, this dynamic 38-year-old businessman had been tired, lacked energy, and been unable to complete some of his business projects. He had been divorced twelve months previously but said he was over that ordeal and involved in a new relationship.

"Ted had really changed his eating pattern over the past year. Since no one made his breakfast for him each morning, he had simply quit eating it. Instead, he grabbed a sweet roll or doughnut at midmorning. At lunch he ate out with clients, usually choosing the restaurant 'special.' For supper, he stopped for fast food such as a hamburger, fries, and a malt. He drank two to three cans of Pepsi-Cola daily and frequently snacked on candy bars or cookies.

"Clearly, Ted was eating no whole grains or fruits, and he had a vegetable only rarely. His sugar intake was very high. I asked Ted if he would be willing to try some radical dietary changes for just two weeks. He said he would do anything, because his business was going to fall apart if he didn't pep up very quickly.

"He began to eat whole-grain cereal, whole-wheat toast, and fruit each morning. At lunch he had a salad, soup, raw vegetables, or a vegetable or tuna sandwich plus fruit. His evening meals were stir-fry vegetables, brown rice, whole-grain spaghetti with tofu or ground beef, various vegetables and pasta dishes, and a couple of fish or lean-meat meals with a potato and vegetable. For snacks, he had low-fat cheese, fresh or dried fruit, and raw vegetables. For a beverage he drank water.

"Ted was slated to return to me in two weeks. On the eleventh day, Ted stormed into my office saying he was canceling his follow-up appointment. He felt better than he had in five years! He told me that his energy level was great and that he had already finished a major paper he had been trying to write for two months."

Stories like this are commonplace. Dr. Manahan describes dozens of similar cases in his book citing caffeine, salt, milk, sugar, fats, and processed foods as the primary troublemakers.

You often hear, that what you eat, as long as you get enough food, does not affect your health. Grocery store foods, it is said, supply all the nutrients a body needs to maintain health. Disease is blamed on heredity, germs, and aging.

If this is so, why is it then, that people afflicted with multiple sclerosis, arthritis, asthma, emphysema, rheumatism, peptic ulcers, chronic migraine headaches, allergies, high blood pressure, heart disease, colitis, eczema, psoriasis, prostate enlargement, Parkinson's disease, candidiasis, kidney disease, gallstones, tumors, sterility, and numerous other degenerative conditions have been able to eliminate these problems by diet alone? Countless numbers of people can attest to the fact that changing their diet, has brought about changes in their health. If they were eating typical grocery store foods before and switched to more natural and pure whole foods, the key must be in the foods.

The quality of the foods we eat has a great deal to do with our health and the ability of our bodies to heal itself and prevent disease. Overeating of poor-quality foods leads to ill health. Not eating enough of the right kinds of foods can cause malnutrition in severe cases like scurvy, beriberi, pellagra, and rickets. These are extreme symptoms of nutritional deficiencies, but many people are living on diets which supply them with barely enough nutrients to survive, let alone be healthy. Poisons in our food also affect our health. Many preservatives are deadly poisons added to foods to kill microorganisms. If these poisons will kill these tiny creatures then they also will kill our cells. And they do. Most preservatives and artificial food additives have been shown to cause cancer or other problems if consumed in large doses. They are added to foods simply because the dose in each package is considered small enough that our bodies can remove them without suffering too much harm. That's like saying it's okay to eat a little cyanide or arsenic or lead because a little won't do you much harm. What about a little in every meal, every day, day in and day out over the course of many years? The cumulative effect can be devastating!

By refraining from consuming all potentially harmful foods and eating only healthy nutritious foods, our bodies have the ability to detoxify and heal themselves. Degenerative disease and infectious illness can be prevented or healed, as well as conditions attributed to aging can be reversed.

With a healthy nutritional program you replace higher quality nutrition-dense foods for lower quality nutrition-poor, toxin-laden ones. "Higher quality" is defined as those that have undergone the least amount of processing. Processing involves removing naturally occurring constituents of the food and adding other material. For example, in making white bread the vitamin and fiber-rich bran is removed and dough conditioners, hydrogenated oils, sugar, preservatives, and other things are added. Whole wheat bread which retains all of its bran and is not loaded up with chemical additives is a higher quality food than white bread. Likewise, an apple is a higher quality food than apple juice which is higher than apple pie.

The way food is grown also affects it quality. Fruits and vegetables grown in artificially fertilized soils or minerally depleted soils are less nutritious than those grown in rich, organic soils. Organically grown foods are produced in naturally fertilized soils and are not contaminated by pesticides, so they are a higher quality than non-organic foods.

Meat from a grass fed, organically raised steer is higher quality than one from an animal kept in a stockyard, fed corn and soy, and pumped up with antibiotics and artificial hormones. Meat from either one of these sources is better than that found in processed meats such as hot dogs which are loaded with preservatives and other additives and incidental contaminants.

Excessive or improper cooking and preparation can lower quality. Cooking not only destroys nutrients, but high heat, as used in frying, changes the molecular structure of some foods, transforming them into substances unusable by the body and often making them very difficult to digest. This is true for both produce and meats. Even raw, dried meat (such as jerky) is superior to cooked meat. To retain the quality of foods, they should be eaten raw or only moderately cooked. Oils, and particularly vegetable oils, when heated to high temperatures, as in deep frying, become carcinogenic. This is true even for a relatively healthy oil like olive. Raw and moderately cooked, organically grown vegetables, fruits, nuts, and seeds are the highest quality foods we can eat. The highest quality meats, eggs, and dairy are those from animals that have been allowed to roam and eat outside (referred to as free-range or grass fed) and are free of drugs and hormones.

BUILDING BLOCKS FOR THE BODY

The body is built from the materials we supply it. If we eat high-quality food, the body will be healthy. If we consume poor-quality food, drugs, and manufactured chemicals, our bodies are forced to use whatever substances are available to build tissue and maintain life.

Most drugs and food additives are toxic to the body. In small amounts, the body is able to eliminate a great deal of these. In larger quantities, they are poisonous and cause sickness and even death. Food and drug manufacturers assume that if taken in small doses, these poisons can be cleared from the body without ill effect. This is generally true—if the body is healthy and the toxins are taken in small quantities. Yet, nowadays, the vast majority of the food sold in stores and restaurants is contaminated with harmful toxins. As a result, we are consuming dangerously high doses of poisons daily. Contamination comes from food additives, improper cooking and preparation, and even the growing process from pesticides. Unsanitary food preparation introduces bacteria and other contaminants, requiring cooking to kill microorganisms before consumption. Synthetic packaging materials can leach out and contaminate the food. Have you ever tasted water from a plastic container that tasted like plastic? You were drinking contaminated water. Milk, juices, and other beverages also leach out chemicals from plastic and Styrofoam containers, but we do not always notice it because the flavor of the beverage masks the taste. Almost everything we eat is contaminated, putting a tremendous strain on our immune system. As a result, the whole body is weakened.

Studies have shown that traces of man-made chemicals can remain in body tissue for decades. These can be

recreational drugs, prescription drugs, over-the-counter drugs, and drugs found in foods (such as coffee, chocolate, soft drinks, etc.) as well as growth hormones (such as steroids fed to cattle), antibiotics (routinely mixed into feed given to beef and poultry), pesticides (a residue which remains on and in commercially grown produce), and chemical food additives (e.g., preservatives, artificial colors, conditioners, etc.).

Although most of these substances are flushed from the body, a residue is incorporated into the tissues and cells. Genetically weak organs and damaged tissue will accumulate greater amounts of these toxins than other parts of the body. Poor eating habits will, in time, create a buildup of toxins in these areas of the body, causing disease. In one person these toxins will affect the joints first, leading to arthritis; in another person it will affect the circulatory system, leading to hardening of the arteries or heart disease; and in another they will build up in the colon leading to colon cancer. The type of disease is determined by the types of food consumed, heredity, and presence of unhealed injuries. Inherently weak organs accumulate the most toxins and are the first to show signs of degeneration and disease. Thus people who have a history in their family of cancer, heart disease and other serious conditions are at high risk when they live on the typical modern diet.

Commercial food preparation and processing not only introduces toxins into our food, but destroys nutrients necessary for good health. Cooking, canning, freezing and the processing of whole grains destroy nutrients necessary

Artificial Food Dyes

Dye	Uses	Toxicity Effects
Red 3	Candy, pastries	Thyroid tumors
Red 40	Candy, pastries, drinks, pet foods	Lymphomas
Blue 1	Candy, pastries, drinks	Chromosomal damage
Blue 2	Candy, drinks, pet foods	Brain tumors
Green 3	Candy, drinks	Bladder tumors
Yellow 5	Drinks, pastries, pet foods	Tumors, allergies
Yellow 6	Drinks, pastries, candy	Tumors, allergies

for good health. The body then must work to eliminate a constant influx of toxins without receiving all the nutrients necessary to do the job. Lack of adequate nutrients and too many toxic substances in our food leads to disease.

Poor-quality foods cause the body to excrete mucus along the gastrointestinal tract. If this mucus formation is constant, it builds up and hardens, coating the walls of the intestines. Most people, who subsist on a diet of poor-quality foods, have old dried mucus and fecal matter in their intestines which has been accumulating for years. Because of this hard fecal casing on the intestinal walls, much of the vitamins and minerals which come through are pushed on and eliminated before they can do any good. Because these nutrients are not absorbed efficiently, the body is malnourished and signals the brain that more vitamins and minerals are needed. People then develop food cravings and eat more, gorging themselves by consuming far more food than the body would normally require. Along with this food comes additional fats and toxins which do more harm than good. In the process, these people wear out their bodies trying to get sufficient nutrients. This leads to weight problems, constipation, and colon disease.

Overeating can also affect the health of every other organ in the body. As the blood circulates through the colon attempting to withdraw nutrients, it will pick up toxins absorbed from putrefied waste and spread them throughout the body. This constant input of poisons puts the immune system under heavy strain. A healthy bowel will eliminate at least one to three times a day. Any less than that signals digestive and nutritional problems.

Eating good quality food will cut down on mucus production and allow the body to wash out accumulated waste. When the bowel is cleansed, the food is readily assimilated and a person can sustain good health on much less food than formerly, and with more vitality and energy.

Eliminating poor-quality food and replacing it with natural healthy food will aid the body in flushing out toxins and rebuilding healthy uncontaminated tissue. Years of dietary abuse, however, cannot be corrected overnight, but may take months and even years of proper eating to correct. Eating healthfully is a lifelong process. Dietary habits must be formed, poor-quality food avoided, and healthy food consumed on a regular basis.

BALANCED NUTRITION

"Let thy food be thy medicine and thy medicine be thy food," said Hippocrates (460-377 B.C.), the father of medicine. The old adage "you are what you eat" holds more truth than most people realize. The food we eat supplies the building blocks for our cells and tissues. The quality of the food we consume determines the quality of our health. Long ago in Asia, doctors discovered the connection between health and nutrition. They effectively treated disease simply by adjusting their patients' diets. It is a form of healing that relies on the body's remarkable capacity to repair itself when given the means to do so—that is, when given balanced, natural, whole foods free from contamination.

Malnutrition is one of the primary causes of disease. Advanced stages of malnutrition can exhibit themselves in a number of characteristic diseases such as scurvy, beriberi, marasmus, and others. Such conditions leave the body vulnerable to infections, depress immunity, and stifle healing, normal growth, and bodily functions. In Third World countries, malnutrition is primarily due to famines, poverty, and politics. In more affluent countries the problem is masked by the abundance of foods and medicines. In order for symptoms of malnutrition to manifest themselves, a diet must be lacking in essential nutrients for an extended period of time. The body maintains reserves of essential nutrients to protect itself during periods when foods are less readily available. It can take months for signs of malnutrition to become evident. Methods of diagnosing deficiency diseases require malnutrition to be in a relatively advanced stage before it can be detected.

Subclinical malnutrition is a condition where a person consumes just enough essential nutrients to prevent full-blown symptoms of severe malnutrition, but the body is still nutrient deficient and prone to dis-ease. This condition can go on indefinitely unnoticed. In Western countries the problem of subclinical malnutrition is epidemic. Our foods are sadly depleted of nutrients. We eat, and even overeat, but we can still be malnourished because our foods do not contain all the essential nutrients our bodies need to function optimally. As a result, the body cannot fight off infections as well, the immune system is chronically depressed, toxins build up, and disease slowly consumes the body. This process is usually attributed to "aging." We are supposed to degenerate and fall apart as we get older and are told there is nothing we can do about it. Often medications are prescribed to mask the symptoms, but taking drugs only adds more chemical toxins to the body.

Subclinical malnutrition is a major problem as it prevents our bodies from removing toxins as it normally should and accelerates the degeneration of the body by toxic buildup. The first thing you should do to prepare yourself for detoxification is to provide the body with the nutrients it needs to do the work of detoxification. A detox program will be of little use if the body is malnourished and can't function properly. Before you start any detox program, you must first make sure you are getting the proper nutrition. Juice fasting for example, one of the most popular forms of detoxification, would not be recommended for anyone who is malnourished as it can make the condition worse. The same is true for heat therapies which sweat toxins from the system. Vital salts and minerals would also be lost in the sweat of a malnourished individual. So it is with most other detox programs.

ESSENTIAL NUTRIENTS

So what are the nutrients that are essential to good health? Water, carbohydrate, fat (fatty acids), protein (amino acids), vitamins (including phytochemicals), and minerals are the nutrients the body uses for the growth, maintenance, and repair of its tissues. From these six categories of nutrients, our bodies get all the building blocks to grow and maintain life and health. There are dozens of different vitamins and minerals necessary for good health. Some vitamins can be synthesized by the body from other nutrients. Some nutrients are classified as "essential" because the body cannot make them in sufficient quantities to meet its needs and so must obtain them directly from the diet. All minerals, many vitamins, a few amino acids, and some fatty acids are considered essential nutrients.

The nutrients can be divided into two categories: energy-yielding (carbohydrate, fat, protein) and nonenergy-yielding (water, vitamins, and minerals). The energy-yielding nutrients are our primary food source. They provide the energy that every cell and every organ needs to function. Without continual replenishment of energy, you would quickly die. The amount of energy released by these nutrients is measured in calories, a term with which everyone is familiar. The body burns calories (i.e., uses energy) during exercise. People often think of calorie as a element of the food but, actually, it is a measure of energy provided by food.

When broken down in the body, a gram of carbohydrate provides the same amount of calories as a gram of protein. A gram of fat, however, provides more than twice as many calories as either carbohydrate or protein. The energy content of food, therefore, depends on how much carbohydrate, fat, and protein it contains.

After a meal, if your body doesn't use all the food energy received to fuel metabolic and physical activities, it rearranges the excess nutrients (and the energy they contain) into compounds such as body fat, and stores them for use between meals. If you consume more energy than

you use, no matter from which of the three energy-yielding nutrients, the result is an accumulation of body fat and an increase in weight. Too much fish (a protein-rich food) is just as fattening as too many potatoes (a carbohydrate-rich food). But too much fried potatoes or deep fried fish is a great deal more fattening than their baked equivalents. Fats and oils, having more calories per gram, will contribute more to the development of body fat and weight gain than either protein or carbohydrate.

Weight conscious people often blame sugar for their weight problems. Sugary foods are really no more fattening than fish or potatoes. Cake, for instance, is made of flour, a carbohydrate-rich food, and sugar, which is almost pure carbohydrate. Cake frosting, however, is fattening, not because of the sugar content, but because of the fat. Sugary foods are usually fattening because most of them are also high in fat. Sugar makes foods taste good, so overcomsumption is easy. Sugar has many other health risks associated with it other than contributing to body fat. Sugar is a highly refined carbohydrate or *simple* carbohydrate. This is in contrast to the *complex* carbohydrate found in fruits and vegetables. Simple carbohydrates are absorbed almost immediately into the bloodsteam, causing great stress on the pancreas and other body organs as well as drug-like effects on the mind and emotions. Complex carbohydrates, on the other hand, are digested slowly and feed a steady, more manageable stream of energy to the blood.

All natural foods contain mixtures of each of the three energy-yielding nutrients. Often, foods are classified by their predominant nutrient; beef is considered a protein, bread a carbohydrate, and cream a fat. This is inaccurate. Beef also contains a lot of fat as well as protein. Carbohydrate-rich foods like bread also contain fat and protein. And cream contains not only fat but protein and some carbohydrate.

A hundred grams of food may contain only ten or so grams of energy-yielding nutrients, the rest being water, fiber, and other non-caloric materials. What isn't immediately used in energy to fuel metabolism or movement is stored in the body. Indigestible material, like fiber, is excreted as waste.

Water

Water is our most important nutrient. We can live for weeks without other nutrients, but deprived of water we would die of dehydration in a matter of days. Approximately 60 percent of our body weight is from water. Water lubricates our joints, protects our brain, facilitates digestion and elimination, and provides the medium for our red and white blood cells to circulate throughout the body, carrying nutrients and removing toxins. All of our cells are filled with and continually bathed in water solutions. It is the medium in which metabolism and all other chemical reactions in the body occur. All of the other nutrients need water in order to fulfill their functions.

Pure clean water, without contamination, is necessary every day. On average we should drink about six to eight 8-ounce glasses of water a day. Children should take less according to their body size, and larger individuals a little more.

Vitamins and Minerals

Vitamins are vital to life, but do not yield energy. They help the body break down energy-yielding nutrients and extract usable energy from them. They serve as helpers, making possible the processes by which the other nutrients are digested, absorbed, and metabolized. Minerals are inorganic elements that the body needs in small amounts and, like vitamins, play an important part in many bodily functions.

Vitamins and minerals are the nutrients most lacking in our diet. Both are either removed or destroyed in food processing. Refined products and highly processed foods are depleted of these vital nutrients. To make matters worse, vitamins and minerals are also leached out of the body by sugar, alcohol, tobacco, drugs, and other chemicals (food additives and pollutants). As a consequence, a diet of poor-quality, contaminated food contributes to malnutrition or, more commonly, subclinical malnutrition and nutritive imbalances. Such a condition can lead to the deterioration of health and increased susceptibility to disease.

Food manufacturers try to overcome part of the problem of the loss of nutrients in processing by adding some vitamins and minerals back into their finished products. Vitamin and mineral supplements are also taken to supply necessary nutrients lacking in typical diets. The vitamins added to processed foods and the vast majority of supplements available are synthetically manufactured. Although not normally harmful if taken in reasonable doses, synthetic vitamins and minerals have a very limited effect on the body. Synthetic supplements will prevent gross deficiency disease such as scurvy, which is caused by a lack of vitamin C, but by themselves can only do so much. Synthetic supplements are combined with fillers and other ingredients such as sugar. Some are over 75 percent sugar. All chewable supplements contain either sugar or artificial sweeteners. Some supplements are actually worthless, because they are not effectively dissolved or absorbed by the body. X-rays have revealed pills completely intact

in the colon on their way out of the body. Companies that handle the sanitation of portable toilets report that during the cleaning process, they come across a great deal of undissolved vitamin and mineral tablets. Some supplements do dissolve, but are not absorbed and are flushed out of the body unused. The quality of vitamin and mineral supplements varies greatly. A calcium supplement may provide 1000 mg of calcium per tablet, but 80 percent may be unabsorbable, so that taking one of these supplements provides not 1000 mg but only 200 mg of calcium. For

Essential Nutrients

Water	**Amino Acids**
	Isoleucine
Carbohydrate	Leucine
	Lysine
Fats	Methionine
Linoleic acid	Phenylalanine
Linolenic acid	Threonine
Arachidonic acid	Tryptophan
	Valine
	Arginine*
Minerals	Histidine*
Calcium	
Chlorine	
Chromium	**Vitamins**
Cobalt	Ascorbic acid (vitamin C)
Copper	Biotin
Iodine	Cobalamin (vitamin B_{12})
Iron	Folic acid
Magnesium	Niacin (Vitamin B_3)
Manganese	Pantothenic acid
Molybdenum	Pyridoxine (vitamin B_6)
Phosphorus	Riboflavin (vitamin B_2)
Potassium	Thiamine (vitamin B_1)
Selenium	Vitamin A
Sodium	Vitamin D
Sulfur	Vitamin E
Zinc	Vitamin K

A deficiency in any one of these nutrients can lead to ill health. Scientists are just now learning that in addition to those nutrients listed above, another 44 trace minerals and thousands of phytochemicals, many yet undiscovered, may play an important part in our health.

* Needed for growth in children but not essential for adults.

adults, the Recommended Dietary Allowance (RDA) for calcium is 1000 mg. Thus a person in need of calcium may think he is getting enough by taking a mineral supplement, but still be seriously deficient. Relying on vitamin pills to meet nutrient requirements will give you a false sense of security. That is why fortified, processed foods are not good substitutes for natural, whole foods. Dietary supplements are not a replacement for sound dietary habits.

The most bioavailable supplements are those derived from natural plant sources—fruits, vegetables, herbs, and the like. For example, rose hips are a natural source for vitamin C and nutritional yeast (which is a fungus) is a natural source for the B complex vitamins. Natural sources are important for two reasons: (1) they are bioavailable—that is, easily absorbed into the body, and (2) they include a synergistic host of other vitamins and phytochemicals that activate and support the beneficial qualities of the vitamins and minerals. Plant foods are all rich in a variety of essential nutrients.

Phytochemicals are "plant chemicals" such as flavonoids which have been shown to have antioxidant and other health-promoting effects. There are thousands of phytochemicals, most of which have not yet been identified, let alone studied. What is known about phytochemicals is that they work with vitamins to promote health and stop or reverse degenerative conditions like cancer. Vitamins by themselves have limited ability as evidenced by studies using synthetic vitamins. But vitamins derived from natural sources, which are always accompanied by an assortment of phytochemicals, can have remarkable detoxification and healing qualities.

A similar situation exists with minerals. Minerals come from the earth—the rocks and soil. In their natural form in the earth, they are difficult for the body to utilize. Plants extract them from the ground and incorporate them into their cell structure. In plants, minerals are transformed into a form that our bodies can readily use. The vitamins and phytochemicals found in natural sources combine to make these plant minerals more absorbable and more potent. Minerals also work better in combination with other minerals. In fact, taking mineral supplements can be detrimental to health as they can actually leach other minerals from the body. For example, too much zinc will leach copper and too much phosphorus will pull out

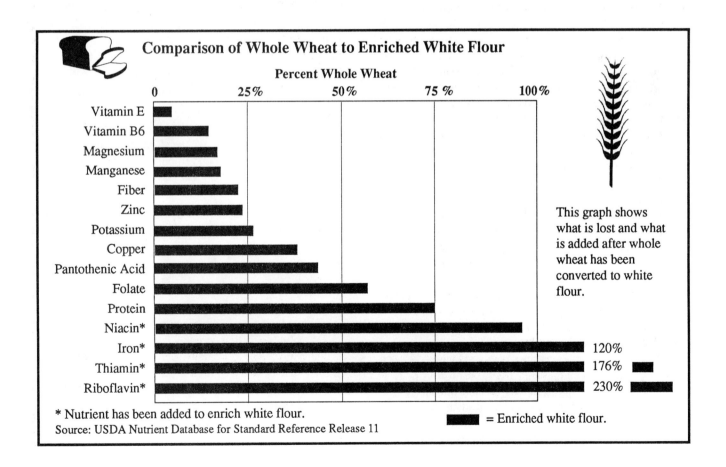

Comparison of Whole Wheat to Enriched White Flour

Percent Whole Wheat

Iron*	120%
Thiamin*	176%
Riboflavin*	230%

* Nutrient has been added to enrich white flour.

Source: USDA Nutrient Database for Standard Reference Release 11

= Enriched white flour.

This graph shows what is lost and what is added after whole wheat has been converted to white flour.

calcium. Consuming too much of any particular mineral from supplements or even the diet can cause deficiencies in other minerals. So a whole spectrum of minerals must be taken to avoid deficiencies. Manufactured foods often have unnatural mineral balances. Soft drinks have high concentrations of phosphorus (in the form of phosphoric acid) which depletes the body's reserves of calcium and contributes to deficiencies such as osteoporosis. Natural plant sources of phosphorus are always buffered with calcium so none of this mineral is lost from the body's reserves.

The best and most complete source for vitamins and minerals is food. Supplements are just that—supplements to the diet. They are not supposed to replace a good diet. Some people believe that by taking supplements or eating "vitamin-fortified" foods they can get by with a poor-quality diet. With high-quality foods you get a complete spectrum of vitamins, minerals, and phytochemicals necessary for maintaining good health. That is the way nature intended it.

Carbohydrate

Carbohydrate is the body's preferred energy-yielding nutrient. Sixty percent of the calories in our diets should come from carbohydrates, which means that the bulk of our diets should consist of foods high in carbohydrates. For this reason, you should build your meals around carbohydrate-rich foods—fruits, vegetables, grains, nuts, and seeds. Natural carbohydrate-rich foods also contain all the protein and fat the body needs, so it isn't necessary for you to add high-protein or fatty foods. Carbohydrate-rich foods are also high in fiber which is crucial for good health. Refined foods such as white sugar and white flour have many nutrients and most all the fiber removed, and so do not supply balanced nutrition.

Complex carbohydrates are composed of chains of sugars or simple carbohydrates. The body converts carbohydrate into blood sugar (glucose), which is the body's form of fuel. During digestion, the body breaks complex carbohydrates into simple carbohydrates which are then absorbed into the bloodstream. All sugars are simple carbohydrates.

When blood glucose level rises too high, serious health problems can result, so the body works to prevent this. If glucose is slowly added to the bloodstream, as it does when digesting complex carbohydrates, the body is capable of keeping the blood sugar level under control. Refined and even natural sugars, however, are absorbed almost immediately into the bloodsteam. This produces a major surge in blood sugar, causing wide and dangerous swings in glucose levels. For this reason sugar, whether refined or natural, should be consumed in moderation.

Starch is the highest quality complex carbohydrate. Chemically, it consists of long chains of glucose molecules. Grains are the richest food source of starch. Wheat, rice, corn, millet, rye, barley, and oats are the most widely used. A second important source of starch is the legume family (beans and peas) including peanuts and dry beans (kidney beans, black-eyed peas, soybeans, etc.). A third major source of starches are tubers such as potato, yam, and cassava. Most human civilizations throughout history have relied on grains or other carbohydrate-rich foods as their staple food source. In Asia it's soy and rice; in Latin America it's beans and corn; in North America and much of Europe it's wheat and potatoes. Wheat is the most popular carbohydrate and food staple used throughout the world. It is for this reason it has been called the "staff of life."

It has been observed that people who center their diets around high carbohydrate foods such as the Filipinos, Chinese, and Japanese (who eat mainly rice and vegetables) suffer little from obesity, heart trouble, breast cancer, and other serious health problems. People who switch from a meat-based diet to one high in complex carbohydrates lose excess weight and become healthier. You can eat the same volume of food, not get hungry, and still lose weight because you only get about a quarter of the calories. Also, you get fewer calories from the fat associated with meat.

Protein

We all know that we need protein, the source of amino acids, for growth and to build muscles. The highest protein food sources are meat and dairy products. People

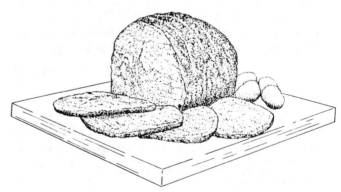

Meat is not the only source of protein.

make an effort to eat steak, chicken, fish, eggs, and cheese to get the protein they feel they need to build strong bodies. Meat has almost become synonymous with protein. When told to reduce our meat consumption, our immediate concern is: where will we get our protein?

Although meat and other animal products are high in protein, they are certainly not the only sources. Many plant foods contain significant amounts of protein. Produce can supply you with all the protein your body needs. Animal protein is not necessary. Protein from meat has been way overvalued, and most people eat far too much meat and protein.

In the United States the Recommended Dietary Allowance (RDA) for protein is set high enough to cover the estimated needs of about 99 percent of the population, including those with unusually high protein requirements such as athletes. Still, most people consume much more protein than the RDA. For an average-sized person, the RDA set by the United States and the World Health Organization (WHO) is only about 50 grams a day. Many people easily consume this much in a single meal.

There is protein in all natural foods—grains, beans, nuts, seeds, and vegetables. The only foods that lack it are processed and refined foods. Such foods have had the protein stripped away. Every living cell, animal or plant has protein. You can get all the protein you need even from a strict vegetarian diet. The gorilla gets all the protein it needs from fruits and vegetables. Likewise, cows don't eat other cows to get their protein. Nor do they drink milk after weaning. It is, in fact, very difficult not to get enough protein.

Plant foods that provide a good source of protein include grains, beans, potatoes, nuts, and seeds. The first three are especially important because they are also rich in carbohydrates.

The main problem with protein is not that we are failing to get enough, but we are getting too much. Our protein intake typically soars to two, three, and even more times what is necessary. Excess protein in the diet, like excess carbohydrate, is converted to body fat.

Dietary Fats

Fatty acids, or dietary fat, is an important part of our diet. We must have some fat in order to be healthy. Vitamins A, D, E, and K are found in the lipid (fat) component of vegetable and animal foods. Foods rich in fat are red meat, chicken, fish, dairy, eggs, nuts, and seeds. Leafy green vegetables also supply some fat. Vegetable oils are derived from nuts and seeds.

By far the most abundant and the most important of the dietary fats are the triglycerides which are composed of fatty acids. The three categories of fatty acids are saturated, monounsaturated, and polyunsaturated.

All naturally occurring fats and oils consist if a mixture of all three. There is no such thing of a naturally occurring fat that is totally all saturated or 100 percent polyunsaturated. Even olive oil which is considered a monounsaturated oil contains both saturated and polyunsaturated fat. Beef fat, which is considered a saturated fat actually contains 44 percent monounsaturated fat as well as 4 percent polyunsaturated fat. Chicken fat which most of us think of as saturated contains only 31 percent saturated fat. It would be more accurate to describe the fat as monounsaturated because it comprised 47 percent of the fat. The rest (22 percent) is polyunsaturated.

People have been eating fat, even saturated fat, for thousands of years without heart disease or hardening of the arteries. It's only been over the past century that fat consumption has become a problem. Studies show that we haven't increased our animal fat consumption, in fact, animal fat consumption has decreased while heart disease has increased. But the fats we eat nowadays are different from what our ancestors ate.

Most of the animals from which we get our meat, dairy, and eggs are raised in confinement and given regular doses of antibiotics and artificial growth hormones. The feed they are given is high is pesticide residue. Most of these chemicals that the animals are exposed to are fat-soluble and, therefore, accumulate in the fatty tissues of the animals and their products (milk and eggs). Animal fat nowadays is chemically contaminated. When you eat animal fat (in meat, dairy, and eggs) you are consuming residual drugs and pesticides. These contaminates can and do have an impact on your health. Why is it that an Eskimo in Greenland, a Masai tribesmen from Africa, or a North American Plains Indian can live on a diet of nearly 100 percent meat and be completely free from heart disease? The animal products they eat were not contaminated by drugs and pesticides. Medical records on the Eskimos of Canada show they had little disease when they lived off the land, but once they moved into permanent settlements and began eating commercially prepared foods, which included meat and dairy with contaminated fat, their disease rate skyrocketed.

Toxins from the environment (pesticides, heavy metals, industrial pollutants, etc.) and those purposely fed to the animals (antibiotics, hormones, etc.) collect and are stored in fatty tissues. When we eat meat we are also consuming these toxins in the fat. No meat, no matter how lean, is free from fat because fatty tissues are intermingled within the muscle fibers of the meat. All commercially raised meat is contaminated. Our bodies were designed to handle natural fats, but the animal fats we have today are dangerous. The only safe animal fats are from organically raised animals.

MEAT AND HEALTH
The Hidden Danger of
High Protein Consumption

High protein foods—meat and dairy products—are high in fat which act as storage tanks for harmful toxins. But fat is not the only problem with animal products. Protein, if overconsumed, can lead to health problems as well.

Protein is an essential nutrient. We must have it in order to build our own tissues. The problem is that we consume far too much and run the risk of protein poisoning. Anything can become toxic if consumed in excess. Even vitamins and minerals, which are necessary for proper body functions, can become poisonous if taken in excess of body needs. A good example is arsenic. The body needs this mineral in minute quantities, but even very small amounts over the body's need can become deadly. For this reason, it is often used as the active ingredient in poisons for rodents and other pests. Likewise, excess protein has a damaging effect which leads to a condition called acidosis which can be fatal.

The body can become dangerously toxic by becoming too acidic (acidosis), or more correctly less alkaline and, consequently, minerally depleted. One of the requirements for the healthy survival of the body is the maintenance or quick restoration of the acid-base balance of its fluids. What this means is keeping the concentration of hydrogen ions in body fluids relatively constant or in

The three graphs on pages 48 and 49 show the relationship between death rates to fat consumption by different populations. The more fat eaten, the higher the death rate. More important than the amount of fat, however, is the type of fat. The people in those countries that consume the most fat eat primarily polyunsaturated and hydrogenated vegetable oils in the form of convenience and prepared foods as well as contaminated animal fats. The type of fat eaten in the countries with the lowest death rate are natural fats both saturated and unsaturated. (Adapted from B.S. Reddy, Advances In Cancer Research, *32:237, 1980.)*

balance. This is of vial importance. If the hydrogen ion concentration deviates even slightly, normal cellular chemical reactions are disrupted and survival is threatened. The acidity or alkalinity of a solution is expressed numerically on what is called a pH scale. Acid-base balance is also known as pH balance.

Most all body fluids (blood, saliva, interstitial fluid, cytoplasm, etc.) are slightly alkaline (basic). Stomach juices are an exception. In the stomach, juices are acidic, a necessity for proper digestion. If the stomach acid were not strong enough, even by a very small degree, certain foods could not be digested or assimilated into the body. Likewise, if blood pH varies only slightly, all body functions could be affected which could lead to disease and even death. Because of the importance of maintaining pH at normal levels, the body constantly works to keep the acid-alkaline balance.

The acid-base balance of the body is influenced by the food we eat. Some foods have an acidifying effect and some an alkalizing effect. A few are neutral. The pH balance of our bodies and consequently our health, depends greatly on the types of foods we eat.

When food is metabolized in the body, it leaves an ash-like residue. This ash is what is left over after most of the usable nutrients have been removed. The elements comprising the ash are either absorbed into the body or eliminated. All food leaves an ash residue. This ash can

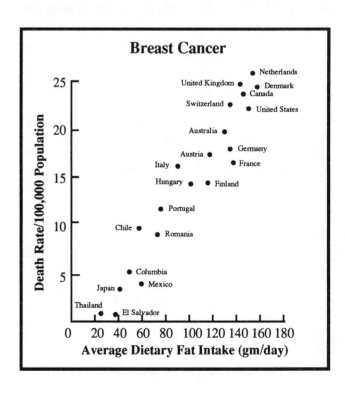

have an acidic, alkaline, or neutral effect on the body's chemistry. Alkaline ash leaves alkalizing minerals which the body can use to neutralize excess dietary acid. Alkaline ash is good because our bodies are supposed to be slightly alkaline. Acid ash, on the other hand, leaves minerals that must be neutralized before the body can dispose of them. Foods high in sulfur, chloride, nitrogen, and phosphorus have an acidifying effect. The residue contains strong acids, such as sulfuric acid and phosphoric acid, that must be neutralized and eliminated by the kidneys. Nitrogen intake beyond the body's needs is converted to urea and removed by kidneys as urine or by the skin as sweat. Some foods have a higher percentage of acidifying minerals than others. Protein, especially animal protein, is high in these elements.

Acidifying elements must be neutralized in order to maintain acid-base balance. Alkaline minerals such as sodium, calcium, potassium, and magnesium serve this function. These elements are found most abundantly in plant foods. The body will store these minerals to maintain pH balance. Bones are the primary source of calcium, potassium, and magnesium.

The body is capable of handling moderate amounts of acidifying foods. However, if most of the food eaten leaves an acid ash, the body will be continually pulling alkalizing elements from its reserves, depleting itself of vital minerals, and acidosis results. If the body is constantly struggling to

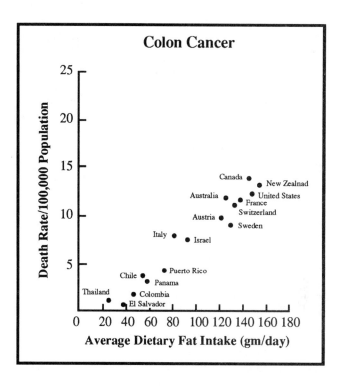

neutralize acid, health will suffer. Chronic acidosis can lead to cellular degeneration.

A great many people suffer from subclinical or mild-stage chronic acidosis. They don't die immediately but hang on the edge, suffering gradual degeneration. Their symptoms are not strong enough to classify them as life threatening. But body chemistry is at its limits, continually struggling to maintain balance, leaching calcium from bones. Body chemistry is in turmoil and health is going downhill year after year.

Acidosis leads to loss of calcium and weakening of the bones (osteoporosis), degeneration of joints (arthritis), precipitation of calcium in body tissues (kidney stones and gout), and development of painful bone spurs. Body chemistry is constantly on the edge of its limitations, which creates tremendous stress and encourages degeneration of tissues, weakening the immune system, increasing susceptibility to disease, and affecting normal bodily functions.

In general, foods which have a high protein content leave an acid ash residue (see chart on following page). Foods which have the greatest acidifying effect are meat, fish, poultry, dairy, and eggs—animal products. Most grains, nuts and legumes, which are good sources of plant protein, also leave an acid ash residue. With few exceptions, fruits and vegetables leave an alkaline ash residue. Eating a diet consisting primarily of animal products and flour

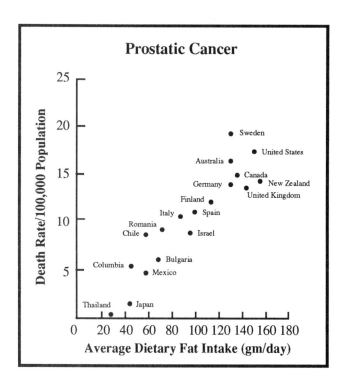

Alkaline Ash and Acid Ash Foods

Alkaline Ash Foods		Acid Ash Foods		Neutral Ash Foods
Almonds	Lettuce	Bacon	Peanuts	Sugar
Apples	Lima beans	Barley	Peas, dried	Corn oil
Apricots	Limes	Beef	Pike	Olive oil
Avocados	Millet	Blueberries	Plums*	
Bananas	Molasses	Butter	Pork	
Beans, dried	Mushrooms	Carob	Prunes*	
Beets	Muskmelon	Cheese	Rice	
Blackberries	Onions	Chicken	Salmon	
Broccoli	Oranges	Codfish	Sardines	
Brussels sprouts	Parsnips	Corn	Sausage	
Cabbage	Peaches	Cranberries*	Scallops	
Carrots	Pears	Currants	Shrimp	
Cauliflower	Pineapple	Eggs	Squash, winter	
Celery	Potatoes	Haddock	Sunflower seeds	
Chard	Radishes	Honey	Turkey	
Cherries, sour	Raisins	Lamb	Walnuts	
Cucumbers	Raspberries	Lintels, dried	Wheat	
Dates, dried	Rutabagas	Lobster	Yogurt	
Figs, dried	Sauerkraut	Milk*		
Grapefruit	Soy beans, green	Macaroni		
Grapes	Spinach, raw	Oatmeal		
Green beans	Strawberries	Oysters		
Green peas	Tangerines			
Lemons	Tomatoes			
	Watermelon			

*Leaves an alkaline ash but has an acidifying effect on the body.

In general, fruits and vegetables leave an alkaline ash residue while meat, dairy, grains, and nuts leave an acid ash residue.

Although citrus fruits such as oranges and lemons contain citric acid and may have an acid taste, thy are not acid forming when metabolized. The acid-forming potential of a food is determined largely by the chloride, sulfur, and phosphorus elements found in the noncombustible mineral residue or ash after metabolism of the food has occurred. Acids such as those found in citrus fruits are normally fully oxidized by the cells during metabolism and leave no mineral residue.

Source: M. Ted Morter, Jr., *Your Health Your Choice*, pages 85-86.

(bread, crackers, pasta, etc.) will lead to acidosis. This is one of the key reasons why vegetarians or near vegetarians are so much more healthy then nonvegetarians.

Calcium is one of the primary alkalizing minerals. We are told by dairy industry and others that milk and other dairy products are good for us because they contain calcium. Calcium is necessary for bones as well as its alkalizing effect in maintaining the acid-base balance. Milk is promoted as one of our best sources of calcium. But is it really?

At the age of 36, Roseanne considered herself healthy. She had a few aches and pains, but she reasoned, doesn't everybody? While casually walking across her front lawn she stepped on a raised clump of grass, twisted her ankle and fell. Ordinarily such an accident would cause little concern for a young healthy person. The pain, however, was so intense she couldn't move, let alone walk. On seeing a doctor, she learned the "twisted" ankle was actually broken. X-rays also showed she was losing calcium from her bones, and even slight stress, like a twisted ankle, exerted enough force to cause a fracture. Her doctor recommended that she drink more milk and to take calcium supplements, but offered no other dietary advice.

Roseanne's sister also had suffered from osteoporosis, but was doing very well now. She told Roseanne not to increase her milk consumption or take the calcium supplements. Instead she told Roseanne to cut down on meats and eat more fruits and vegetables. It seemed to work for her sister so she followed the same advice. For the next year she remained on a low-protein diet. During this time, pain she had been experiencing from arthritis for a couple of years disappeared. She revisited the doctor and new x-rays showed the bones had become more dense. Roseanne reversed the effects of osteoporosis and the pain of arthritis by reducing the amount of milk and meat in her diet. She got essentially all of her calcium from plant foods as well as getting her body chemistry back into balance. Her story is not unusual. Others in similar circumstances have discovered that the best source of bioavailable calcium is not found in milk, but in fruits and vegetables.

While milk is rich in calcium, it is also high in protein and has an acidifying effect on the body. A study on calcium reported in *The American Journal of Clinical Nutrition* verified the results experienced by Roseanne. In this study, subjects who were given 1,400 mg of calcium (nearly twice the recommended daily amount) along with 142 grams of protein, suffered a mean calcium *loss* of 84 mg. When protein was reduced to 47 grams the subjects retained 10 mg of calcium. This study showed that too much protein in the diet causes more calcium to be lost than is consumed. When the subjects were given approximately 1 percent less protein than the recommended amount, their bodies started to retain calcium.

Another study on protein-induced hypercalciuria (excessive urinary excretion of calcium) was conducted by the Department of Nutritional Sciences at the University of California, Berkeley, which was also reported in *The American Journal of Clinical Nutrition*. The results of this study showed that high calcium consumption does not offset the calcium loss caused by a high-protein diet.

In the study, the subjects were put on a controlled formula diet that contained high levels of protein and 1,400 mg of calcium. The researchers found that the more protein the subjects ate, the more calcium they lost. They also found that adding calcium did not increase the amount that was absorbed into the blood. When fruits and vegetables were added to the high-protein diet, the calcium balance did not improve. The conclusion that can be drawn from this and the previous study is, that no matter how many fruits and vegetables or milk and calcium supplements you take, diets high in protein will still cause a net loss of calcium.

Milk, although high in calcium, because of its protein content, is not necessarily a good source for calcium. However, calcium from milk may be beneficial *if* total protein intake is limited to 47 grams. Calcium supplements nor milk will do any good if protein intake is high (over 47 grams according to the study). Milk is high in protein—8 grams per cup. One glass of milk equals about 2½ cups containing 20 grams of protein. Just three glasses of milk provides 60 grams of protein, far over the limit at which calcium is not leached from the body. If any other food, including fruits and vegetables, is also eaten more protein is added to the body and calcium leaching is intensified. Drinking more than three glasses of milk a day then may actually weaken the bones.

All food grown in nature contains protein. If you eat a variety of foods, you will get all the protein you need, even if you eat a strict vegetarian diet without meat, fish,

foul, dairy, or eggs of any type. We have been led to believe that only animal protein provides a complete protein. Actually, plants also have complete protein and you can get all the protein elements you need from plant foods.

The recommended amount of protein is approximately 50 grams a day for an average-sized person. This amount of protein can be obtained easily without even realizing it. If you started breakfast with one egg and a glass of milk, at lunch you had a garden salad with a little cheese sprinkled on top, and for dinner you ate one chicken leg with another glass of milk, you would have far more than 50 grams of protein just from the dairy and meat. Any bread, vegetables, or other foods would provide additional protein.

How many people eat just one egg for breakfast? Or one chicken leg for dinner? Or just a sprinkle of cheese on a lunch salad? Ordinarily people eat two or more eggs along with bread or pancakes (also good sources of protein). At dinner one small piece of chicken isn't going to satisfy anyone except a small child. Often, people will devour three, four, and even more pieces of chicken as well as rolls, potatoes, and other side dishes, all of which also contain protein. The protein intake soars to two, three, and even four times more than what is necessary. In affluent societies, our diets are based on meat and dairy products. That is the way we were raised and the only way most of us know how to eat.

Some researchers have recommended that the daily intake of protein should be lowered to about 20 grams. This is easily accomplished on the most strict vegetarian diet. Remember, cows don't eat meat to get their protein, nor do they drink milk after weaning.

People have died from consuming too much protein by way of protein supplements, a popular fad among misguided body builders and athletes. Kidneys can become overworked, excreting nitrogen, a component of all protein, and be the cause of kidney failure and death. Osteoporosis can result from eating too much protein. Diets high in protein promote the excretion of calcium, depleting the bones of this important mineral, thus leading to the development of osteoporosis. Eating large amounts of protein doesn't help the athlete or body builder add muscle. It is exercise that builds muscle, not dietary

We will never understand disease until we understand foods.   —Hippocrates protein. The amount of protein stated in the RDA provides more than enough to satisfy the need of athletes.

Do You Need To Become a Vegetarian?

Most natural health diets recommend limiting or even forbidding meat and meat products. Does eating healthfully mean you must give up eating meat and dairy products? No, it does not. Animal products provide many nutrients beneficial to maintaining good health. The problem is eating the right kinds of animal products and eating them in moderation.

Just because someone is a vegetarian does not guarantee good health. There are many malnourished vegetarians who have pale sickly looking complexions!

Some vegetarians are still affected by colitis, colorectal cancer, and other diseases often considered caused by poor dietary habits. The question some ask is: "If vegetarianism is so healthy, why are these people developing degenerative diseases like meat eaters?"

Just because someone claims to be a vegetarian, doesn't mean he is eating healthfully. Many healthy people have been predominantly meat eaters (e.g., Eskimos and early American Indians). However, the meat they ate was organically grown (wild game) and they did *not* overeat. They also ate internal organs (which have the most nutritive value), and exercised (a very important element in achieving good health).

Many vegetarians feel that just refraining from eating meat and dairy will automatically make them healthy. Wrong! They may eat lots of produce (probably coated

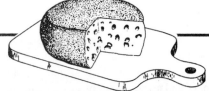

How Much Protein Do You Eat?

Dietary guidelines generally recommend that our protein intake contribute about 12 percent of the total calories consumed. Sixty percent of calories should come from carbohydrate, and 30 percent or less from fat (1 gram of protein = 4 calories, 1 gram of carbohydrate = 4 calories, 1 gram of fat = 9 calories, so 1 gram of fat contributes more than twice as much energy as 1 gram of either protein or carbohydrate). Most people in affluent cultures eat much more protein than 12 percent. Protein need depends on a person's muscle mass and bone structure. Larger people (not fatter) need more protein than smaller people. On average 50 grams a day is recommended as ample protein for most people of average size. Some health authorities believe this figure is far too high and should be closer to 20-30 grams a day. 50 grams a day is very easy to obtain even on a strict vegetarian diet. In fact, most people eat far more than 50 grams of protein a day. A single meal with protein-rich foods such as meat and dairy products can easily supply all the protein a person needs for an entire day. If you eat meat and/or dairy two or more times a day, you are running the risk of protein overload. A diet like this day after day leads to acidosis and all of its accompanying health risks. Because some vegetable foods, such as soy, dried beans, rice, and pasta, are good sources of protein, even vegetarians can get too much protein in their diets. This is one reason why fruits and vegetables are so important.

The Committee on Dietary Allowances of the Food and Nutrition Board of the National Academy of Sciences states the RDA in grams of protein per kilogram of body weight per day. They consider that a generous protein allowance for a healthy adult would be 0.8 grams per kilogram of *appropriate* body weight per day.

Most adults need between 2,000 and 3,000 Calories a day to fuel metabolism and daily activities. These figures vary depending on muscle mass and bone structure. A larger more muscular person requires more calories. Men generally require 500 to 800 more calories than woman. An average-sized woman would need 2,100 and average sized man about 2,900 calories.

The following chart lists the amount of grams in common foods. Use this list to determine your daily protein intake. What was your protein consumption yesterday? Write down all the foods you ate and the approximate serving size, include all meals and snacks. For foods not listed on the chart make an estimated guess. For example, if you ate two handfuls of potato chips you could approximate that as being equivalent to ½ potato which would amount to 2½ grams of protein.

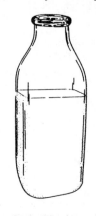

Continued on next page

with waxes, pesticides and other contaminants) as well as refined processed foods such as white bread, sugar, processed honey, chocolate, coffee, etc. It is no wonder why these vegetarians end up with colitis, arthritis, cancer, etc. They are in reality eating no better then anyone else.

Strictly speaking, vegetarianism is not a detoxification diet and will not cleanse your body or make you healthy!

Most people's bodies are overacidic. And a diet of produce helps to bring the pH level of the body back to normal. Too much of a good thing, however, can be just as harmful. Remaining on a strict fruit diet or an all raw foods diet many months can have an over-alkalizing effect. Such a condition can cause alkalosis or too high a blood pH. This can be just as damaging to the health as low pH or acidosis. For optimal health, you should eat a balanced diet of all foods. The alkalizing effect of fruits and vegetables

should be balanced by the acidifying effect of grains and even some wholesome meat, eggs, and dairy.

You don't need to become a vegetarian to be healthy. But you do need to watch the amount of animal products you eat and make sure you do not consume more than about 50 grams of protein a day. What meat (including dairy and eggs) you eat should always be organically raised to avoid contamination by residual drugs, hormones, and pesticides.

VARIETY—THE SPICE OF LIFE

Variety is not only the spice of life but is essential to good health in our modern world. This is particularly true nowadays because overworked soils are often depleted of essential trace minerals. Toxins in the environment also

A cup of fruit juice would be approximately equivalent to 1 cup fruit or 1 gram protein. One apple would also be equivalent to about 1 cup fruit. A hamburger patty is about 3 oz. You can estimate meat portions using the chart below as a guide.

Food	Amount	Protein Content
Wheat bread	1 slice	3 (grams)
White bread	1 slice	2
Pasta (white)	1 cup cooked	7
Pasta (wheat)	1 cup cooked	8
Cornmeal	1 cup dry	10
Rice (brown)	1 cup cooked	5
Rice (white)	1 cup cooked	6
Rice (instant)	1 cup cooked	3
Dried beans	1 cup cooked	15
Tofu	1/2 cup	10
Meat (all types)[1]	1 oz	7
Egg	1 egg	6
Vegetables[2]	1/2 cup	2
Fresh fruit	1 cup/each	1
Potato (without skin)	1 potato or 1 cup	3
Potato (with skin)	1 potato or 1 cup	5
Milk[3]	1 cup	8
Yogurt (plain)	1 cup	12
Cheese	1 oz/slice	6
Nuts	1 oz	3
Fat	1 teaspoon	0
Sugar	1 tablespoon	0

(1) Includes fish and fowl, lean or high fat. (2) Except potatoes. (3) Nonfat, low-fat, or whole.

Using this list you can determine the amount of protein in a typical fast food meal consisting of a cheeseburger, fries, and milkshake. One 3-ounce ground beef patty provides 21 grams of protein; one bun (two sides) has 4 grams of protein; condiments, including dressing, tomato, lettuce, pickle, etc. equal about 1 gram. A single 1-ounce slice of cheese adds 6 grams. The total amount of protein in just the cheeseburger comes to 32 grams. Combine that with a 16-ounce milkshake (16 grams) and fries (4 grams) and you have a grand total of 52 grams of protein, enough for the body for an entire day.

The serving sizes used here are average, not the large portions typically ordered. Two regular cheeseburgers, one large order of fries, and milkshake would provide 84 grams of protein, far in excess of dietary needs for most individuals, including large physically active people. It is very easy to get too much protein, as well as fat, by eating fast foods.

Below are protein figures for some common fast foods:
Arby's regular roast beef sandwich 22g
Burger King Whopper 27g, Whopper w/cheese 31g
Long John Silver's fish and fries, 3 pce 43g
KFC chicken breast 1 piece 24g, thigh 18g
McDonald's Big Mac 25g
Taco Bell beef burrito 22g, bean burrito 13g, regular taco 10g

have created an increased necessity for adequate mineral intake. Toxins leach trace minerals from our bodies causing even a greater deficiency.

Eating the same types of foods over and over again can lead to the development of allergic reactions or food sensitivities. Rotating the types of foods you eat helps to prevent the body from developing food intolerances. Most intolerances are the result of contamination in the foods—pesticides, insect droppings, processing chemicals, heavy metals, mold, etc. If a certain food is eaten constantly, these toxins build up and cause sensitivities. When sensitivities develop and the food is eaten, it will cause adverse reactions whether or not it is contaminated. This happens because the body has developed a conditioned reflex to that type of food—it associates that food with certain toxins and immediately initiates a reaction. People who have adverse reactions to wholesome foods like wheat, nuts, and soy most likely became that way by eating the same contaminated foods over and over. Often food intolerances develop in children who were given solid foods too early in life. This is especially true if they were not breast fed.

Although eating clean foods will improve your health and may reverse numerous degenerative conditions, you must also eat a nutritionally balanced diet in order to obtain optimal health. There are people who avoid poor-quality foods and eat mostly organic foods, but still have health problems. The reason for this is that they do not eat foods that provide them with all the essential nutrients their bodies need. Too little or too much of certain minerals, for example, can cause deficiencies or imbalances that affect bodily functions.

Our bodies require approximately 90 nutrients—amino acids, vitamins, fatty acids, and minerals. In order to get a combination of all the nutrients and avoid deficiencies, you need to eat a variety of foods containing these nutrients. No single food or group of foods can supply you with all the nutrients your body needs. A diet that consists of the same foods will limit your intake of necessary nutrients and may eventually cause health problems.

People may think they are getting all the nutrients they need if they eat only vegetables (even organic vegetables). They probably aren't. Even if they eat primarily fresh raw fruits and vegetables supplemented with occasional beans, nuts, and grains, they probably do not have a balanced diet. Just eating good foods doesn't guarantee that you are getting all the nutrients you need. Apples are good food, but if that is all you ever ate, you would soon have poor health. As good as apples are, they do not contain all the nutrients your body needs to function properly.

The protein in meat and meat products provide a complete source for all of the amino acids our bodies need. But if you do not eat meat products, the necessary amino acids can be derived from protein-rich plant sources such as legumes. No single variety of bean, however, supplies a complete source of essential amino acids, as meat does. Beans can provide all of the essential amino acids, but you need to eat different types of beans. By eating a variety of beans, and other foods rich in vegetable protein, you can supply the body with the source of all the amino acids it needs. Eating a variety of foods is an important key to good health. Beans, grains, and potatoes are all good sources of plant-derived protein. Animal protein is not necessary in the diet.

Some nutrients are more important than others and must be eaten in larger quantities. Some we need in only trace amounts but are vital to good health and without them we become either sick or the body malfunctions causing degenerative conditions to exist. Nutrient deficiencies can be very dramatic such as beriberi (vitamin B_1 deficiency), scurvy (vitamin C deficiency), and pernicious anemia (vitamin B_{12} deficiency) which are life threatening. Some deficiencies can go almost unnoticed because they do not put the body in immediate danger. Symptoms associated with nutrient deficiencies are often overlooked as genetic or environmentally caused, or just the result of advancing age. These may include thinning hair, psoriasis, varicose veins, fatigue, diminishing eyesight, cataracts, arthritis, senility, skin blemishes, slow healing, depression, insomnia, and numerous other conditions.

Meat and grains are the source of the essential nutrient niacin (vitamin B_3). Corn, although a grain, lacks significant amounts of niacin. People whose diets consist primarily of corn and corn products, can develop a vitamin B_3 deficiency known as pellagra. Symptoms include dermatitis, diarrhea, dementia, muscular weakness and swollen tongue. Pellagra can also afflict people who do not eat an adequate amount of grains or meat products (the two main sources of vitamin B_3), and essentially suffer from malnutrition.

Minerals are also of importance. Consuming too much of any one mineral may cause deficiencies in other minerals. Zinc is a necessary mineral, but zinc reduces the availability of dietary copper, another essential mineral. Eating Zinc supplements or foods high in zinc (such as meat) without increasing copper intake may cause a copper deficiency. Symptoms associated with copper deficiencies include wrinkled skin, hernias, varicose veins, aneurysms, anemia, hypo- and hyperthyroidism, and learning disabilities, among others. It is better to have too much copper than not enough, as the body can eliminate the excess.

Deficiencies in certain minerals will cause the body to use other minerals as substitutes if it can. Sometimes these substitutes are detrimental to health. Lead, for example, is a highly toxic metal. It can replace iron in the hemoglobin molecule. Hemoglobin, which is part of the red blood cell is vital in transporting oxygen to all the cells in the body. When lead replaces iron in this molecule, the blood cell becomes dysfunctional. If iron is lacking in the diet and lead is available, lead will be used in the synthesis of hemoglobin which can lead to fatal results. As long as the body has access to all the minerals and other nutrients it needs, potentially harmful elements are, to some extent, prevented from causing harm. The excess is simply removed from the body.

Legumes are a good source for iron, but a poor source for calcium. Grapefruit is a good source of vitamin C but a poor source of magnesium. Apricots have lots of vitamin A but little calcium, iron, or phosphorus. So it is with all foods, they are rich in some essential nutrients but lacking in others.

People who exclude all animal flesh can get the nutrients this source provides by eating products produced by animals such as eggs, cheese, and milk. In contrast, the person who eats no animal flesh, not even fish, needs an alternative source of iron, zinc, and some of the vitamins offered by meat; for this person, the liberal use of legumes is recommended. The person who uses only plant foods has to plan with still more care. For example, one nutrient, vitamin B_{12}, is found only in animal foods, so this person has to eat *naturally* fermented foods such as sauerkraut, tamari sauce, or miso which also provide B_{12} from the bacterial cultures which develop in the fermentation process. Vitamin B_{12} is needed in only minute amounts, so a vegetarian can get all that is necessary by occasionally eating fermented foods. Eating it every day is not necessary. The body apparently can store B_{12} to some degree and, although it is an essential nutrient, most people need not be concerned with eating enough. If they don't eat fermented foods, they should take a vitamin B_{12} supplement or regularly use products such as soy milk which has been fortified with vitamin B_{12}. As for people who attempt to eat only fruit, no vegetables or grains, there is no way they can maintain their health for long.

All produce varies in its nutrient content even among the same type. A russet potato will have slightly different constituents than a red potato. Two red potatoes grown in different soils may vary nutritionally. You would think one potato would be the same as another. But that is not so. The soils in which they were grown have a significant bearing on their nutritional content. A potato grown in soil with adequate magnesium, will have more of that mineral than one grown in magnesium-poor soil. This is true for all produce.

Minerals are vital to good health. There are about 60 minerals that are believed to have physiological value. In fact, not a single function in the human body can take place without at least one mineral cofactor. Even enzymes would be useless without them. Some minerals are needed in only trace amounts, but they are needed, and if they are not supplied in the food, health will suffer.

It is a well-known fact that because of repeated use, most agricultural soils have been depleted of vital trace minerals. Mineral depletion has affected not only North America, but Europe, Australia, and Asia as well. Laboratory tests prove that the fruits, vegetables, and grains do not contain the nutrients they had a few generations ago.

Produce that normally would provide rich sources of minerals are now mineral deficient. Even eating a "healthy" diet composed of fresh vegetables, fruits, and grains could be woefully lacking in necessary trace minerals. Organically grown produce is generally no better. The soils they have been grown in are also minerally depleted. Although they may not be contaminated by pesticides or chemical fertilizers, they would still be lacking in necessary minerals. If the minerals were not in the soil, the plant cannot extract them. Unlike vitamins, minerals cannot be created or destroyed. They are a natural resource. Minerals come from the earth. The only way to get minerals into the soil is to put them there. Minerals in the soil come from the decay of rocks. Rocks are aggregates of minerals and are made up entirely of minerals. As they weather and deteriorate, these minerals are released into the soil. Plants, which may also help break apart the rocks, absorb the minerals. We, in turn, eat the plants and utilize the minerals. We cannot utilize most minerals directly from the soil. The plants convert them into a form which make them bioavailable. So we must get most of our mineral needs from plants or mineral supplements.

The minerals that are available in the soil are dependent on the type of rocks in the area. Every rock type is composed of different minerals. Therefore, the mineral content of the soil in one area of the country may be very different than that of another. Although both may or may not be deficient in trace minerals. So, wheat grown in one area of the country may have a different mineral content than wheat grown in another part. The same is true with tomatoes, onions, green beans and other produce.

In order to get a variety of nutrients, you should eat a variety of foods grown from a variety of locations. In this way you can achieve a reasonably balanced diet.

Nutritionists generally agree that people should not eat the same foods day after day, except for staple foods such as grains. Even then it is best to vary the types of grains and buy from different producers so you get grains grown from different localities. You should switch brands or varieties of all produce. Variety permits you to take advantage of the fact that some foods are better sources of some nutrients than other foods. Also, a monotonous diet may deliver unwanted amounts of undesirable food constituents, such as contaminants (pesticides, pollutants, heavy metals, etc.). In a diet with variety, each food's ingredients are diluted by the bulk of all the other foods eaten and even further diluted if several days are skipped before it is eaten again.

Whole grains are our most important food. Throughout history they have been quite literally the staff of life for the vast majority of cultures in the world. There is good reason for this. Grains provide a rich source of nutrients, including complex carbohydrates—the body's preferred food. Carbohydrates are broken down during metabolism to provide the energy the body needs to perform all other functions. Bodily functions such as temperature regulation, muscle movement, digestion, and even immunity are dependent upon the energy derived from the metabolism of carbohydrates. Although the body can break down fat and protein, it will metabolize carbohydrates first.

Grains should comprise the bulk of your diet, as they have for cultures throughout history. Use a variety of whole grains—wheat, rice, corn, millet, spelt, etc. Legumes also contain much of the nutritional value of grains and have been used as a staple in the diets of many peoples. Meals should be built around grains or legumes. Generous portions of fruits and vegetables should round out your fare. Meat and animal products should be used sparingly, primarily just to add flavor to vegetable and grain dishes. Animal products should not be eaten as the main course, as is commonly done in affluent countries. All animal products should be organic—free from steroids, antibiotics, and other drugs. Produce, likewise, should be organically grown to ensure it isn't contaminated with pesticides and other chemical residues. Eat a wide variety of produce grown in different locations to get the greatest combination of nutrients. If you follow this guideline, you will have a clean, balanced, nutritious diet—a diet that will enable your body to function as it was designed to—with health and vitality.

A diet filled with variety will enhance your enjoyment of natural, wholesome foods. As you eat these foods, you will enjoy them more and not miss the sugar, meat, and processed foods you probably grew up on.

 **ADDITIONAL RESOURCES**

Brain Allergies: The Psychonutrient Connection. Philpott, William H., M.D. and Kalita, D.K., Ph.D. New Canaan, CT: Keats Publishing, 1987.

Diet for A Poisoned Planet. Steinman, David. New York: Ballantine Books, 1990.

Empty Harvest: Understanding the Link Between Our Food, Our Immunity, and Our Planet. Jensen, Bernard, Ph.D. and Anderson, Mark. Garden City Park, NY: Avery Publishing Group, 1990.

The Hidden Addiction: And How to Get Free. Phelps, Janice, K., M.D. and Nourse, A.E., M.D. Boston: Little, Brown & Co., 1986.

Is This Your Child?: Discovering and Treating Unrecognized Allergies. Rapp, Doris, M.D. New York: William Morrow and Co., 1991.

Lick the Sugar Habit. Appleton, Nancy, Ph.D. Garden City Park, NY: Avery Publishing Group, 1988.

Nutritional Influences on Illness. 2nd Edition. Werbach, Melvyn A., M.D. Tarzana, CA: Third Line Press, 1992.

Chapter 4

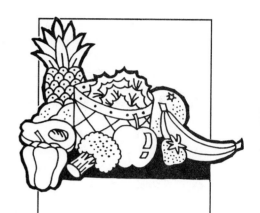

NATURAL FOODS DIET

FOODS AFFECT OUR HEALTH

David came home from school, dragged himself into his room, clinching a package of chips and a coke, and flopped onto his bed to rest. For months David had been coming home fatigued, unusual for a growing teenager who should be full of energy and enthusiasm. All ambition and energy seemed gone. He spent much of his time in his room eating chips, cookies, and drinking Coke. Often that is all he would eat because he wasn't hungry for dinner.

Some months earlier he had noticed a bulge near his groin. At first he ignored it, too embarrassed to mention it to his parents. But it was getting noticeably bigger and he became concerned and told his Dad.

David's father took him in for tests. A biopsy revealed cancer. The doctor called it a neuroblastoma, and warned it was highly malignant. Stage 4. The worst. The mass in David's abdomen was the size of a grapefruit. Finger-like tentacles extended out from the tumor toward his kidneys and liver. The doctor gave him only a 20 percent chance of survival.

David and his parents could not understand why he, a teenager, would have cancer. "It must be genetic," the doctors speculated. But neither of his parents had signs of cancer. Although his grandfather had suffered with prostate cancer, maybe that was the link. He was the unfortunate victim of genetics.

David immediately started an intense program of chemotherapy. If the tumor shrank, then surgery or a bone marrow transplant could be considered. The chemotherapy drained David of his strength and health. "We almost lost him a couple of times because of internal bleeding," recalled his mother.

The chemotherapy program lasted nearly a year. The tumor, however, remained. The doctors decided that David's only hope was to remove the tumor. The treatments made him embarrassingly bald and sapped his strength. David became more withdrawn, went through several periods of deep depression, and stayed in his room consoled only by his chips and Cokes which became a daily routine.

David's operation was performed by a renowned surgeon from the Mayo Clinic. But one look at the extensive growth and he knew that little could be done for the boy. The medical team made an attempt, but were only able to remove a small portion of the mass.

"We've done all we can for him," the doctor told his parents. "You better prepare yourselves. I don't think he has more than six months to live."

"I cried," recalls his mother. "David was too young to die from a disease like this." There was nothing else that could be done for him.

Man is what he eats.
—Goethe

To a greater extent than most of us are willing to accept, today's disorders of overweight, heart disease, cancer, blood pressure, and diabetes are by and large preventable. In this light, true health insurance is not what one carries on a plastic card, but what one does for oneself.
—Lawrence Power, M.D.

Hypertension is a disease of civilized life. Growing up in New Guinea or the northern forests of Brazil is a fine way to avoid the disease.
—Harvard Medical School Health Letter

"After we brought David home," said his mother, "a friend handed us a book he thought might help." The book was about using nutrition to combat disease. It contained accounts of how others had regained their health through dietary changes. "Could this be the answer?" she wondered. The doctors gave them no hope for recovery. It was worth a try.

When she told the oncologist that she planned to put David on a strict diet, the doctor was angry. She had already made arrangements with a specialist to try some experimental drug treatments and ridiculed them for believing in an unconventional (and less expensive and less dangerous) nutritional approach.

"I wasn't about to let them experiment on my son. He had suffered enough with the chemotherapy."

The first stage of David's nutritional program was to eliminate all junk foods, including the daily chips and Coke he was accustomed to. All meat and dairy products were also removed from his diet. His meals consisted primarily of whole grain foods, fruits, and vegetables. He drank carrot and apple juice every day. "It was too difficult to make two separate meals for the family," David's mother says, "so we all ate pretty much the same types of foods. I believed this helped encourage David to eat well, knowing that we were all doing this together."

Six months after the doctors pronounced his death sentence, David was alive and doing well. Just three months after beginning their nutrition program the doctors were amazed. They even called it a miracle. Under chemo and radiation treatments his cancer counts kept going up. When he switched to nutrition, the counts went down to normal. And now they can't even find the tumor! David feels great. His energy has returned and his zest for life has been renewed. His hair has grown back and a once severe acne problem that troubles most teenagers is now virtually unnoticeable. An added benefit resulting from the change in diet is that all the family members report an increased sense of well-being and health. "It not only helped David," says his mother, "but it helped us all gain better health."

Diet is the center of all detoxification programs. What goes into our mouths has the most effect on our health, both good and bad. By eliminating the foods that contribute to toxification of the body and eating foods that help clean the body, better health will result. All other detoxification programs will fail if we continue to eat contaminated and nutrition-poor foods. Following the Natural Foods Diet, which is explained in the following section, will provide the nutrition the body needs to be healthy, and will help remove and keep toxins out. It provides the foundation for all of the detoxification programs outlined in this book.

THE NATURAL FOODS DIET PLAN

When we hear the word "diet," we often think of a temporary restriction on certain foods for the purpose of losing weight. There are low-calorie diets, low-fat diets, low-carbohydrate diets, high-protein diets, and on and on, ad nauseam. These diets are all temporary measures to reduce unwanted weight. They are, in fact, fad diets. Once the weight is lost, old eating habits resume, and weight returns.

Fad diets can do more harm than good. Many of these diets are nutritionally unbalanced and don't eliminate harmful toxins from being consumed. In some instances they replace natural substances with artificial ones or with overprocessed "low-calorie" prepared foods which lack nutritive value. In an effort to reduce sugar, for instance, chemicals like saccharin and Nutrasweet are used, which for most people are much more harmful to their health. Although sugar is a very refined processed food that can cause health problems if eaten too frequently, at least it is a food. Saccharin and Nutrasweet are not foods. They are man-made chemicals, and the body has greater difficulty dealing with them.

All fad diets are considered temporary measures to reduce weight or improve health. Once that goal is reached, old eating habits gradually return and the benefits gained are soon lost. In order to get lasting benefit from a diet, it should be a true diet—a diet that will provide necessary nutrition and become a way of life.

The Natural Foods Diet is not a temporary fad to be indulged in simply to lose weight or to quickly regain health. It is a lifestyle change that should last your entire life. And as long as you follow it, you will avoid the substances that lead to ill health, disease, and premature death.

In this diet only clean wholesome foods are consumed. There is no limit on the amount that can be eaten nor is there any calorie counting. You eat until you are satisfied and as often as you are hungry. As long a you only eat the foods allowed, you will lose excess weight, eliminate harmful toxins, strengthen your immune system, and achieve health and well being. Your resistance to disease and illness will increase, your endurance will improve, your mind will become sharper, you will have more energy and accomplish more.

Because the Natural Foods Diet is limited to only pure, wholesome foods, changing from a typical diet of prepared, processed foods, junk food, and other poor-quality food will bring a cleansing change into your life. Eating a Natural Foods Diet will allow the body to detoxify. The detox programs discussed in the following chapters will bring about quick detoxification and should

> We need to get it into our heads that foods have the chemicals needed for tissue repair. Foods, including juices, build tissue, and when a sufficient amount of cleansing and building has taken place, the body heals itself by virtue of natural laws.
> —Bernard Jensen, Ph.D.

be used along with the Natural Foods Diet to speed the detoxification of the entire body.

For the remainder of this chapter, you will learn which foods can be considered "natural" and which ones are not. Lists will identify the major foods or substances which you should or should not eat. Please note that lists flagged with two stars (☆☆) indicate the best choice. Those flagged with one star (☆) indicate foods that may be eaten, but in moderation only. The foods on lists which have no star should be avoided entirely.

FOOD ADDITIVES

Nearly all packaged, canned, or prepared foods, condiments, and beverages contain additives. Some of these additives are made from natural sources and are generally harmless. Others are chemically manufactured and can be deadly. Additives are used to improve taste, appearance, and texture and make foods more appetizing, as well as to extend their shelf life.

There are some 3,000 additives routinely used in our foods. On average, a person consumes nearly 150 pounds of additives each year. Some of these additives, like beet juice or vitamin A have no adverse effects in the amounts given. Others, like refined sugar, salt, and MSG can have detrimental side effects on people who are sensitive to these substances. Many additives, such as sodium nitrite, BHT, and sulfur dioxide can be poisonous in even small amounts and should be completely avoided. The most harmful additives are the ones that are synthesized chemically. The body does not recognize them as natural substances and has difficulty neutralizing and eliminating them. Consequently, some of them tend to accumulate in fat tissues and other metabolically depressed areas of the body. This accumulation, which may take many years, can lead to toxic reactions.

Types of Additives

Sweeteners. The most common food additive is sugar. Sugar is used in a multitude of products, not just sweet foods or desserts. Sauces, fruits, packaged dinners, as well as treats contain sugar. Even frozen and canned fruit often has sugar added. Fruit is routinely picked before ripening because it can be transported to market or processed before spoilage occurs. Because unripe fruit lacks flavor and sweetness, sugar and sometimes artificial flavors are added to enhance taste. There are three basic types of sweeteners (1) Natural—raw honey, raw maple syrup, molasses, sucanat, raw sugar cane juice, rice syrup, etc. (2) Processed—white sugar, brown sugar, corn syrup, sucrose, fructose, maltose, dextrose, whey, processed honey, processed maple syrup (Grade A), etc. (3) Artificial—saccharin, aspartame (Nutrasweet), and cyclamate (banned in the United States and some other countries).

Flavorings. Although sweeteners are the most frequently used additive, flavorings comprise the largest number of additives. There are over 2,000 different types of flavorings. About 500 are natural and the rest synthetic.

Natural flavorings consist of extracts, oils, and spices. Most of these are considered safe if consumed in moderation. Synthetic flavorings are made from so many different types of chemicals that they are listed simply as "artificial flavor" or "imitation flavor" on packaging.

Colorings. Dyes and coloring agents are added to foods to enhance their appearance and make them more appetizing. They generally do not affect taste or quality but are used solely as a means to increase customer appeal and, consequently, sales.

Natural colorings such as beet juice, annatto, carotene, and paprika are safe to use. Artificial colors are chemicals synthesized from petroleum and coal-tar products. Artificial colorings have been of great concern because they have been fingered as the culprits in many physical and emotional health problems. Throughout the years many commonly used dyes have been withdrawn because of adverse affects, including cancer, which they have produced in humans.

Chemical colorings are usually listed by number such as Yellow #1 or Red #5. Often they may be listed only as "artificial colors." They are used in most packaged and prepared foods as well as in medications, synthetic vitamins, candies, and drinks.

Preservatives. Preservatives by their very nature should cause you to think twice about ingesting them. Preservatives are added to foods to prevent oxidation and kill or retard the growth of microorganisms. They are poisons added to our foods to destroy unwanted organisms. Logically, you may ask, if they kill other organisms, what are they doing to me? Preservatives are poisonous to humans too. However, the amount that is added to foods is so small it does not induce an immediate reaction and is thus considered safe. Larger doses or frequent small doses of these chemicals are unquestionably dangerous. The concern is that most ordinary foods contain preservatives and so people eat preservative-laced foods for breakfast, lunch, dinner, and snacks day after day, year after year. It does not take a genius to recognize the danger in this, yet food manufacturers keep telling us it is safe to consume preservatives in small amounts. Ingesting a tiny amount of arsenic may not kill you immediately either, but would you still want to do it? And would you do it day in and day out for years on end?

There are about 100 different chemicals used to prevent spoilage. There are three main types of preservatives: antioxidants, mold inhibitors, and sequestrants. Antioxidants, such as BHA, BHT, and benzoic acid are used to retard oxidation of fats in foods. Oxidation causes rancidity and alters taste. Mold inhibitors are commonly used in baked goods to prevent the growth of mold. Some common preservatives include sodium proprionate, calcium proprionate, sodium diacetate, sorbic acid, and lactic acid. Sequestrants prevent physical or chemical changes to the color, odor, flavor, or appearance of the food. Commonly used in dairy foods, examples are sodium citrate and EDTA.

There are a few natural preservatives such as salt, vinegar, and citric acid (vitamin C) that can be used without the danger associated with these other agents.

Nutritional Supplements. Because food processing often removes or destroys natural nutrients, vitamins and minerals are often added back. The nutrients added to processed foods are almost always synthetic. Although synthetic vitamins are identical to natural vitamins, they do not have the phytochemicals, such a bioflavonoids, that always accompany natural vitamins. Many vitamins require phytochemicals in order to achieve all the benefits offered by them. Beta carotene, long touted for its cancer-fighting ability, has been shown to be worthless in this respect if synthetic vitamins are used. Beta carotene from natural sources, which is always accompanied by numerous phytochemicals, work synergistically together and has shown to be of benefit as a cancer fighter. There are thousands of phytochemicals, most of which have not been identified. The only way to get them is from natural vitamin sources, not synthetic chemicals.

Minerals, likewise, when added to foods may not be of great value. Many mineral supplements as well as mineral additives are not readily absorbable by the body. Colloidal and chelated minerals are absorbed best.

Although synthetic vitamins and minerals added to foods are not generally harmful, and may do some good, they are not as beneficial as the natural elements that were

CAFFEINE

A study conducted at Johns Hopkins School of Medicine confirms that caffeine is indeed as addictive as cigarettes, alcohol, or intravenous drugs. Eliminating caffeine from the diet suddenly causes withdrawal symptoms similar to those observed for other addictions, such as headaches, lethargy, and depression.

Caffeine is the world's most popular mind-altering drug. More than 80 percent of all adults consume it in some form, whether in coffee, tea, sodas, or in stay-awake pills. Many experts claim that if it were coming to market today, it would be classified as a prescription drug. Its pervasiveness in our culture and its historical acceptance do not necessarily mean it's safe.

Effects and Findings:
- Heavy intake may cause symptoms of schizophrenia.
- Caffeine stimulates the central nervous system. It can increase the heartbeat and the metabolic rate.
- Caffeine intake may exaggerate the effects of premenstrual syndrome.
- Caffeine can increase the production of stomach acid and may aggravate ulcers.
- Common problems associated with caffeine include anxiety, insomnia, diarrhea, heart palpitations, malabsorption of iron, and headache.
- It takes several days for caffeine to leave the body.
- One study has shown that caffeine users are more apt to develop osteoporosis.
- Rats given caffeine had a 20 percent birth-defect rate.
- Some studies have found connections between caffeine and various cancers.
- More than 1 cup of coffee per day is likely to decrease fertility in women.

Source: Copley News Service

extracted from the foods in the first place. Nor do the few that are added back replace the dozens that may have been removed.

Other Additives. There are numerous other additives like acids, alkalis, buffers, bleaching and maturing agents, moisture controllers, activity controllers, emulsifiers, texturizers, processing aids, and clarifying agents. Some are derived from natural sources but most are synthetic chemicals.

The Dangers of Food Additives

All synthetic and many so-called "natural" food additives have been shown in animals or humans to be detrimental to health. Effects include: tumors, diarrhea, leaching essential vitamins and minerals from the body, stunted growth, retarded mental development, growth of kidney stones, lowering of nutritional value of foods, preventing absorption of vital nutrients, encouraging growth of harmful intestinal bacteria, glandular dysfunction, headaches, gastric distress, metabolic changes, epileptic-like changes in brain activity, cirrhosis of the liver, brain lesions, alteration of natural hormone production and secretion, allergic reactions, adverse effects on sexual development and function, heart arrhythmia, mutation of DNA and, of course, cancer. This is just a partial list of health problems associated with food additives; many more conditions too numerous to list have been reported. Despite what you may hear from the food industry, some food additives do cause cancer, saccharine being the most notable example. Many food additives become carcinogenic when combined with other chemicals and so are not classified by themselves as a cause of cancer.

Many of the chemicals in our foods become even more toxic when combined with other food additives, environmental pollutants, drugs, or with substances naturally produced by the body. In laboratory tests on animals, chemicals can show mild toxic effects, but when combined with other food additives, alcohol, tobacco, drugs, or human body chemistry, they can become deadly. An example of this is the formation of trihalomethanes, many of which are carcinogenic. These substances form when chemicals, such as chlorine or fluorine (common additives in drinking water), combine with an organic hydrocarbon (food dyes, waxes, plastic wrap, etc.). Another example is the nitrosamines which are also carcinogenic. These are formed when nitrites and nitrates in foods (common in lunch meats, frankfurters, ham, etc.) react with other organic acids in our body or in the foods we eat.

Food manufacturers, whose purposes are profit motivated, admit that additives cause health problems, but they justify their actions by claiming that the small amount put into foods poses little threat to health. Yet, every year thousands of people suffer adverse effects directly from food additives. Over the years many of the most troublesome additives have been removed from the market. But most additives have a cumulative effect and should be avoided.

What Food Additives Can You Eat?

Not all food additives are potentially toxic. Those made from wholesome natural products are the least dangerous. Synthetic chemicals and highly processed food derivatives are not found in nature and are foreign to our bodies; they all have been shown to cause health problems in animals or humans. Even some additives from natural sources can have adverse effects. These substances contribute to the toxic load in our bodies, depress our immune system, and irritate tissues.

You should avoid all foods containing chemical additives. Often, you cannot tell from reading the ingredients on a label if they are natural or not. A simple rule of thumb is if the ingredient is a long multi-syllable word, it is probably a man-made chemical or a highly refined plant or animal extract and should not be eaten. Avoid all foods that contain ingredients you cannot identify. The best foods to eat are those that are as close to their natural state as possible. The more processing foods undergo, the longer the ingredient list becomes, and the more chance for not only the addition of chemical additives but of contamination from processing (cleaning fluid residue, insect droppings, plastic leaching, etc.). It is best to avoid most products that have more than a half dozen or so ingredients.

Below are two lists of commonly used additives. One contains additives that are generally safe to use. Most of these additives are derived from natural sources and are harmless when used in moderation. The other list shows additives that should be avoided. The additives in the second list are all synthetic or highly processed and denatured. These lists are nowhere near complete, but give you an idea of what types of additives pose little harm and which ones you should avoid.

Additives Generally Safe to Use ☆

Annatto
Beet juice, beet powder
Beta-carotene or carotene
Citric acid
Gelatin
Herbs and spices (cloves, peppermint, ginger, etc.)
Lactic acid
Lecithin
Minerals (iron, calcium carbonate, etc.)
Natural oils and extracts (vanilla, almond, etc.)
Natural sweeteners (raw honey, raw maple syrup, molasses, etc.)
Pectin
Sea salt, natural rock salt
Sodium bicarbonate
Sorbic acid
Vegetable glycerin
Vitamins (thiamin, riboflavin, niacin, folate, etc.)
Yeast

Additives to Avoid

Aluminum salts
Artificial colors
Artificial flavorings
Artificial sweeteners (aspartame and saccharin)
Bisulfite
BHA
BHT
BVO
Caffeine
Carrageenan
EDTA
Hydrogenated vegetable oils (including margarine and
    shortening)
Metabisulfite
MSG
Natural smoke flavor
Olestra
Processed and refined sweeteners
Propylene glycol
Propyl gallate
Salt (with aluminum silicate added)
Sodium benzoate
Sodium nitrate and nitrite
Sodium propionate
Sodium sulfite
Sorbitol
Sulfur dioxide
THBQ
Xylitol

Incidental Additives

Incidental additives are those substances in foods that do not appear on package labels. Most of these come as part of other ingredients, for example, ordinary table salt almost always has aluminum silicate added to prevent caking. Aluminum silicate is one of the chemical additives that should be avoided. Whenever "salt" is listed in the ingredients it means ordinary table salt, *including* aluminum silicate. Aluminum silicate is not listed as an ingredient because it is an ingredient of the salt. Sea salt or natural rock salt do not normally contain aluminum silicate and would constitute more natural ingredients. Many substances used as ingredients that appear "clean" may in fact be adulterated with chemical additives that are not listed on the food label.

Another source of incidental additives is from contamination during processing and packaging. These include pesticides, herbicides, fungicides, petroleum based waxes, and other synthetic chemicals used in the prepara-

tion of foods. Some are purposely added, like pesticides and waxes others are residues from cleaning or processing. Iodine which is used as a disinfectant, and can be poisonous to humans, is routinely used to rinse out empty milk canisters at dairies. Iodine residue remains in the containers when they are refilled with fresh milk. Formaldehyde, benzene, and carbon tetrachloride—all carcinogens—are used to extract vegetable oil from seeds. Lye, a strongly caustic and poisonous alkali, is used to extract fatty acids. It is also used in the preparation of canned fruits. Peaches, for example, are immersed in lye bath solutions to cause the skins to fall off easily. The chemicals used to process these foods are never completely removed. Small, but measurable amounts, remain in our foods and collect in our bodies. Virtually all canned and packaged foods, even many health store brands, contain chemical contaminants.

Packaging materials often leach into foods. PVC (polyvinyl chloride) from plastic bottles and plastic wrap contaminate numerous food products. How many foods in your local grocery store are packaged in plastic containers? Virtually all meat is wrapped in plastic as well as many other items such as water, cheese, margarine, lunch meats, and frozen foods. Next time you go to the grocery store, look at the number of foods stored in plastic containers. Heat increases the release of PVC into food it is in contact with. People often microwave foods in a plastic container or cover it with plastic wrap, which increases the food's exposure to this harmful chemical. PVC is only one packaging contaminant; chemicals from paper and metal packaging materials can also leach out into foods. Many companies now are lining the inside of their canned goods in plastic to prevent the metal from leaching into the food, but the plastic they are using is leaching PVC.

Most of the time you will not be able to taste these contaminants in the foods as they are masked by the flavor of the food. Sometimes you will be able to taste them if they are particularly strong or the food has a mild flavor. If you can smell or taste the packaging material on the food, you can be assured that it is contaminated. Water, distilled or spring, which is often bottled in plastic containers, frequently has a plastic taste. Plastic molecules from the bottle have contaminated it. Essentially you're drinking part of the plastic from the container and clogging your body with an unnatural material that may find its way into the bloodstream.

Processed foods can be grossly contaminated, but drugs can be even worse. Drugs contain many chemical additives that could be harmful beside the drug itself. Charles T. McGee, M.D. in his book *How to Survive Modern Technology,* describes an analysis of Premarin, a

---

Fake Fat

Olestra, a fake fat which has no calories, is finding its way into many foods, particularly snack foods. The FDA says olestra is safe but will require a lable because research shows that olestra "may cause abdominal cramping and loose stools," and it could inhibit the absorption of needed nutrients—specifically vitamins A, D, E, and K. To counter this loss, products using olestra must be enriched with those vitamins. Olestra also reduces absorption of beta carotene and other carotenoids (nutrients that may help prevent heart disease and cancer). The long-range effects of consuming olestra are still not known, but like other chemical food additives, it appears to have the potential of contributing to many of the health problems of modern society.

---

commonly used female hormone medication. Premarin is an estrogen drug made from pregnant mares' urine. It is usually given to menopausal women. Estrogens are used to relieve menopausal symptoms. (Severe menopausal symptoms, by the way, are generally an unnatural response in an overly toxic body. Hormonal medications only add to the toxic load.) Premarin, like other drugs, may appear to help relieve some symptoms, but can and does cause many additional symptoms. An analysis of this product showed that samples of Premarin contained not only estrogen but twenty-five other chemicals among which were: talc, polyethylene glycol, shellac, edible black ink, carnauba wax, sucrose, corn starch, propyl paraben, Yellow Dye #5, and sodium benzoate. Most pharmaceutical drugs, especially children's flavored tablets and liquids, contain many chemicals and contaminants besides the medications.

Packaged Processed Foods

The foods which contain the most additives, both intentional and incidental are packaged, processed, convenience foods. A simple item like crackers could contain as many as 25 ingredients. Even whole foods such as canned or frozen fruit and vegetables can contain a dozen additives.

Not only are convenience foods contaminated with additives and processing residues, but nutrient value is often of low quality. Processing removes or destroys much of the original nutritional value. Heating, freezing, chemical baths, refining, and such, all lower the nutritional quality of foods. When you eat convenience foods, you are eating high-calorie, toxic-filled, nutritionally poor foods.

Most packaged processed foods are considered convenience foods—they can be eaten right out of the package or simply be heated and served. Most canned, frozen, and many packaged foods are convenience foods. The first step towards removing toxins from the body and preventing new toxins from entering the body is to eliminate convenience foods from your diet.

Eat nothing that contains preservatives, artificial colorings, flavor enhancers, or chemical food additives. Read the label on everything you buy. Even so-called packaged "health" foods sold in health food stores often contain sugars and other chemical additives, and are overprocessed so that the nutrient value has been destroyed. Although they may be somewhat cleaner than packaged foods sold in grocery stores, most of those should not be eaten on a regular basis. Processing destroys nutrients, and chemical additives, which have no food value, are not food and are, therefore, not meant to be consumed. They only burden the digestive and immune systems, slow down intestinal motility, encourage excess mucus production, and clog the gastrointestinal tract. Just removing problem foods from your diet will greatly improve your health and energy.

Included on the list of refined, processed foods are white bread (and all products made from white flour: donuts, crackers, cookies, cakes, pasta, etc.), breakfast cereals, frozen convenience foods (e.g., TV dinners, pot pies, sandwiches, pizza, burritos, etc.), canned or packaged foods (e.g., soup, quick noodle mixes, chili, ravioli, etc.), and all similar foods. You should avoid them all.

The less a food has been processed, the better. The best foods are natural organically grown foods that have gone through as little handling as possible. The foods you should eat are fresh fruit and vegetables, nuts, seeds, whole grains, and freshly ground flours. Make your own meals from healthy, clean products. It takes a bit longer to make meals from scratch, but you know everything that goes into them. This way you can keep them clean, free from contamination and dangerous food additives. For convenience, you can make enough for several meals at the same time and freeze the rest for later use.

SUGARS AND SWEETS

Sugar, in one form or another, is the most common food additive and is a key ingredient in many foods. Sugar imparts a naturally pleasing taste to foods. In the United States and Canada people consume on average 100 pounds of sugar a year. People in other Western countries consume similar amounts. Much of the sugar we eat comes from sweet foods and desserts, but a large portion is found in everyday foods such as bread, barbecue sauce, frozen and canned fruit, peanut butter, spaghetti sauce, breakfast cereal, etc. In fact, it is hard to find any packaged convenience food without some form of sugar. Our love affair for sugar is natural, but, if not kept within reasonable limits, can become addicting and extremely detrimental to our health. Unfortunately, most of us eat far too many sugary foods.

There are many different types of sweeteners—some relatively natural, some highly processed, and some artificial. Packaged foods contain a variety of these sweeteners. Sweeteners have a variety of names not often recognized as such. A packaged food can look low in sugar because the word "sugar" is not listed or is listed only as a minor ingredient, but total sugar content can constitute a major portion of the product. An item can have ten ingredients, five of which are sugar, all indicated by different names. If you are not familiar with all the different forms of sugar, you can be fooled into believing many of the foods you buy have little of it.

All sugars are simple carbohydrates and affect the blood sugar level of the body, even natural sugars. They weaken the immune system and cause stress on organs, particularly the pancreas which struggles to maintain constant blood sugar levels. Sugars also leach essential vitamins and minerals from the body, depleting vital nutrients and contributing to malnutrition. As a consequence, sugar not only contributes to many health problems, but lowers the body's ability to remove toxins from the body.

Refined sugars are the worst health hazard, for they provide no nutritive value other than calories and create a great deal of stress on the body. Natural sugars, having undergone less processing, retain some vitamins, minerals, and phytochemicals and are, therefore, less stressful on the body. However, all sugars, even natural sugars, create stress. For this reason, foods made with refined sugar should be completely avoided and natural sweets should be eaten only in moderation.

Sugar consumption dramatically inhibits immune function. The ingestion of 100 grams of sugar in any form—table sugar, fructose, honey, etc.—significantly reduces the ability of white blood cells to destroy bacteria. This amount of sugar is what is in two sixteen-ounce sodas or a slice of cherry pie. Sugar begins to suppress the immune system within thirty minutes after you eat it, and the effects last for over five hours. Impairing the activity of immune system leaves the body vulnerable to increased numbers of infectious organisms and reduces its ability to remove disease-causing toxins. People who eat sugary foods at mealtime and for snacks constantly keep their immune systems depressed.

In an effort to avoid the health problems associated with high sugar consumption, sugar substitutes have been created. The most widely used is aspartame (trade name Nutrasweet). Artificial sweeteners may help to avoid problems caused by excess sugar consumption, but create health hazards of their own. The risks of consuming sugar substitutes can be far greater than sugar. Artificial sweeteners also keep a person's craving for sweets alive, so they do nothing for helping people break away from their sugar habit. In fact, the opposite is generally true, artificial sweeteners encourage excessive eating. People get a false sense of security, believing that eating foods with artificial sweeteners is not harming them, so they eat more.

Refined Sweeteners

Refined white sugar is almost 100 percent sucrose. It is the most widely used sugar. It is made from sugarcane and sugarbeets.

Brown sugar is often considered to be "raw" sugar and, therefore, a natural product that is less harmful than white sugar. Brown sugar is not raw sugar, it is white sugar with a tiny bit of molasses added to give it color and flavor. Turbinado sugar has also falsely been called raw sugar, but is nearly as refined as white sugar.

Most honey and maple syrup sold in stores are highly refined products. Vitamins, minerals, and enzymes have been removed and so they are no better than white sugar. All honey, even natural raw honey, is primarily sucrose. A cup of honey is sweeter than a cup of white sugar, not because it is chemically different, but because in its liquid state it is much more dense and, therefore, you get more of it for each cup.

Because of the name similarity, "fructose" is often called "fruit sugar" and is promoted by manufacturers as a natural, and therefore harmless, sweetener. Fructose, however, is far from being a natural sugar and is definitely not harmless. Fructose, in fact, is more highly refined than sucrose and, like sucrose, is made from sugarcane and sugarbeets, not fruit. Table sugar (sucrose) is composed of equal parts of fructose and glucose. Sucrose must be refined further to remove the glucose so as to produce pure fructose. To call fructose a "natural" sugar is an out and out lie.

Because all refined sugars provide no nutritive value, other than calories, and because they contribute to many health problems, they should all be avoided. Natural sweeteners, which retain some nutritive value include: raw honey, unrefined maple syrup, sucanat (raw sugar from sugarcane), chopped dried dates, fruit juice, barley malt, brown rice syrup, and molasses. Molasses is a by-product of sugar production. It is what remains from raw sugar when most of the sucrose is removed. It contains all the vitamins and minerals from the raw sugarcane and sugar beets and, for this reason, is one of the most healthful sweeteners.

All sweeteners should be used sparingly. Sugar, no matter what its source, has a detrimental effect on the body's immune system. It has been shown that even eating natural sweeteners lowers the body's ability to fight infection and remove toxins. As the body becomes used to eating whole natural foods without excess sugars and flavor enhancers, the tastebuds become more sensitive to flavors and sweets so that less sweetening will be necessary for "sweet" foods to be enjoyable.

Natural Sweeteners ☆
Barley malt
Brown rice syrup
Date sugar
Fruit juice
Molasses (blackstrap or barbados)
Raw honey
Sucanat
Unrefined maple syrup

Refined Sweeteners
Brown sugar
Corn syrup
Dextrin
Dextrose
Fructose
Glucose
Honey
Maltodextrin
Maple syrup
Sucrose (white sugar)
Turbinado

Artificial Sweeteners/Sugar Substitutes
Aspartame (Nutrasweet)
Mannitol
Saccharin
Sorbitol
Xylitol

MEAT AND DAIRY PRODUCTS
Meat

Eating excessive amounts of meat and other animal products can cause numerous health problems. Too much protein in the diet can lead to acidosis, which, in turn, can adversely affect all body functions. Animal protein also causes mucus to be excreted in the gastrointestinal tract. Eating too much meat causes an excessive amount of mucus to form, clogging the intestines and hampering digestion. As a result, fecal matter can become encrusted along the walls of the colon preventing absorption and hampering proper elimination. A sluggish colon sets up an environment favorable for the propagation of pathogenic bacteria, fungi, and parasites, leading to various infections and illnesses that can affect not only the colon but spread throughout the entire body.

One of the major health concerns with eating animal products is the high fat content. Animal fat is a major source for the toxins which enter our bodies. It is in the fat cells that chemical residues are stored, including growth hormones, antibiotics, and environmental toxins to which the animals are exposed.

All meat contains fat. You can trim off much of the obvious fat, but it is impossible to remove most of it as fat is intermingled with the muscle fibers and can be undetectable. Even lean cuts of chicken and beef contain a great deal of fat. Pork and pork products are the worst. Not only because of the fat content, but because pork is often infested with parasites. These animals eat garbage, often referred to a "slop." When we eat pork, we ingest residue from slop that has been stored in the pig's tissues.

Uncontaminated fish is perhaps the best animal food because it contains essential fatty acids our bodies need. Unfortunately, much of the fish nowadays is contaminated by pollutants from industrial waste and sewage. Seafood from the bay waters is perhaps the most hazardous as many countries dump toxic waste into the ocean and much of the toxins are absorbed by the sea life. Freshwater streams near manufacturing plants are not any better. Shellfish, catfish, and other scavengers are the most polluted types of fish. They are the garbage collectors of the deep and consequently acquire a great deal of toxic debris in their bodies.

Because meats of all types and meat products are all contaminated by chemicals and pollutants, you should avoid them all. The only exception are those products that are organically raised. These animals are not contaminated with chemicals and drugs. But because they are high in protein they should be consumed sparingly.

Dairy

Dairy products (milk, cream, cheese, etc.) are also highly contaminated with drugs and toxins. Milk is touted as a highly nutritious food source rich in calcium, protein, and vitamins A and D. The vitamins are added to the milk after processing. All milk has been pasteurized (heated to kill bacteria) and homogenized. These two processes destroy much of the value of the milk. In the process of pasteurization, milk is heated to kill bacteria and in so doing nutrients are also destroyed. This is one of the reasons vitamins A and D are added. Homogenization is probably the biggest concern with milk. Homogenizing involves breaking the milk fat into tiny particles so that the fat is evenly distributed throughout. This gives it a smooth even texture. It is possible that this process interferes with the body's ability to digest and utilize this fat in its homogenized form. The increase in cardiovascular disease has been correlated with the rise in the use of homogenized milk. Studies have shown that newborn calves given a diet of pasteurized and homogenized milk, will die of malnutrition. Is milk good for the body? In its raw form milk is a good nutritious food. But unless you raise your own dairy cows, you are not likely to get it this way.

Milk and milk products do add a great deal of flavor to foods. The least harmful, and possibly even beneficial, dairy products are butter and soured milk (buttermilk, cottage cheese, and yogurt). Butter, which is made from whole milk through a churning process, is mainly the milk fat. It is two-thirds saturated fat with some vitamins and minerals, including vitamin B_{12}, which is not obtainable in plant foods. Butter is recommended over margarine. Margarine is a hydrogenated oil foreign to the body and harmful to health. Butter is natural and can be digested and used by the body. Only organic butter should be used.

The cultured or soured milks are the end products of fermentation. Fermented milk is more stable and resistant to spoilage than fresh, and can aid digestion. Fermented milk contains bacteria (some brands, however, do not, so look on the label) that partially digests the milk, making it easier for our bodies to process, and reinforces the "good" bacteria in our intestines. Cheese made from organic milk can be used in moderation.

Many fruit yogurts have sugar or corn syrup added along with the fruit. It is best to use plain yogurt and combine it with fresh unsweetened fruits or use it as a topping on vegetable dishes.

There are alternatives to cows' milk. The most healthful natural milk is goat milk. Goat milk is the closest commercial dairy product to human milk in content and usually lacks chemical additives. Other alternatives are nut, rice, and coconut milks.

Eggs

Eggs, like meat, are also contaminated by hormones and drugs fed to the chickens. Chickens also are given arsenic in their feed which makes the eggshells harder. Residues from all these chemicals are found in the eggs. Some people who have allergic reactions when they eat eggs show no adverse effects when they consume organic eggs. This shows that the chemical residue in commercial eggs does have an effect on our health and should be avoided.

Eat Organic

Animal products do contain many nutrients beneficial to our bodies. But you need to choose what you eat carefully. If you want to eat meat or dairy products, eat only that which is organically grown. You will avoid consuming residual drugs and chemicals fed to most animals. You will also get a biologically healthier product. Animals that have been raised without confinement, exposed to fresh air and health-giving sunshine, and eating natural foods will have more minerals, less fat, and be healthy. Most animals raised for food are kept locked up in cramped confined cages all their lives and fed meat and other fatty foods to make them heavier. They become so sickly that antibiotics are routinely added to feed to keep sickness to a minimum. Such conditions do not make healthy animals, but it does make tender meat.

Organically raised beef, chicken, turkey, buffalo, and most game animals like deer, elk, and pheasant are comparatively clean and all right to eat. Eggs should be from free-range chickens.

Dairy products should be from organically raised animals. Pasteurization and homogenization lessen the food value so raw milk is best. Only organic milk should be drunk. Soured milk such as yogurt, cottage cheese, and buttermilk is best as it contains enzymes and bacteria that are beneficial to digestion. If you must eat cheese, make sure it is organic; better yet, use goat milk and goat cheese. Goat products have a distinctive taste and may take some time to get accustomed to.

White fish (those that have fins and scales) are generally acceptable for food. Avoid any fish from polluted waters. Nowadays, much of the ocean is becoming dangerously polluted and many fish also contain mercury and other pollutants, particularly those living in bays and along the coast. Fish harvested from the ocean away from land and from high mountain streams are the safest to eat since they are farthest from industrial pollution. Shellfish should be avoided entirely as they are generally highly acidifying and contain numerous environmental pollutants.

All animal products should be eaten fresh. Canning and preserving adds harmful chemicals and destroys nutrients. Never eat hot dogs, baloney, pepperoni, ham, and other prepared meats. These meats contain preservatives such as nitrates and nitrites which are known to cause health problems.

The key to eating meat, fish, and dairy products is to eat them sparingly. Eat modest quantities. Limit yourself to no more than a few organic eggs and a pound or so of organic meat or fish a week. Your body does not need any more than this and can do well on much less or none at all. Never sit down and eat a large portion of meat, like a thick steak, by itself. Don't get into the habit of eating meat as the main dish. Meat should be eaten only as a complement to add flavor to other foods. Use it in soups, bean dishes, casseroles, and such. A half pound of meat for a meal which serves a family of four is ample.

Animal Products ☆☆
Game meats (deer, elk, pheasant, etc.)
Organic beef, chicken, turkey, lamb, and buffalo
Organic eggs
Freshwater fish*
Deep sea fish*
Raw organic goat and cow milk
Organic soured milk products
Organic cheese
Organic butter
*Fish with fins and scales from unpolluted waters.

Animal Products to Avoid
Red meat (beef, pork, ham, sausage, etc.)
Lunch meats (frankfurters, pepperoni, cold cuts, etc.)
Fowl (chicken, turkey, etc.)
Eggs
Shellfish (crab, lobster, shrimp, scallops, etc.)
Bay water fish
Catfish and other scavengers
Cow milk (all conventional dairy products)

FATS AND OILS

Most people think fat is bad. Foods in store aisles loudly proclaim they are low-fat or non-fat. Excess consumption of fat can be bad, just as the excess consumption of any one thing can be. But fat is an important and essential part of our diet. It is through the fatty portion of our foods that we get the fat-soluble vitamins, such as vitamin E which is essential to good health. Beta-carotene is another fat-soluble nutrient that has received praise as an antioxidant and cancer fighter. If all fats were stripped from our foods we would soon die of vitamin deficiency. Natural fats for the most part are good, in moderation. Fat becomes bad only when it has been artificially altered or damaged in processing. Unfortunately, most of the fats we eat nowadays are unhealthy.

Some fats are so important they are classified as "essential" nutrients. The three essential fatty acids are linoleic, linolenic, arachidonic. They are considered essential because the body cannot manufacture them, so we must get them from our diet. Linoleic and arachidonic acids are classified as omega-6 fatty acids. Linolenic acid is classified as an omega-3 fatty acid. Omega-6 is abundant in fresh produce, vegetable oils, and even meats. Omega-3 is less common. Omega-3 fatty acids play an important role in lowering blood pressure thus reducing risk of heart disease. Omega-3 fatty acids are found abundantly in fish and to a lesser extent, leafy green vegetables and some seed oils (flax, canola, walnut).

The best sources of essential fatty acids are fish, fresh vegetables, nuts, and seeds—not pure oils. The problem with vegetable oils is that they go rancid quickly.

Processing radically affects the quality of the oil. The majority of vegetable oils are highly processed or refined. In the refining process, the oil is separated from its food source with petroleum solvents and then boiled to evaporate the solvents. The oil is refined, bleached, and deodorized which involves heating to temperatures over 400 degrees Fahrenheit. Preservatives are frequently added to retard oxidation. The resulting product lacks color, aroma, flavor, and nutritional value.

Hydrogenated oils go a step further. Hydrogenation chemically converts unsaturated vegetable oils into artificial saturated fats called *trans fatty acids*. Unsaturated oil (monounsaturated and polyunsaturated) is liquid at room temperatures. Saturation hardens oil so that it can form a thick buttery texture. This chemically altered oil has no nutritive value whatsoever and increases health risks. Preliminary studies have suggested links of hydrogenated oils to degenerative diseases like Alzheimer's. It clogs arteries more than any other fat, and unlike natural saturated fat, cannot be used by the body for any useful purpose.

Margarine and shortening are hydrogenated oils. Fried foods sold in grocery stores and restaurants are usually cooked in hydrogenated oil because it gives a crispness people enjoy. Many frozen, processed foods are cooked or prepared in hydrogenated oils. French fries, biscuits, frozen pies, pizzas, etc. are all prepared with hydrogenated oils. Baked goods such as cookies, crackers, and muffins are prepared with hydrogenated oil as is peanut butter, cake frosting, and many other common foods. All foods containing hydrogenated oils should be eliminated from your diet.

Instead of margarine or shortening, use organic butter. Organic butter, without additives, is relatively easy to digest and can be used in your diet.

The less processing an oil undergoes, the less

damaging it is on health. The most natural oils are extracted from seeds by mechanical pressure and low temperatures, and without the use of chemicals. Oils derived by this process are referred to a "expeller pressed" or "cold pressed." These oils contain no colorings, preservatives, or chemical additives. The term "cold pressed" is not really accurate. In reality, all oils are subjected to some heat in processing. Expeller pressed oils are processed at lower temperatures than refined oils (160 degrees F as opposed to temperatures up to 470 degrees F).

Look for oil labeled "expeller pressed" or "unrefined." Store unrefined oils in the refrigerator to prevent rancidity. Some oils will solidify at refrigerator temperatures, but this will not harm the oil.

All oils, whether cold pressed, saturated, unsaturated, or hydrogenated, are degraded or oxidized when heated.

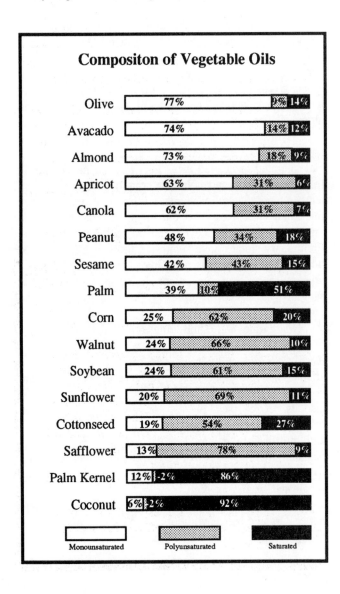

High temperatures, such as deep frying, destroys the nutritive value of oil and alters its chemical structure. Deep-frying oxidizes all types of fats especially monounsaturated and polyunsaturated vegetable oils. Unsaturated vegetable oils are less stable than saturated fat or hydrogenated oil and, therefore, degrade more quickly. Oxidized oils have been found to induce damage to interstitial tissues and blood vessel walls and cause numerous organ lesions in animals. They have even been identified as contributing to the development of atherosclerosis and heart disease. The logical conclusion is to avoid using oils that have been heat processed and do not use polyunsaturated oils in cooking. It makes no sense to buy a cold pressed oil and use it to cook with. The cooking temperate oxidizes the oil and makes it just as bad as conventionally processed oils. Polyunsaturated oils generate toxic free radicals when heated, even at moderate temperatures. Polyunsaturated oils should only be used cold, such as in a salad dressing.

The more unsaturated a fat is the more easily it is destroyed by heat and the more quickly it becomes rancid. Monounsaturated oils (such as olive oil) can be heated to low or moderate temperatures, but they, too, will oxidize and form destructive free radicals if heated at too high a temperature or for too long. Olive oil should be used at temperatures below about 325 degrees. Saturated fats are much more tolerant to heat and can be used in cooking without fear of creating dangerous free radicals. The best fats for cooking are organic butter, ghee, and coconut and palm oils.

Many people refrain from using butter or ghee (clarified butter) thinking that it is bad for them because it contains saturated fat. Recent research, however, has shown that butter contains significant amounts of short-chain and conjugated linoleic fatty acids, both of which have been shown to help *prevent* numerous degenerative health problems, including heart disease. Population studies, for example, have shown that when people remove butter from their diet and replace it with margarine their rate of heart disease increases!

You can't say one oil is better than another simply because it is more unsaturated. Polyunsaturated vegetable oils are really no more healthy than any other fat. This comes as a surprise to most people because we have been told that polyunsaturated vegetable oils are better than saturated fat and, therefore, good to eat. Polyunsaturated fats, however, have been shown to contribute to blood fat levels leading to cardiovascular disease, and to increase the risk of developing cancer and other degenerative diseases.

One vegetable oil that has become popular in recent years is canola oil. Canola oil comes from the rapeseed plant. Rapeseed oil contains an undesirable fat known as erucic acid. Erucic acid is highly toxic to the heart muscle. Natural rapeseed oil contains as much as 45-50 percent erucic acid, making it very dangerous. Because of erucic acid's toxic effects, laws limit the amount of this fatty acid in oils used for human consumption. Through the process of genetic engineering the erucic acid content has been reduced to less than 1 percent. To distinguish this genetically altered oil from the original, it is give the name canola (Canada oil). This genetically modified oil is the canola found in our foods. Being genetically engineered, it is not an oil that is found in nature and contains small amounts of a fatty acid that is known to be unhealthy. I recommend you avoid it.

Saturated fats, such as those in meat and milk, are often avoided because they can raise blood cholesterol levels and high cholesterol is considered a risk factor for heart disease. But not all saturated fats are alike. Recent studies have shown that saturated fats from some plant sources have the opposite effect—reducing total fat concentration in the blood, thus helping to prevent cardiovascular problems. The saturated fat molecules in these vegetable oils are shorter than those in animal fats, which gives them drastically different chemical properties.

The most common vegetable oils that have the shorter saturated fat molecules are the tropical oils—coconut, palm, and palm kernel oils. Once considered bad oils because of their high saturated fat content, nutritionists are now recognizing them as some of the healthiest.

By far the best cooking oil you can use and one of the best all-round oils is coconut oil. Coconut oil has a high saturated fat content, more than lard or butter, making it a good cooking oil because it doesn't oxidize like monounsaturated and polyunsaturated fats do when heated. And, unlike saturated fat from meat and dairy, it does not contain environmental toxins, raise blood cholesterol, or contribute to cardiovascular disease. In fact, studies show it can *reduce* the risk of cardiovascular disease.

Non-hydrogenated, cold processed, coconut oil is perhaps the healthiest all-round oil you can use. Palm oil and palm kernel oils are also high in good saturated fat, but not as easily available as coconut oil. Currently palm and palm kernel oils used in North America and Europe are mostly all hydrogenated and therefore should not be eaten.

The Best Oil ☆☆
Coconut (nonhydrogenated)
Organic butter and ghee
Extra virgin olive oil

Oils Okay to Use Occasionally ☆
Vegetable oils (cold pressed)

Oils to Avoid
Non-organic animal fats (beef tallow, lard, butter)
Hydrogenated oils
Margarine
Shortening
Vegetable oils (conventional)

PLANT FOODS

Your diet should consist primarily of vegetables, fruits, whole grains, legumes, nuts, and seeds. These foods contain all of the proteins, carbohydrates, fatty acids, vitamins, minerals, and phytochemicals your body needs for good health. Eat them both raw and cooked. Eat fresh raw fruits, vegetables, nuts, and seeds. Make a variety of fruit and vegetable salads. You may also make nutritious soups and baked dishes as well as steamed or roasted vegetables. And, of course, eat baked goods of all types using a variety of grains.

The produce you use should be organically grown to avoid pesticide residue and chemical contamination. Organically grown produce doesn't always look as nice as the other. Chemical fertilizers enhance appearance and pesticides prevent minor bug damage common with organic produce. Consequently, organic produce may have

Minimizing Risks Associated with Pesticides

- The best solution is to eat organically grown foods.
- Meat, dairy, and eggs should be avoided. Even animals raised under free-range conditions that are considered "organically raised" carry some contamination. If you must eat animal products make sure they are organic. Trim the fat from meat, and remove the skin from poultry and fish; discard fat produced during cooking.
- Wash fresh produce in water.
- Discard the outer leaves of leafy vegetables such as cabbage and lettuce.
- Peel fruits and vegetables, especially if they are waxed; waxes don't wash off and can seal in pesticide residue.

Fruits and Vegetables Preserve Health

Eating plenty of fruits and vegetables significantly lowers the risk of stroke. Researches surveyed 832 men in an ongoing heart study. The men had no cardiovascular disease and were 45 to 65 years old when enrolled in a dietary assessment study which began in the late 1960s. The participants were monitored for the next 18 to 22 years for, among other things, any episodes of strokes. The results: there were 97 stroke-related incidents, and researchers found a substantial decrease in stroke risk among those who had consumed higher quantities

AN APPLE A DAY KEEPS THE DOCTOR AWAY!

of fruits and vegetables. For each increment of three half-cup servings a day, there was a 22 percent decrease in stroke risk. (The average number of servings among participants was 5.1.)

"These results," the researches conclude, "provide support to programs aimed at widespread increases in the consumption of fruits and vegetables. If successful, such programs may have beneficial effects on the incidence of stroke as well as other chronic diseases."

—American Medical Association

some minor blemishes, but is healthier. Grown in organic soils, free from man-made chemicals, you get produce as nature intended.

The less processing produce undergoes, the better. The best foods are eaten right off the vine or tree. This isn't always possible, so choose foods that are in as natural a state as you can get. Canned fruits and vegetables are nutritionally depleted and often highly contaminated. Frozen foods are generally better than canned, but may still contain food additives and contaminants. Stick with fresh produce. Freeze or can your own if you want them to keep when out of season.

Some foods can be eaten either raw or cooked. Others are better eaten cooked. These include grains, legumes, and tubers (potatoes, yams, etc.). Cooking can destroy some of the nutrients, but it will also release nutrients locked in the cellulose of the plant that would otherwise pass through the body unused. That is why it is best to eat both raw and cooked foods.

Grains provide a major portion of the world's diet. Generally, when we think of grains we think of wheat and sometimes corn and rice. These are good foods, if eaten whole—no white flour or polished rice. But there are numerous other grains to choose from: oats, spelt, barley, rye, millet, quinoa, amaranth, and buckwheat. From these grains you can make an assortment of breads and baked goods, casseroles, and other nutritious dishes.

The following list shows the wide variety of plant foods available for us to eat. Eliminating junk foods does not restrict the variety of the foods we can enjoy. Actually it opens up a new world of delicious and nutritious foods you may have otherwise never considered eating before.

Grains* ☆☆
Whole wheat
Kamut
Brown rice
Corn
Oats
Spelt
Barley
Millet
Quinoa
Amaranth
Buckwheat/kasha
Rye

Vegetables* ☆☆
Potatoes
Tomatoes
Onions
Peppers
Cabbage
Artichokes
Beets
Carrots
Eggplant
Cucumber
Rutabaga
Brussels sprouts
Collards
Kohlrabi
Celery
Parsley
Chard
Mustard greens

Cauliflower
Endive
Garlic
Kale
Leeks
Lettuce (all types)
Broccoli
Parsnips
Radishes
Spinach
Sprouts (all types)
Squash (all types)
Turnips
Watercress
Shallots
Asparagus
Bok choy
Avocados
Jerusalem artichoke
Yams/Sweet potatoes
Okra

Legumes* ☆☆
Kidney
Garbanzo
Pinto
Black beans
Black-eyed peas
Soybeans (fermented)**
Lentils
Split peas/green peas
Green beans/wax beans
Snow Peas

Fruits* ☆☆
Apple
Apricot
Banana
Papaya
Mango
Peach
Guava
Nectarine
Persimmon
Plum
Pear
Fig
Date
Cherry
Blueberry
Raspberry
Boysenberry
Blackberry
Gooseberry
Cranberry
Currant
Strawberry
Mulberry
Melon (all types)
Pineapple

Kiwi
Pomegranate
Grape
Orange
Lemon
Lime
Grapefruit
Mandarin
Kumquat

Nuts and Seeds* ☆☆
Almond
Sesame
Pumpkin seed
Sunflower
Filbert/Hazelnut
Chestnut
Walnut
Black walnut
Brazil nut
Cashew
Pecan
Peanut
Pistachio
Macadamia
Coconut
Pine nut

*Organic
**Fermented soy includes soy sauce, miso, and tempeh. For details about the health aspects of soy go to www.soyonlineservice.co.nz

Nonorganic Plant Foods ☆
Same foods as organic if thoroughly washed or peeled

Plant Foods to Avoid
Dried or dehydrated fruit that has been bleached or
   sulfured
Canned fruit and vegetables
Packaged or frozen fruit and vegetables with food
   additives
White flour
Polished white rice

WATER AND BEVERAGES

Water forms a major part of almost every body tissue. It is the medium in which chemical processes occur in our body. Drinking pure clean water is vital to achieving and maintaining good health.

Lack of adequate water slows down metabolism which therefore inhibits healing, toxin removal, removal of old cells, and replacement of new tissue, and hampers the function of cells and organs. The body cannot effectively remove toxins if the body is dehydrated.

With the following formula you can calculate the minimum amount of water you need to consume each day. Bodyweight (in pounds)/2= X. Drink X ounces of water. Example, 140 pounds/2=70 ounces of water or 9 eight-ounce glasses a day. A 140 pound person should drink 9 eight-ounce glasses of water a day. Keep in mind this is a minimum, you can drink more.

You should drink one glass before going to bed at night and another immediately upon arising. During sleep, the body heals and cleanses itself. It is not busy digesting, thinking, or working, so all energy is channeled to repair and cleaning. As the body accumulates toxins, it needs water available for their removal. Water in the morning replenishes that which is removed in the morning and helps keep the body's fluid level in balance.

Water must be pure and clean—coffee, soda, juice, milk, and other beverages do not count. The water in these drinks contains substances that must also be cleaned and removed from the body. An analogy to this is the dump truck concept—an empty dump truck can remove more junk than a partially filled one. Pure water can remove more garbage than water already loaded with dissolved solids. Some beverages, especially those that contain alcohol or caffeine, promote dehydration because they have a diuretic effect. So you can drink 10 cans of soda a day and still be dying of dehydration.

Most tap water is contaminated with chemicals (chlorine, fluorine, etc.) and environmental pollutants. Although the water may look and taste clean, these chemicals can cause a great deal of distress for the body. Drink distilled or filtered water.

Before drinking tap water or using it for cooking, let it run for at least 30 seconds if it hasn't been used for several hours. Water sitting in pipes can pick up lead from pipes. Do not use hot water for drinking or cooking because it leaches lead from pipes faster than cold. To disinfect water, boil it for three to five minutes. That also evaporates chlorine and some volatile chlorination byproducts.

You may consider using bottled water. Many people, in an effort to avoid contaminated tap water, buy bottled water. This, however, is no guarantee that the water you get is "clean" and may be just as bad or even worse than your own tap water. One-fourth of all bottled water is actually just tap water. All water, whether it be artesian, filtered, or distilled, is contaminated if it is stored in a plastic container. Plastic molecules leach into the water and plastic, as you have learned from Chapter 1, can have adverse health effects.

The best solution is to use a home filtration device or distiller. Filters come in a variety of sizes and styles. Shop for a unit certified by NSF International, an environmental-quality and public-health organization. Not having the label doesn't mean a device won't work, but having it assures that it removes the contaminants for which it's certified. To obtain a list of the drinking-water treatment units it currently certifies, write NSF International, 3475 Plymouth Road, Ann Arbor, Michigan 48105, USA.

Activated-carbon filters remove bad tastes, odor and many organic compounds, including pesticides, chloroform, and solvents—but not bacteria, nitrates, sodium, fluoride, or heavy metals. A typical under-sink model with a cartridge about three inches in diameter and six to ten inches tall will give you a generous flow of water on demand. You'll need to replace the cartridge after about

500 gallons—a year's drinking and cooking supply for a family of four. Carbon can harbor bacteria, so flush the system for 30 seconds to a minute after it sits unused for more than a few hours. Some special filters can remove nitrates and heavy metals. A system that is bacteriostatic will prevent the reproduction of bacteria that are trapped by the filter element. Any home filter has to be cleaned or changed regularly to work right and keep from becoming a health hazard in itself.

If you want almost complete removal of lead—along with arsenic, asbestos, parasite cysts, and nitrates—you might look into reverse-osmosis filters. But they're slower, fussier to maintain, and more expensive than carbon filters. They waste quite a bit of water as well. It takes five gallons of water run through a reverse-osmosis filter to produce one gallon of clean water.

The Elixir of Life

The importance of water in maintaining good health was accidently discovered by Dr. F. Batmanghelidj while he was serving time at Evin Prison in Iran. In 1979 a violent revolution swept a new government into power. Almost all professional and creative people who had stayed in the country were rounded up and jailed as political prisoners. Dr. Batmanghelidj was one of these.

Because he was a doctor he was given the responsibility of caring for the sick. He wasn't there long when one night, an inmate suffering from excruciating stomach pain, was brought to him. The man was suffering from peptic ulcer disease and pleaded for something to stop the pain. Dr. Batmanghelidj had nothing at his disposal that would help. In desperation he gave him two glasses of water. To his surprise within minutes the man's pain disappeared. He told the patient to drink two glasses of water every few hours. The man remained free from pain and disease while in prison.

This was Dr. Batmanghelidj's introduction to the role water can play in health and healing. Dr. Batmanghelidj started researching the effects water has

on health. For nearly three years he treated countless numbers of patients for a variety of illness using ordinary tap water and nothing else. When he was released from prison. He came to the United States where he continued his research and wrote a book titled *Your Body's Many Cries for Water*. Dr. Batmanghelidj claims that many of the degenerative illnesses we suffer from today are to a large extent caused by chronic dehydration. He has treated many thousands of patients with water and has witnessed complete recovery of those suffering from an assortment of conditions such as high blood pressure, migraine headaches, arthritis, asthma, back pain, chronic constipation, colitis, heartburn, chronic fatigue syndrome, and obesity.

Dr. Batmanghelidj claims that every single one of these conditions can be caused by dehydration. Severe dehydration is so destructive it causes quick death. But chronic low-grade dehydration causes disease and a slow death. Health deteriorates so slowly we don't realize what's happening. We attribute it to age. He maintains that most of us are chronically dehydrated because we don't drink enough water. Dehydration causes damage to cells which leads to inflammation, swelling,

and pain. Each individual's response to dehydration differs depending on their own chemical and physical makeup. For some it manifests itself first as arthritis in others migraine headaches. Arthritis occurs when joints become dehydrated and tissue damage occurs. Back pain occurs when discs between vertebra become dehydrated causing bones and muscles to twist out of alignment causing stress.

The recommend amount of water is a 2-3 quarts a day. This is the amount the body loses from perspiration, respiration, and elimination every day. This is the minimum amount you should consume each day for the rest of your life. If you are chronically dehydrated then you need to increase this amount to replenish your reserves.

Chronic dehydration isn't something that happens in a day. It is a slow process that occurs over weeks, months, and years. Consequently, rehydrating the body isn't a one time event. You can't drink a gallon of water and cure chronic dehydration. The body isn't a sponge that immediately soaks up water. The body must adapt and adjust to an increase in water consumption. Injured cells and tissues must have time to repair themselves. This takes time.

Home distillers are the most thorough water cleansers you can buy. They will remove nearly all contaminants and provide you with pure clean water. The downside is that distillers cost more than filters, use up electrical energy, and require distilling time.

Filtered and distilled water have most all trace minerals removed, as a result, they tend to wash out and deplete the body's mineral reserves. You need to replenish these mineral salts. You can do that by taking a daily trace mineral supplement and/or adding more sea salt to your diet. Sea salt is preferred over regular salt because it contains important trace minerals.

In addition to the water you need daily, you may also drink herbal teas if made with distilled or filtered water. Fresh organic fruit and vegetable juices are also fine. Avoid coffee, black tea, alcohol, carbonated sodas, frozen and processed fruit juices, cocoa, and other chocolate drinks. Avoid any beverage with artificial additives or sweeteners.

Beverages ☆☆
Fresh mineral or artesian water
Filtered or distilled water
Fresh organic fruit and vegetable juices
Herbal tea

Beverages Okay to Use Occasionally ☆
Soy, rice, and nut milks
Coffee substitutes (Roma, Postum, etc.)
Tap water

Beverages to Avoid
Bottled artesian and distilled water (if stored in plastic containers)
Soft drinks
Alcoholic beverages
Coffee
Black tea
Chocolate milk
Juices with additives
Prepared mixes (including fruit-flavored powders)

DIET SUMMARY

The Natural Foods Diet is just that—"natural foods" without chemical additives or contaminants and with as little processing as possible. The best foods are organically grown and come straight from the garden to the dinner table fresh, clean, and pure.

The Natural Foods Diet consists basically of all the foods listed in this chapter which are flagged by one or two stars. Your diet should be centered around the two-star

foods and supplemented with *minor* amounts of the one-star foods. Avoid completely all the foods listed without a star.

Certain foods or food additives are particularly troublesome. Simply avoiding them will bring about marked improvement in health. The biggest troublemakers are: caffeine, sugar, fat, non-organic meat and dairy, and processed convenience foods. Unfortunately, these are the things most people love and overindulge in.

The healthiest diet is one based on organically grown vegetables, fruits, whole grains, legumes, nuts, and seeds eaten as close to their natural state as possible. Which means, foods are best prepared from wholesome raw ingredients instead of devitalized packaged products. Homemade bread is preferred to store bought. A home cooked burrito is preferred to the frozen, packaged variety, even if the store bought variety is made with wholesome ingredients. The more processing and handling foods get, the more contaminated they become. Make as much of your own meals from basic foodstuffs as you can. Eat lots of homemade soups, baked and steamed vegetables, salads, and fresh produce, and the like.

Use packaged or prepared foods (eat only those which have no chemical additives) and animal products like cheese, frozen vegetables, sweets, butter, etc. sparingly. Strictly avoid the big troublemakers listed above and any foods with chemical additives.

This does not mean you can never eat an ice cream cone, although you would be better off without it. If your body is clean and healthy, it can remove the junk from an ice cream cone eaten on rare occasions. One of the drawbacks with eating foods like this is that they are habit forming. Sugar is addictive and can cause numerous health problems. The best thing to do is to avoid it entirely. If you want to have a "treat," eat a more healthful treat, one made with natural ingredients. It may not be particularly good for you, but it may be a whole lot better than ice cream.

How can you tell when your body has cleansed enough to eat an occasional treat? Are headaches, joint pains, acne, and other conditions gone? Are allergies no longer a problem? If not, then the body is still toxic, and eating any foods with toxins or that clog the gastrointestinal tract will only cause harm. If you eat a relatively clean diet, but still indulge frequently in unhealthy treats, toxins will build up, slower than in those who eat poor foods on a daily basis, but they will build. Degenerative disease will eventually catch up with you. You will enjoy better than average health for a longer time then most people, but instead of getting cancer, diabetes, or heart disease when you are 40 or 50 years old, you may get them at 60 or 70. You have a good chance of avoiding them altogether by remaining on a clean diet permanently.

The Danger of Biomagnification

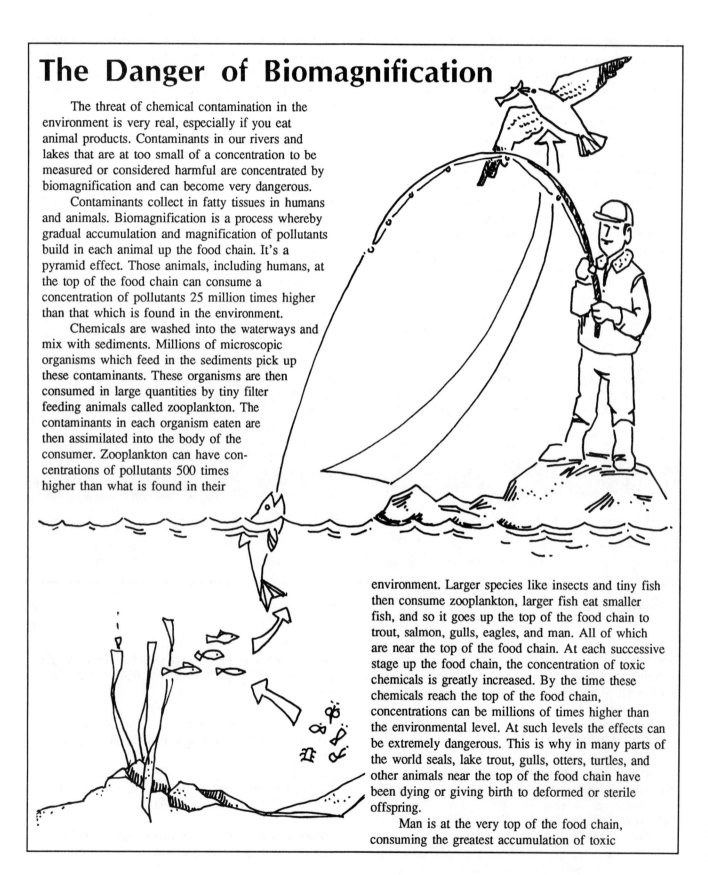

The threat of chemical contamination in the environment is very real, especially if you eat animal products. Contaminants in our rivers and lakes that are at too small of a concentration to be measured or considered harmful are concentrated by biomagnification and can become very dangerous.

Contaminants collect in fatty tissues in humans and animals. Biomagnification is a process whereby gradual accumulation and magnification of pollutants build in each animal up the food chain. It's a pyramid effect. Those animals, including humans, at the top of the food chain can consume a concentration of pollutants 25 million times higher than that which is found in the environment.

Chemicals are washed into the waterways and mix with sediments. Millions of microscopic organisms which feed in the sediments pick up these contaminants. These organisms are then consumed in large quantities by tiny filter feeding animals called zooplankton. The contaminants in each organism eaten are then assimilated into the body of the consumer. Zooplankton can have concentrations of pollutants 500 times higher than what is found in their environment. Larger species like insects and tiny fish then consume zooplankton, larger fish eat smaller fish, and so it goes up the top of the food chain to trout, salmon, gulls, eagles, and man. All of which are near the top of the food chain. At each successive stage up the food chain, the concentration of toxic chemicals is greatly increased. By the time these chemicals reach the top of the food chain, concentrations can be millions of times higher than the environmental level. At such levels the effects can be extremely dangerous. This is why in many parts of the world seals, lake trout, gulls, otters, turtles, and other animals near the top of the food chain have been dying or giving birth to deformed or sterile offspring.

Man is at the very top of the food chain, consuming the greatest accumulation of toxic pollutants whenever animal products are eaten. Fish, ordinarily considered healthy, can be very contaminated because they live off of smaller animals. But biomagnification can also affect cows, pigs, and other animals raised for food. These animals are routinely fed fish meal and ground carcasses of dead livestock. Feeding them the pulverized bodies of other animals makes them gain weight, which increases profits. Not only do livestock get concentrated environmental toxins from dead animals, but they also get all the antibiotics, hormones, pesticides and other chemicals these other animals had accumulated in their lifetime. Even feed is often grown on land heavily sprayed with high levels of pesticides.

All nonorganically produced beef, pork, chicken, milk (including yogurt, cheese, etc.) and eggs have highly concentrated levels of contaminants. In fact, foods of animal origin, not fruit or vegetables, are the major source of pesticide residues in our diet. Studies indicate that of all the toxic chemical residues in the diet, almost all, 95 percent to 99 percent, come from meat, fish, dairy, and eggs. The smartest way to reduce toxic exposure is to eat lower down on the food chain, or in other words, fruits, vegetables, seeds, and grains.

An analysis published by the *Pesticides Monitoring Journal* determined that grains and root vegetables had the least pesticide contamination. Next came legumes, fruits and leafy vegetables, in that order. These were followed by fats and oils. Even in plants toxins accumulate greatest in fat cells from which vegetable oils are made. Dairy products contained about three times as much pesticide residue as vegetable oils. Meat, fish, and poultry had two and a half times as much contamination as dairy.

Fish has been recommended as a "healthy" alternative to red meat because of its lower saturated fat content and the presence of omega-3 fatty acids— considered essential to good health. Fish, however, is some of the most polluted food you can eat. In fact, 47 states in the United States currently have fish consumption advisories that warn about eating certain species. They cover 1,740 rivers and lakes and large chunks of coastal areas.

Clean fish is still a better choice over other meats. Most fish caught in the United States are used to make fish meal and fed to cattle. Thus cattle are even more toxic than fish. Large fish like fresh tuna and swordfish have the highest levels of contaminants. The least dangerous fish to eat are smaller, deep-ocean fish that do not live or spawn near the coast, such as cod, halibut, and pollack, or freshwater fish from high-altitude streams that are not contaminated from industrial or agricultural runoffs or dumping. But even these fish will carry some pollutants.

 ADDITIONAL RESOURCES

Beyond Pritikin: A Total Nutrition Program for Rapid Weight Loss, Longevity and Good Health. Gittleman, Ann Louise, M.S. New York: Bantam, 1996.

Diet for a New America. Robbins, John. Walpole, NH: Stillpoint Publishing, 1987.

Dr. Dean Ornish's Program for Reversing Heart Disease. Ornish, Dean, M.D. New York: Ballantine, 1990.

The Coconut Oil Miracle. Fife, Bruce, N.D., New York, NY: Avery, 2004.

Dr. Wright's Guide to Healing with Nutrition. Wright, Jonathan V., M.D. New Canaan, CT: Keats Publishing, 1990.

Transition to Vegetarianism. Ballantine, Rudolph. Honesdale, PA: The Himalayan International Institute, 1987.

Staying Healthy with Nutrition. Haas, Elson M., M.D. Berkeley, CA: Celestial Arts, 1992.

Vegan Nutrition—Pure and Simple. Klaper, Michael, M.D. Paui, HI: Gentle World, 1987.

Chapter 5

THE HEALING PROCESS

THE CLEANSING CRISIS

Every year people come down with colds and flus. We are told that these seasonal illnesses are caused by viruses and are easily spread from person to person. Some people get sick several times a year, while others rarely do so. People can work side-by-side exposed to the same germs yet some get sick and others don't. Why is this? Why don't all those who are exposed to the cold virus catch colds?

Contrary to popular opinion, exposure to germs is not the reason why people catch colds. Bacteria, viruses, fungi and other pathogenic organisms are constantly in and on our bodies. They are everywhere and everybody is exposed to them. The rhinovirus, for example, which causes the common cold is always present, but we don't all have colds because it is kept under control by our immune system. Rhinovirus can only proliferate and cause problems when the immune system becomes weakened by a toxic overload or by physical or mental stress. It is a well-established fact that cold temperatures do not cause colds nor does exposure to other sick people. Colds are passed around only among those people who have weak immune systems. Healthy people with strong immune systems come in contact with those who have highly contagious diseases without "catching" their illnesses.

Colds are usually more prominent during the winter because people are less healthy at this time. They eat fewer fruits and vegetables, don't get as much exercise, and they are cooped up in buildings without healing sunlight and fresh air. Stress also is accentuated in these conditions. When our bodies become overloaded with toxins and our immune system is overworked, we become susceptible to the cold virus. When a cold strikes, our bodies attempt to purge the virus and other accumulated filth. Sickness is, in effect, a cleansing process. If the body has the strength and nutrients it needs, then the illness is overcome and the body regains health. And because of the cleansing, we may be healthier immediately after the sickness than before. A condition that causes the body to expel toxins is referred to as a cleansing crisis. Thus, a cold is a cleansing crisis. As you will learn later, cleansing crises can also occur without sickness.

If the body is too weak, or adequate nourishment is not provided to fight off the invading germs and cleanse toxic substances, the illness will be prolonged. Nutrients vital to good health may be used up in the process and, if not quickly replenished, the deficiency will lead to some degree of malnutrition and all of its accompanying consequences. The person will still feel sick even after the major symptoms have subsided. These are the type of individuals who are at greatest risk from potentially deadly viruses and bacterial infections.

The symptoms associated with common illnesses are part of the body's natural cleansing process. When our bodies become dangerously overloaded with toxins, our immune systems weaken and we become vulnerable to infectious organisms. When we become sick, our body is telling us to rest so it can focus its healing energies on housecleaning (detoxification). Symptoms of sickness— runny nose, fever, diarrhea, nausea, sneezing, coughing, loss of appetite, etc.—are all processes of cleansing.

When we have a fever, for example, body temperature is elevated as a means to kill invading organisms and sweat out byproducts of the cleansing process. An increase in mucus production, which causes a runny nose and sinus and throat congestion, is an elimination process. The mucus is carrying away harmful debris cleansed from the body. Coughing is a means by which the body removes garbage from the lungs. Vomiting and diarrhea are processes by which the body cleans out the digestive system. Loss of appetite, aching muscles and joints, and fatigue are symptoms which encourage the body to slow down and rest while the cleansing process is taking place. Rest is necessary as the body needs to focus on purification. Pain tells us that there is a problem in the body that needs attention. A sprained ankle will be painful if used normally. The pain causes enough discomfort that we stop using it or treat it carefully to avoid as much pain as possible. In so doing, the body can properly heal the injury. If pain were not present, even though we knew the ankle was injured, we would probably continue to use it, preventing the ankle from healing properly, and possibly causing further damage.

Symptoms we associate with illness are actually beneficial. They are not degenerative, but constructive processes. Suppressing symptoms with medications only retards the body's healing processes. For example, when pain is present there is a problem that needs to be corrected, not ignored or suppressed by drugs. If you took pain relieving drugs for a sprained ankle and then continued to walk on the ankle, you would only be suppressing the symptoms and doing greater harm to the ankle. The pain may, or may not, eventually go away, but the ankle will be weakened and perhaps permanently damaged and cluttered with scar tissue. Because it was not allowed to heal properly, it will be vulnerable to further injury. It may continue to cause irritation throughout life. How many people complain of "old" injuries? "My old football injury in my knee was acting up" or "I hurt my back a few years ago and it aches when I sit for a long time," etc. These are all injuries that were not allowed to heal properly and as a consequence give trouble throughout

life. Not only are these tissues or organs weakened physically, but their ability to function and remove metabolic waste and toxins is diminished, thus leading to a buildup of poisons that aggravate surrounding tissue which may eventually lead to dis-ease.

Just as the suppression of pain will lead to incomplete healing and additional problems in the future, suppression of other symptoms will have a similar effect. When drugs are taken to relieve the symptoms of a cold or the flu, poisonous waste is not eliminated as effectively, the illness lasts longer, and toxins accumulate in the tissue of weak organs or damaged tissues of the body. Toxic accumulations in these organs may lead to more serious disease in the future, resulting in surgical removal of the infected tissue. For example, colds treated with drugs will drive toxins deeper into the body where they accumulate. Over time these toxins build up until the body has another period of cleansing, but this time the cleansing is expressed as influenza where a more severe cleansing must occur. But if drugs are taken to stifle the removal of toxins, they again are driven back into the body and later give rise to a more severe condition like bronchitis. If toxins are still prevented from discharging, then emphysema may develop. In many instances, after suppressing symptoms with drugs for some time, the person's conditions worsens to the point where surgery is performed to remove the most offending affected organs. This may save the person from death temporarily, but now the body is permanently crippled, denied a valuable part of the anatomy necessary for optimal health. This imbalance may lead to problems with other organs which now must compensate for the lost organs. Surgical removal of a lung will reduce the amount of oxygen delivered to the blood and the rest of the body. The entire body then becomes oxygen starved. As a result, it cannot clean out toxins as well, and toxins accumulate faster, increasing degeneration of other inherently weak or damaged organs. All of this can be avoided by allowing the body to eliminate toxins naturally.

BREAKING ADDICTIONS

One of the first steps towards detoxification and improved health is to begin eating a Natural Foods Diet. If you have been eating like most people do nowadays, you probably eat a lot of packaged, processed, and convenience foods. When you switch to the Natural Foods Diet, you will notice some distinct changes in your health. Be prepared to feel good, bad, and sick. That's right sick. Before you get better, you will get worse—temporarily.

Ultimately you will be healthier than you have ever been in your life and feel great both physically and

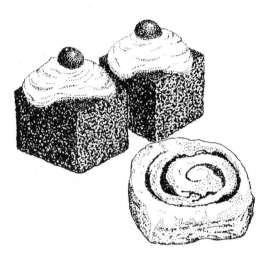

Sugary foods can be addictive.

mentally. Mental and physical capacity will improve, energy will increase, you will be happier and more positive about yourself and about life. You will lose unwanted fat, improve blood circulation, and look healthier. But before you reach this stage you will experience some physical and psychological changes that may seem unpleasant.

Some food additives, like caffeine and sugar, are physically and psychologically addictive. After eating them for a time, our minds and bodies begin to crave them. It's similar to drug or alcohol addiction. Cravings are one sign of addiction. If we just *have* to have a Pepsi or a candy bar, it is not the body saying it needs the nutrients in these substances, it's the addictions we have to them that initiate this response. Suddenly cutting them out of your diet can cause withdrawal symptoms such as headaches and mild depression or anxiety, which may last a few days. If you regularly eat or drink foods containing caffeine such as coffee, soda, and chocolate or sugary foods of any type, you will probably experience withdrawal symptoms when you stop consuming them.

Meats as well as food additives stimulate the body and the senses. Meat has a stimulating effect which forces the heart to beat faster than normal, producing a sense of exhilaration. When these foods are reduced or eliminated from the diet, the heart and body slow down to a normal pace, which registers in the mind as relaxation or a decrease in energy. This initial letdown, or feeling of lack of energy, will last from one to two weeks. After the body has had time to adjust, you will have a feeling of increased strength and greater well-being as a result of the recuperation and cleansing which follow. Some people will half-heartedly try to improve their diet for a few days or even a week and then quit. They complain that they felt better on the old diet because the new one makes them feel weak or gives them a headache. These people fail because they don't give their bodies time to adjust to the new diet. If they would have kept with it longer, they would feel better and improve their health.

Processed foods with additives and flavor enhancers tend to be more stimulating than natural foods. The first negative thing you will experience when you switch to a more natural diet is cravings for the highly flavored foods you have grown accustomed to. Our sense of taste has been overly stimulated as a result of eating too much salt, sugar, meat, fat, flavor enhancers, artificial flavorings, etc. Eating the comparatively bland diet of fresh fruits and vegetables, without additives, can seem dull and at first perhaps even monotonous (although there are numerous ways to prepare a variety of delicious-tasting, natural meals). As you become accustomed to eating naturally, your sense of taste will improve and you will no longer need salt to enhance flavor. Rich foods you may have craved before will no longer hold power over you.

The food cravings, possible headaches, temporary drop in energy level, and the perceived blandness from the lack of stimulation from food additives are difficult for some people to handle. Eliminating favorite junk foods is probably the most difficult challenge. It is important to keep a positive mental attitude. If you eat a healthy diet begrudgingly and torture yourself with dreams of cakes, ice cream, and steak, you will only make yourself miserable! Tell yourself that you don't miss those unhealthy foods and you don't want them. Look for ways to prepare what you can eat so that it satisfies your taste. Eventually, you will begin to enjoy and even prefer natural foods.

THE BODY'S POWER TO HEAL

Curtis was in near shock. The lab tests verified his doctor's suspicion—colon cancer. Curtis had been experiencing abdominal pain and constipation for some time. He knew something was wrong, but he didn't think it would be cancer. No one else in his family ever had cancer.

His doctor recommended surgery to remove the cancerous tumor that was growing in his colon, encouraging him to have it done before it progressed any further. The doctor was persistent, "It's not going to get any better, the sooner we operate the sooner you can recover."

"Will surgery remove all the cancer?" Curtis asked.

"We can remove the tumor," the doctor said, "but there is no guarantee that the cancer hasn't spread to other parts of your body. The concern right now is removing that growth."

"You mean, Doctor, that even if the tumor is removed, I may develop cancer again?

"Yes, but we will put you on a program of radiation and chemotherapy to inhibit additional growth."

Curtis wanted time to think about it. The prospect of having surgery as well as radiation and chemotherapy did not set well with him.

"Don't wait too long," the doctor warned, "it will only get worse."

With the encouragement from a friend, Curtis sought a second opinion from a doctor who believed in and practiced natural therapies. Curtis indeed did have cancer, but this doctor told him he could get rid of it without surgery, without radiation, and without chemotherapy. Cancer could be expelled throughout his entire body so that he wouldn't need to worry about a recurrence. All he had to do was to watch what he ate and follow a special diet program, a diet that consisted of whole natural foods. Eating "health" foods was a much more pleasant prospect than the dangerous and expensive treatments the first doctor recommended.

The first thing Curtis cut from his regular diet was meat, dairy, and products made with refined sugar and white flour. His new diet consisted primarily of whole grain breads and cereals, fruits, and vegetables. All processed and packaged foods containing food colorings, preservatives, and other chemical additives were out.

He had been warned that removing these poor-quality foods from his daily diet and replacing them with nutritious natural foods would have a dramatic effect on his health and well-being. He should not expect immediate recovery. The body needs time to heal. As it cleans and pulls out toxins, he was told, he may experience some discomfort, symptoms similar to sickness. This would not be an adverse reaction caused by eating the healthy foods he was now consuming, but a result of the body purging toxins from the tissues and cells of his body. It was in fact, a sign that he was getting better, not worse. With that warning, Curtis plunged into his detoxification program.

During the ensuing months Curtis continued to experience pain and constipation that were caused by the tumor. Two months after starting his new diet he became ill. He had a fever, was vomiting, experiencing abdominal cramping, and diarrhea. At first, he assumed he had caught the flu. He became worried when he saw blood in his stool. He called the doctor, thinking perhaps the cancer was getting out of hand. His doctor reassured Curtis that as long as he was following his dietary recommendations, he was okay. The "flu" he was experiencing was actually a "healing crisis" in which the body purges poisons from the system. Expelling these stored-up toxins can be done through any and every orifice in the body. Thus, the vomiting and diarrhea were part of the cleansing process and nothing to be worried about. In fact, it was a good sign because it indicated that the body was getting stronger and healthier. Toxins that had been accumulating in his body for years, as the result of a weakened immune system, were now being pulled out of the tissues and expelled.

Sure enough, the symptoms he experienced subsided and left after a couple of days. The strangest thing happened. Once the symptoms passed he felt better than he had in years. He seemed to have more energy and a renewed sense of well-being. But his ordeal was not over. The tumor was still there.

Three months later he came down with a severe "cold" with its accompanying sinus congestion, cough, fatigue, headache, and nausea. He had heavy mucus discharge from his lungs and sinuses. Again, the doctor told him not to worry, for it was just another healing crisis. When these symptoms cleared Curtis noticed an interesting development in his health. Hay fever which had always bothered him during the summer months was no longer present. He felt better than he had for a long time. Maybe, he thought, the diet was doing him some good. The tumor, although still present, at least had not gotten any bigger.

In the following months Curtis experienced several minor healing crises, including a skin rash that broke out over much of his body and lasted several weeks. During this time, his doctor had him go on periodic juice and cleansing fasts and take herbal supplements to accelerate detoxification and healing. Most of his juice fasts lasted from three to seven days. His last fast extended to 36 days and was accompanied by daily enemas.

One morning he woke up with a severe diarrhea and agonizing abdominal cramping. His head was pounding and body burned with a fever. During that day he passed, through his bowels, a fleshy tumorous growth the size of his fist covered with long stringy tentacles. This was the tumor that had caused him so much trouble, the tumor the first doctor wanted to remove by surgery. His body removed the tumor on its own as verified by subsequent examination.

Curtis was freed from the cancer that attacked his body and threatened his health. Not only was the cancer gone, but so was his hay fever, persistent psoriasis which had plagued him for the past several years, and chronic lower back pain. His bowel movements also became regular and easy. His blood pressure, at one time high, was now normal. He also said his eyesight had improved. He had much more energy and didn't tire as easily as he had just a year before. His whole body, it seemed, was rejuvenated. He felt like he was 20 years younger.

The interesting thing about Curtis' story is that his body was able to heal and repair itself—it didn't take medications or surgery. His body did it on its own when harmful substances were removed from his diet and when he was supplied with nutritious foods. If his body knew how to heal itself from cancer and other degenerative conditions, then your body has the same ability. Our bodies are all designed alike. If someone else has been able to overcome a debilitating illness, so can you. Stories like Curtis' are not rare. People are ridding themselves of disease all the time in similar fashion.

THE HEALING CRISIS

All those who have lived on processed and packaged foods, meat, and dairy products sold at grocery stores and in restaurants will go through what is called a "cleansing crisis" when they begin to eat healthfully. The cleansing crisis can also be initiated after following a detox program, such as those described in the following chapters. The cleansing crisis is the most pronounced part of the cleansing process. You may feel great for a while and then come down sick—headaches, stomach cramps, skin eruptions, aches and pains throughout the body. This cleansing crisis may occur within a couple of weeks after you start a cleansing diet or may not show up for several months. The crisis may repeat itself several times followed by periods of increasing better health.

This is an area of confusion for many people. After eating healthfully they would expect to get better, not sick. The diet is supposed to make them healthy; why then, are they getting sick? These symptoms of illness are actually indications of improving health!

As the body stores fat, the chemistry of the fat reflects the internal environment of the body at the time of formation. If you are taking medications, traces of those drugs will be incorporated into the fat tissue. If you have a viral or bacterial infection, these too may be trapped in or around the developing fat cells as well as other body tissues. Here these toxic agents may lie dormant until the fat is dissolved. Researchers have identified drugs that have been trapped in body tissues for decades.

At times people suffer from diseases that have lain dormant in their cells for many years. Shingles, as an example, is caused by the chicken pox virus. About three percent of the population will suffer from shingles at some time in their lives. In most cases the disease results from reactivation of the chicken pox virus that lay dormant for years after the original chicken pox infection. It usually resurfaces in older adults during times of stress, when undergoing radiation therapy, or when taking immunosuppressive drugs.

In the gastrointestinal tract, mucus is secreted to carry toxins out of the system. When you have a stuffy nose from a cold, the mucus carries off dead cells and toxins harmful to the body. If too much mucus-forming food is eaten (e.g., meat, dairy, gluten, grease, etc.), the mucus becomes thick and cannot easily drain out of the body. It loses moisture, especially in the colon which absorbs water, and the mucus encrusts itself on the lining of the intestine along with all the toxins it is carrying. In the colon this could also include fecal matter which is trapped and begins to putrefy. Old mucus and putrefying fecal debris may be caked on the walls of the intestine and colon for years, slowly building up year after year. Accumulation of 5 to 20 pounds of encrusted putrefying feces is not uncommon.

During the cleansing process, excess fat and hardened mucus and toxic wastes in the body emulsify and wash out into the bloodstream to be discarded. This influx of toxins into the system brings on symptoms of sickness. People who have had problems with skin rashes or eruptions will frequently eliminate poisons through the skin and new rashes will develop. The skin, as a cleansing organ, is becoming more active. Since the body does not have to

Drug Detoxification

The body does store many of the byproducts of nearly all drugs. When these drugs are being eliminated from the system, they throw the body into a toxic crisis. Many of the same side effects that the original drug produced may be again experienced: dizzyness, lethargy, or great exhilaration, vivid dreams and nightmares. These are the expected result of drug detoxification. It is important to stick it out and achieve the reward of being free of these toxins. Drugs will be expelled from the body in the same kind of cycle as are other toxins, so one should not be alarmed if the same symptoms are experienced more than one time. Sometimes when drugs are being eliminated, the presence of specific drugs are very evident on the breath. One girl who had had no anesthesia for several years found that on a fast, her breath smelled like anesthesia for a day or two when the drug deposit was being expelled from her liver. One patient on a very severe cleanse went on a six-week drug trip. She had never had anything but medicinal drugs, but she had been on them for many years.

—Stan Malstrom, N.D., *Own Your Own Body*

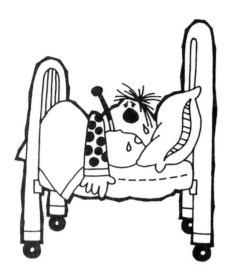

spend energy on hard-to-digest junk food, it's able to remove poisons more rapidly. The symptoms will vary according to the materials being discarded, the condition of the organs involved in the elimination, and the amount of energy you have available. You may experience some constipation, occasional diarrhea, frequent urination, nervousness, irritability, depression, fever, mucus discharge, cramps, cold sores, headaches, muscle pain, boils, skin rashes, infections, swelling, nausea, canker sores, fever blisters, excess gas, tiredness, etc. You will experience discharges from every orifice, as the body purges impurities from the system. This is nature's way of cleansing the body.

One of the biggest misconceptions people face with the healing crisis is the belief that they have caught some hideous infection (i.e., a disease crisis). If they go to a doctor who is not familiar with this aspect of natural healing, he will diagnose it as an allergy or an infection and will prescribe antibiotics or other drugs which will suppress the healing process. Although the drugs may bring temporary relief, the cleansing process will be halted and toxins will remain in the body and be reabsorbed into the tissue. To eliminate these toxins, the person must go through the cleansing crisis all over again.

There is an important difference between symptoms of the disease process and those of the healing process. The first is the result of the body succumbing to disease and the latter is the result of the body overcoming disease. The body has become strong enough to purge toxins and latent microbes from the tissues and, although symptoms of illness manifest themselves, the body is now strong enough to overcome the problem and eliminate the

poisons. As a result of eating wisely, the organs of elimination have become stronger, the immune system has become more effective, and energy level has increased.

These symptoms are part of a curing process and are constructive. Don't try to stop them with medication or even vitamins, which may act like drugs when taken in high dosages. Natural herbal supplements, however, may be beneficial and can even speed healing, but are not necessary. Let nature take its course. If you are eating properly, these symptoms are not deficiency conditions or allergic reactions. The symptoms generally will last only a few days to a week or so. During this time no drugs should be taken, as the body is trying to eliminate toxins. Taking drugs will only hamper the elimination process and just add more toxins into your system.

The more you rest and sleep when symptoms are present, the milder they will be and the more quickly they will be terminated. When symptoms arise, look on the positive side, be happy your body is reacting this way, it indicates you're getting healthier.

A single healing crisis will not purge from your body all the toxins that have accumulated over the years. The healing process works in cycles. You will have feelings of health and well-being separated by periods of discomfort caused by the elimination of toxins. If you have had problems with psoriasis, when you first start your diet, it may greatly improve the condition, although not completely clear it up. You may be relatively free of skin problems for a couple of months and feel the new way of eating is slowly working. Then, red, itching flaking skin will suddenly reappear and become as bad, if not worse, than it has ever been before, even though your diet is clean. Your first thought is that you are having a resurgence of the skin problems you've had for years. It may last a month or more, but then clear up completely along with the dandruff problem you have had for the past 20 years. After this you will feel and look great. The dry flaky skin rash was the body's way of ridding itself of toxic debris. Now that the diet is clean, new toxins are not being infused into the cells and tissues and the body was finally able to purge them from the system.

A few weeks later you may develop a severe case of acne that gets worse over a matter of days, but subsides and clears up in a couple of weeks. Immediately after this, you find that you are free of hepatitis and you feel more energetic than you were before. The acne served as an outlet for the poisons in the liver which produced the hepatitis.

You will continue to feel good for a time, then suddenly become tired and nauseous for a few days. When discomforting symptoms leave, you will feel better than you did before. Still later, you may have a headache, diarrhea, or a fever, but in a day or two you will feel even better than before. Some healing crises are rather mild and may go almost unnoticed. Others may be quite severe and require bed rest for several days. This is how recovery works. The first cleansing crisis is often the worst with each succeeding reaction being milder and of shorter duration than the one before. The body becomes purer, stronger, and healthier with longer periods of symptom-free health, until you reach a plateau where you are relatively free of symptoms and illness.

HERING'S LAW OF CURE

While your body is cleansing, you will reexperience many of the illnesses you have had in the past, all the way back to childhood. This is called the "reversal process." In the 19th century a Hungarian homeopathic physician named Constantine Hering made a discovery which is now known as *Hering's Law of Cure*. He states, "All cure comes from within out, from the head down and in reverse order as the symptoms have appeared in the body." In other words, healing starts from the inside of the body and works outward and from the top of the head and works downward, occurring in the reverse order in which sickness afflicted the body. This law has proven accurate since it was first revealed over a hundred years ago.

From Within Out

Current medical philosophy assumes that if symptoms are absent, the body is healthy and well. Consequently, treatment is focused on eliminating symptoms while ignoring the underlying cause. Symptoms, however, are reactions of the body in an effort to fight off illness or disease within the body, they are not illnesses in themselves. A fever is a symptom, not a disease. Likewise, a runny nose, diarrhea, high blood pressure, skin rashes, menstrual disorders, stiffness in the joints, etc. are all outward signs of disorder inside the body. Treating the symptom will not cure the disease; drugs may mask the symptoms, but the underlying cause goes unchecked and will continue, possibly causing greater problems later. Arthritis, for example, is not a localized problem, but a metabolic or chemical dysfunction of the entire body. In order to get lasting relief from arthritis, the entire body must be put back into chemical balance. Drugs which treat only the area of the joints provide only temporary relief without curing the problem. Treating localized areas with drugs, surgery, or radiation is only treating the symptom and will not bring lasting relief.

Hering's Law states that all cure "comes from within out," which means that in order to get rid of symptoms, you must get rid of the underlying cause. When the body is being healed from the inside, the outward signs (e.g. the symptoms) will disappear. A cleansing diet will strengthen the body so that it can heal itself from the inside out.

In Reverse Order

Hering's Law also states that healing will occur "in reverse order as the symptoms have appeared in the body." What this means is that during the cleansing process, symptoms of illnesses that you have had in the past will return. They will resurface in the reverse order in which they occurred, all the way back to childhood. If you had an infection a year ago, you will reexperience the symptoms, especially if they were suppressed with antibiotics or other drugs.

Your fat cells, encrusted mucus, and fecal debris in your intestinal tract represent the chemistry of the body at the time they were formed. Drugs, toxins, harmful microbes, etc. trapped in this material will be released into the bloodstream as the body cleanses itself. These substances will cause a reoccurrence of symptoms of disease associated with these toxins.

Because toxic material is emulsified in reverse order in which it formed in the body, the corresponding illnesses will reoccur in reverse order from when they first appeared. The most recent being removed first, will be the first to resurface. For example, if a person had a strep infection eight months ago and a bout with the flu two months ago, he will reexperience the flu first and then the strep infection. Keep in mind that the body has already made antibodies to fight these microbes, so if symptoms appear they will be quickly taken care of by the immune system. In many cases, few or no symptoms will occur. However, if the immune system is weak, as it is with many people, symptoms may be as severe as when the infection first occurred, but will eventually subside, without medication. If the body has been cleansing for a while and a healthy lifestyle is being lived, the body will be stronger and better able to repel any resurfacing illnesses.

Typically, when a person who is on a cleansing diet reexperiences an illness, his first thought is that he "caught" another infection. Often, the diet is blamed for weakening him to such a point that he got sick. It must be kept in mind that this infection is not a new one, but a purging of an old infection. The person's body is becoming stronger and is throwing off all remnants of the microbe or chemicals (drugs, poisons, toxins) that caused the illness. The infection will be short lived. Suppressing the illness with drugs, however, can drive the bacteria or toxins back into the tissues as they were before. These agents of disese would again need to be brought out through a cleansing crisis. Drugs often hamper the body's cleansing processes. If an infection resurfaces, it is best treated with natural, user-friendly, medications such as herbs.

Often, as people age their immune systems becomes overworked. Stress, toxic accumulation, and infections may all contribute to weakening the immune system. As a result, old microbes and toxic debris trapped in the tissues of the body are allowed to reinfect the system. These can cause great harm. Unlike the release of toxins during a cleansing crisis when the body has become strong enough to purge the poisons from the system, a degenerating body is weak and a disease crises arises causing repeated illness and continual discomfort. The entire body breaks down and deteriorates, until disease overcomes it. Healing the body through a cleansing process will help keep this from happening.

In his book, *Juicing Therapy*, Bernard Jensen, D.C., Ph.D., relates an experience with a patient who suffered with numerous chronic leg ulcers. She had seen many doctors over the years without success. Dr. Jensen put her on a cleansing diet and detoxification program. Within three weeks her legs were completely healed. She did not go through a healing crisis at this time, but after about three months under his care, this patient lost her sight for two days. At first she could not understand why this should happen and then she remembered an incident a number of years earlier when, as a piano teacher, she had worked so intensely in preparing for a recital that she lost her sight for two days. After the healing crisis, her sight was restored to the state when the disorder began.

Another lady had extreme scoliosis (curvature of the spine). During detoxification she developed what she described as a severe cold. Afterwards her spine was remarkably better and continued to improve. Some people will experience severe back pain for several days or even for a couple of weeks, then after that, the pain will suddenly disappear, their posture will be improved, they will stand taller, and have more flexibility.

If you have had back problems in the past, pain may temporarily return as the body heals and adjusts to overcome structural problems.

A person who suffered dizzy spells and headaches ever since being in a car accident as a teenager reported a disappearance of these symptoms after a healing crisis. Symptoms increased briefly during the crisis, but she reported afterwards that she has remained symptom-free for months.

If you have had dental problems, your teeth may hurt. You may reencounter stabbing pain extending down to the nerve and feel as if it is infected. The body is healing; you

don't need to have dental work at this time. Your teeth are removing bacteria, inflammations, etc. and although swelling may occur, and it may hurt to chew, it will heal on its own in a few days.

Sore feet, aches, arthritis, ulcers, ringworm, and any other problem may resurface or intensify temporarily during the crisis as cleansing is taking place. A full recovery may not happen after one crisis, but symptoms may be improved. If the condition has been present for many years, it will take time to completely correct it. Some people may have to experience dozens of healing crises over several years to cleanse and remove a lifetime of toxic accumulation.

From the Head Down

Tanya suffered from multiple sclerosis (MS), a disease in which the coverings on nerves degenerate, impairing nerve function and muscle control. There is no cure for it. After years of unsuccessful treatment from doctors, Tanya was told to accept her fate and live with it. In desperation, she turned to alternative health care.

First, she cleaned up her diet and discontinued all medications. Then she started a series of detoxification programs to cleanse her body of poisonous accumulations of drugs and environmental chemicals.

While she was following the regimen given her, she became angry, bitter, and stressed for no apparent reason. She snapped at her husband and family and didn't know why, as they had done nothing particularly wrong.

The most surprising part about the cleansing crisis is that in addition to the physical crisis, there is also an emotional crisis. Just as old illnesses return, emotional disturbances will also resurface. Your past feelings, emotions, thoughts, and memories, will be brought to the foreground. "All cure comes . . . from the head down" as stated by Hering.

R. H. Van Wyck, director of the Vancouver Institute of Applied Psychology says, "Each physical state is accompanied by a psychological counterpart, and strictly psychotrauma or heavy emotional material is also reexperienced during the reversal and healing crisis process." He has observed that a patient's ability to improve behaviorally is linked to the level of toxic accumulation. A healing process will clean psychological debris as well as physical toxins from the body.

To be physically healthy, you must also be mentally and emotionally healthy. Our thoughts, actions, reactions, and interactions with others have a great bearing on our physical health. Anger, fear, greed, hate and other negative feelings affect the function of the body and secretion of hormones. Such feelings cause hypertension, stress, nervousness, and the release of too much epinephrine (adrenaline) and other hormones. Excess acid is also produced. The production of too much acid in the body may lead to acidosis. Acidosis creates an environment in the body which is susceptible to numerous degenerative disease conditions.

Toxins from poor-quality food and putrefying fecal matter in the colon poisons the entire body, including the brain. As a result, the emotions are affected. This spawns discontent, anger, moodiness, and impatience which leads to social and family problems. These problems, in turn, aggravate emotional disturbances which increase the acidity and toxicity of the body. Toxins aggravate emotions, which in turn increase toxicity. The cycle feeds on itself, growing worse and worse. Is it any wonder that the divorce rate has risen so high in the past few decades and that violent crime is also at an all time high?

Emotional disturbances or symptoms are often labeled by such terms as PMS, hyperactivity, learning disability, etc. Some people say they just can't understand why a person who at one time was very friendly, has over the years become a grumpy old man or a women troubled with PMS. Children are labeled as hyperactive or learning disabled. Simply cleansing the bowels of toxic debris has brought about remarkable changes in the attitudes in people. A complete cleansing can bring about permanent positive changes.

Emotional disturbances are a threat to good health. The body's innate wisdom knows this and will remove emotional problems during the cleansing process. For those people who have had severe emotional crises in their lives, the thought of reexperiencing them is disturbing. This is the time when people are most apt to break down and resume eating poor-quality foods. Perceptions become distorted, feelings of discouragement arise, common sense is overridden, and priorities are realigned. Going on a food binge is a typical way of trying to cope with these feelings. Good health doesn't seem to matter any more. Once these emotions are removed, good sense returns.

Like physical illness, these thoughts and emotions need to be purged from the mind. This can only be done by faithfully remaining on a clean diet. Eating poor-quality food will drive these emotions back into the subconscious, only to resurface later. Get rid of them once and for all by sticking to your cleansing diet and riding out the discomforts.

Cleansing will bring feelings of well-being, cheerfulness, vitality, and positive emotional feelings. But, the emotional crisis must be passed before this can happen. A person may reexperience many emotional states for them to be completely purged. During this time you may feel anger, envy, or uselessness, become irritable, or lose will power—these are all signs of emotional cleansing.

Spouses and family members must be made aware of these conditions and be especially patient during these times, give encouragement, and be positive and loving to help the person over this trying period. They must not overreact to what may appear to be unjustified criticism, nagging, moodiness, and mental abuse. This is only a temporary phase that will soon pass. Keeping in mind that once this emotional crisis has passed, the person will become more positive, more loving, happier, and much more of a joy to be around than they have been for years, should be motivation to endure the short crisis period. Be aware that you may experience several emotional crises before the body has cleansed completely. On the other hand, since we are all different, you may not encounter any emotional irregularities.

HEALING CRISIS VERSUS DISEASE CRISIS

One of the most often asked questions about the healing crisis is how does one distinguish the difference between a healing crisis and a disease crisis? The healing crisis manifests the same type of symptoms as the disease crisis. In both cases the body is removing toxins and cleansing itself, so both are cleansing crises. In a healing crisis, however, the body is becoming stronger and healthier. While in a disease crisis, the body is struggling to remove toxic levels of poisons and microbial infestation in an effort just to survive.

A disease crisis develops when toxins accumulating in the body have reached a level of concentration where the immune system cannot adequately handle them, and normal bodily functions, and in some cases life itself, are threatened. As a result, the body reacts with a heavy cleansing crisis. Such a crisis is telling the body to stop doing what it is doing and rest. Typically, symptoms of illness include a discharge from one or more organs of elimination along with aches, pains, a lack of energy, and a loss of appetite. Often, just the thought of certain foods will cause feelings of nausea. The reason the body brings on these symptoms is not only as a means to remove toxins, but to tell the mind it needs to take time to rest and to cut down the intake of foods. The body needs rest so that it can focus its energy on cleansing. Food intake needs to be reduced, not only to prevent more toxins from entering the body, but to conserve energy that would be spent in digestion.

The disease crisis comes on after a gradual buildup of toxins from food, drugs, or environmental pollutants. It can

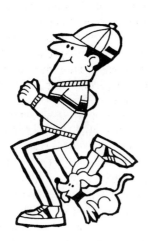

After a healing crisis you will have an increased feeling of vitality and well-being.

also occur as a result of a weakening of the immune system from physical or emotional stress. How often have you caught a cold during a stressful time in your life, finals at school, heavy workload, or family or social troubles? Disease crises occur to save life.

If someone has been on a detoxification program say for six months and becomes "sick," how can you tell if it is a disease crises or a healing crisis? If the person has been removing toxins and diseased tissues for six months and replacing them with strong healthy cells, his body is much stronger and healthier than it has been. His channels of elimination have improved. His immune system has improved. He has more energy. His powers of recuperation are stronger. Remember, a disease crisis occurs when toxic levels build up to a point that the body goes into a state of distress, resulting in massive elimination to prevent further damage. If the person is now stronger, healthier, and has more vital energy than he had before, then the cleansing crisis he encounters most likely is a *healing crisis.*

However, if a person has been on a detoxification program for only a month when he has a crisis, is it a healing crisis or an illness? One month is not long enough to completely clean and repair the body. A person with years of accumulation of toxins and environmental pollutants cannot clean out this mess in just one month. Channels of elimination will still be more sluggish than normal. The immune system will still be overburdened. So, how can you tell?

Even though the body is not completely healthy yet, after starting on the detoxification program, a body has gotten cleaner and stronger. Therefore, the symptoms are

likely due to a healing crisis. When you are doing the right thing, you won't get sick. The body is getting stronger, not weaker. Illness can't easily tackle a body that is growing stronger and healthier.

As you eat right and live right, your body becomes stronger, tissues and cells become stronger, and organs become more efficient. Waste and toxins are removed more efficiently so a disease crisis should not be manifest.

A disease crisis, however, may happen if the person isn't adhering strictly to the cleansing program. He may be sneaking "treats," taking medications, using external chemicals on the skin (e.g., antiperspirants, lotions, shampoos, etc.), or exposed to environmental pollutants. If he has cleaned up his diet and improved his lifestyle, even though he is not doing it 100 percent, he is still improving and gradually getting stronger, but may still be susceptible to infection, especially if exposure is intense or he is under stress. Exposure to a new virus or an increase in stress may lower the body's level of resistance to the point that a disease crisis might ensue.

The body continually works to achieve homeostasis—where every organ functions in harmony with each other to establish a physiological equilibrium. For a healing crisis to develop, the organs have to reach a state of integrity where they can accomplish the functions they were designed for. Every organ has become healthier and elimination has reached an improved level of efficiency. They may not be completely healthy yet, but they are working better than they had before. When all organs are strong enough to do the job of elimination, toxins will be purged. A healing crisis brings on elimination through all five of the eliminating organs—skin, bowel, lungs, liver, and kidneys. The elimination in a healing crisis is greater than in that of a disease crisis because each of these organs is working more efficiently. The colon, for example, in a healing crisis has reached a state of health where it is able handle the task of elimination. During a disease crisis the colon is weak and toxins are not efficiently removed, causing fecal matter to become trapped in the bowels where it putrefies and poisons the system. That is why enemas are often recommended for those who are sick. However, you don't necessarily need an enema during a healing crisis because the colon is healthier and more capable of handling the workload.

Before a healing crisis strikes, the body has been healing and getting stronger. You will feel a sense of well-being. Some say they get a burst of energy and renewed vitality immediately before a crisis strikes. The crisis initiates intense cleansing and rebuilding accompanied with symptoms of elimination and, often, discomfort. After the healing crisis you will again have a feeling of health and well-being. You may experience several healing crises and feel better and better after each one. Disease crises, on the other hand, can linger on and sap your strength for an extended time even after the worst symptoms have faded. You feel no improvement in health after the crisis than you did before.

When a person first encounters a severe healing crisis, it is common for him to worry. Even though he may be well informed about the discomforts of the healing process, he doesn't really believe, accept, or understand it. What often happens is that the person begins to wonder if the crisis he is going through is really a disease crisis. If it is a disease crisis, he may feel a need to get medical attention so it doesn't get worse. After all, medical doctors are very well trained to handle emergencies and life-threatening situations. The discomfort of the crisis may get worse with each day. He worries. He begins to believe that he must be sick and needs medical help. He goes to the doctor. If you go to a doctor what can he do for you? Diagnosing an illness won't cure it. All he will do is give you some drugs to suppress the symptoms.

Symptoms are necessary for the removal of toxins. They are the body's method of healing. During a disease crisis, the symptoms are not the disease, they are the reactions of the body to disease. Stopping the symptoms does not cure the disease. For example, treating a runny nose with a decongestant stops the flow of mucus in the sinuses. You may feel better because you can breathe easier. You will have a false sense of well-being which will allow you to continue on with your hectic lifestyle, never allowing the body to rest and cleanse properly. Mucus forms to remove toxins from the body. If it is stopped with a decongestant, the toxins are trapped inside the body. Some will eventually be removed by other channels of elimination, but many of these toxins will migrate and collect in other tissues of the body which can eventually lead to cellular degeneration and dis-ease.

We have been conditioned all our lives to believe that when we get sick we must go to the doctor so he can give us something to feel better. We are continually blasted with this theology in advertisements. "For fast pain relief get . . . ." "To soothe aching muscles use . . . ." "For relief of upset stomach buy . . . ." There seems to be a "cure" for just about any ailment, or at least that is the concept we are led to believe by the drug companies. We are conditioned to want and expect instant relief. Natural healing doesn't work that way. It takes time. Drugs which suppress symptoms will give a false sense of being cured as a war rages on deep inside the body.

The body was designed to heal itself. You get a cut, there is nothing you can do to heal it. You might put something on to keep out infection, but that is about all you can do. The body does the healing. The same is true for any injury or illness. If you catch a cold or get an infection there is noting you can do to heal the body. There are medications (both natural and chemical) that you can take that may help, but it is the body's innate wisdom and curative power which eventually brings healing.

The body has to heal itself whether it is encumbered with drugs or not. It can do a better job of healing without the added burden of dealing with toxic chemicals. The body does the healing, not the doctor and not the drugs. Taking medications during a cleansing crisis to treat symptoms stops the cleansing process.

If a viral or bacterial infection results from a healing crisis, it is because the infection is being pulled out of the tissues. This means you have been exposed to it before and your immune system has already made antibodies which will eventually overpower and completely eradicate the infectious agents. Drugs aren't necessary.

Even if you were going through a disease crisis, taking drugs may not help. They will suppress the symptoms without treating the cause. So it doesn't really matter whether you are going through a disease crisis or a healing crisis, taking drugs to mask the symptoms will only make matters worse. If symptoms are severe and you feel that you need something, try natural herbal remedies first. They are harmless when taken at suggested dosages and may do you some good.

The time when drugs, such as antibiotics, are useful is during a disease crisis when the body is infected by a dangerous bacteria (not a virus, antibiotics are useless against them) and is in such poor health it cannot otherwise muster the strength to fight off the infection. Unfortunately, most of us have such poor dietary and lifestyle habits that our bodies often need these types of drugs to survive. But practicing preventative medicine by eating healthfully and cleansing out toxins will give the body the strength it needs to fight most infections without resorting to drugs.

The healing crisis must be understood before you try any detox program. You only get better, not sicker. The healing crisis is a sign of improving health and needs no help from medications or other treatments. The reason the crisis has arisen is because the body has become strong enough to throw off the toxins, and remove them from the tissues; and elimination organs have become strong enough to handle the removal. Look forward to the healing crisis and rejoice when it happens. Although you may feel bad physically and perhaps mentally for a while, you will know that you are healing and will have improved health when it is over.

WHAT TO EXPECT AND WHAT TO DO

In order to remove dis-ease from the body and achieve health and well-being, you must go through the cleansing crisis. Prepare yourself mentally for it. Look forward to it. When it comes, be happy in the knowledge that you are healing.

No two people are alike. Everyone eats differently, has different genetic makeup and lifestyle. Everyone has different levels of health when they start on a cleansing program. The symptoms you encounter, their frequency, and severity will be completely different from anyone else's. So you can't compare yourself with others.

The crisis can come without warning, but generally you will know it is close at hand by the way you feel. You will feel wonderful just before the crisis. This is how it usually works. The eliminatory organs become stronger and more efficient, energy level increases and you feel great—better than you have for months. Cleansing and rebuilding are proceeding at an accelerated pace. This explosion of activity can only come about when the body is strong enough to handle intensive housecleaning. Then the bottom drops out. The body pulls out so much junk that has been stored in the tissues that disease-like symptoms appear.

During a crisis there is often an absence of appetite and an onset of tiredness. Drink plenty of clean water and get plenty of rest. Avoid overeating during this time. Eating does not give you strength. It takes energy from the body to digest food and eliminate waste. Conserve this energy by eating lightly, if at all. If you have no hunger, do not eat. It would be good even to fast, consuming only juice, herbal tea, or vegetable broth. Very little energy is needed to digest these liquids, and the nutrients they contain are easily absorbed. Liquid is vital to cleansing because water flushes out the toxins. Drink plenty. Mucus becomes more runny when you are properly hydrated. Mucus which becomes thick is harder to eliminate and can plug the pipes draining sewage from the body.

The first healing crisis will come according to the health of the individual. A young person may have a crisis after only a couple of weeks, while for an elderly person it may take three months. Older people have a buildup of many more years of poor living habits to correct than younger ones. So, generally, the older you are, the more severe and more frequent crises will be.

The detoxification program you use will also determine the speed of healing and cleansing. Fasting, for example, is one of the quickest methods of cleansing the body and can easily initiate a healing crisis. Other detoxification methods can be much slower.

A healing crisis can come as a result of anything you do that improves your health and strengthens the immune system. Converting to the Natural Foods Diet and eliminating your exposure to low-quality foods and environmental toxins can bring on a healing crisis. Any of the detox programs described in the following chapters of this book can initiate the healing crisis. Subclinically malnourished people who take vitamin and mineral supplements have overcome their deficiencies and gone through crises. One supplement dealer commented that he encountered many people who would use his products for a few weeks then stop because they claimed that they made them sick. The supplements didn't make them sick, it made them healthy enough to purge disease-causing toxins from their bodies. They made themselves sick from their lifestyle and dietary habits. They did not recognize the cleansing crisis for what it was and interpreted it as a sickness.

Some people, when they experience their first healing crisis, think it's a disease crisis and give up because "the diet didn't work—I got sicker." You can't expect to clean 40 years of junk and rebuild an entire body in just a few weeks. Some health care workers estimate that it takes seven years to thoroughly clean toxins out of the body and rebuild with new healthy tissues. During this time, periodic healing crises should be expected. To some people, seven years may seem like a long time. But at the same time strength and vitality will continue to improve. While detoxing, you do not grow older and sicker, but younger and healthier. You may see improvements in your health almost immediately. The longer you eat wisely and utilize detoxification methods, the healthier you will be. If you return to habits that burden the body with poisons and pollution, good health cannot be maintained.

 **ADDITIONAL RESOURCES**

Doctor Patient Handbook. Jensen, Bernard, Ph.D. Escondido, CA: Bernard Jensen, 1978.

The Healing Crisis, 2nd Ed. Fife, Bruce, N.D. Colorado Springs, CO: Piccadilly Books, Ltd, 2002.

Chapter 6

FASTING

THE ULTIMATE DETOXIFIER

Fasting is the quickest way to detoxify the body and promote healing. The purest and most intense cleansing program is a distilled water fast. No food or drink is taken into the body except pure distilled water. Although this is the quickest way to cleanse the body, to many, it is the most difficult. Most of us have become addicted to eating, and it's hard to give it up for several days. Miss one meal and the stomach begins to growl and churn. The slightest smell of food sends visions of tasty morsels dancing through our heads. We think after missing a couple of meals that we're starving. Why go through such misery?

Fasting is the most effective method known to draw out poisons from the cells and tissues throughout the entire body. The body's natural cleansing and healing forces are enhanced when you abstain from food. Old and diseased cells are removed. New healthy cells are grown to take their place. The body, in effect, is rejuvenated. Eating nothing could be the healthiest thing you ever did for yourself.

Contrary to popular belief, fasting is not starvation. Many people think that if they don't eat for a day or two they will be starving and doing themselves harm. They may be hungry, but they will be far from starving. We've become used to eating whenever the stomach grumbles. These "hunger pangs" are not a sign of true hunger, but simply an indication that the stomach is empty. An empty stomach is not the same as starvation. There is an important distinction between hunger and starvation. Yes, you will be a bit hungry when you fast, but the body is well equipped to handle even long periods without food. Fasting can continue as long as the body's nutritional reserves can still support itself. Starvation begins when abstinence extends beyond that time and reserves are depleted or have dropped to a low level.

Starvation is the process of dying. You cannot starve yourself into good health. You fast for proper and reasonable amounts of time, allowing the body to focus on healing and cleansing to improve health. You will not starve by going without food for a few days. Your body tissues contain enough reserves to supply most people with all the nutrients they need for well over thirty days without eating any food whatsoever. Water, however, must always be taken.

Fasting is the oldest therapeutic treatment known to man. It is mentioned in the Bible and in medical texts of ancient Egypt and Greece. Hippocrates, the father of medicine, was a proponent of fasting as a means of achieving good health. In almost every culture, fasting has been used to improve spiritual or physical well-being. Moses, Elijah, and Christ each fasted for 40 days. Traditional Asian cultures have long recommended fasting to lighten both mind and body. During the month of Ramadan, Muslims refuse food during daylight hours to cleanse their hearts and souls.

Fasting is natural and, contrary to those who don't understand it, enormously healthful. Fasting is a method nature has intended for us. It is better than all medications and treatments devised by man. Animals instinctively fast whenever they are sick or injured. Even when food is available, they will refuse to eat until their health has improved. This is one way zoo caretakers identify sick animals. By the same means we know when our own pets are sick. Humans, however, ignore this instinct. When sick, we may not feel hungry, which is the body's instinctive signal telling us not to eat, but we are told we must eat something to "keep up our strength." So we load the body up with foods which require energy to digest, energy that could better be used in healing the body. Whenever you are sick, follow your instincts. Your body will heal faster if you cut down on food consumption.

THE MIRACLE OF FASTING

People have recovered from a remarkable number of ailments as a result of fasting. Fasting enhances the cleansing and immune power of the body so that conditions that could not be handled while eating normally, are eliminated and cleared up. Dr. Herbert Shelton, the author of the book *Fasting Can Save Your Life*, was very successful in treating thousands of chronically ill patients with fasting.

One of Dr. Shelton's patients was a 70-year-old man who had been sick most of his life. For thirteen years he had suffered with bronchial asthma and was hospitalized five times on account of it. He suffered even longer with chronic sinus trouble. For six years he had been completely deaf in his left ear. To top it off, he had an enlarged prostate that had been giving him problems.

He had sought the standard medical treatment over the years, but found no lasting relief. He grew worse with time. His conditions were considered incurable and was told he would just have to live with them.

After release from his fifth hospitalization from an asthmatic attack, he went to Dr. Shelton's clinic. He said he had suffered enough and that he was convinced that the regular methods of care offered him no real promise of health. Dr. Shelton had him discontinue all drugs he had been using, which only served to mask his symptoms. "But," he asked, "what shall I do if I have an attack of asthma?"

"You will grit your teeth and clench your fists and suffer through it," was the reply. "You cannot get well if you continue to use drugs."

He was sent to bed and instructed to remain there and take nothing into his mouth but water until he was told that he could resume eating. The treatment will be worse than the disease, he thought. He was weak from years of struggling to get the oxygen he needed and didn't know if he could go without food. He was assured that he would be carefully watched and that no harm would come to him.

About four o'clock in the morning of his first night of fasting, he developed a severe paroxysm of asthma. He was unable to breathe while lying in bed, so he sat up on the side of the bed and rang for assistance. The doctor came and after examining him, said: "You'll be all right in a brief time. It will take about twenty-four hours for you to become free of asthmatic symptoms, and then you'll be comfortable." He was left to endure the cleansing process for the rest of the night.

When the doctor saw him again in the morning, he was feeling so well that he was ready to forgive the seeming neglect he received earlier. He was more than overjoyed when he went on day after day breathing as easily as when he did in his youth with not the slightest sign of asthma. He did not have another single paroxysm of asthma so long as he remained at the institution. His sinuses were still draining and the fast continued. After about six days without food, he was able to void urine without difficulty, something he hadn't been able to do for years. His prostate gland was shrinking back to normal size.

He continued to fast and watched a day-by-day disappearance of symptoms, until his sinuses cleared up and breathing became effortless. On the twenty-fifth day, he asked the doctor if he could break the fast. The doctor told him that this would be premature, he was still detoxifying and was not fully recovered, and it would be best to continue. "You are not in jail," said the doctor. "You cannot be made to fast against your will. But, if you want my best advice, you will continue for a while."

He took the doctor's advice and continued with the fast. What will always seem to him as a miracle was the fact that on the thirty-sixth day of the fast, he regained the hearing in his deaf ear. His hearing was so good that he could easily hear the low ticking of a small watch held at arm's length from his ear. Equally important is the fact that the recovery of hearing was permanent. The fast was continued through the forty-second day, then discontinued. He felt better than he had for years. He was able to breathe effortlessly and had more energy than he did before. He remained at the clinic for a while, then returned home. To his surprise he discovered, after his return, that he was no longer impotent, a symptom he had assumed was a natural consequence of age. He now knew that age was not the cause of any of his ailments and that a person can have a long healthy life without suffering with degenerative diseases.

I have recounted this case, not because it is unusual, but because it illustrates recovery from a variety of conditions that conventional methods were at a loss to cure. The man being seventy years old and chronically ill, was still able to endure a 42-day fast, consuming only water. Even at his age and with several problems, his body's immune system, without the burden of digesting food, channeled the energy to healing and recovery. The most unusual part of this man's recovery was the regaining of his hearing. Although the recovery of hearing, eyesight, and other senses are frequently reported after a fast, some conditions are not remediable because they can be caused by a variety of conditions. Degenerative conditions, for the most part, can be reversed.

The body is a marvelous organism. It can heal itself if given the chance. It was designed to combat all foreign invaders and degenerative conditions. It can do that if not pumped up with poisons or torn down by abuse. A doctor may prescribe medication to combat an infection, but he cannot kill the invading microbe. He may suture and bandage an injury, but he cannot heal the wound. He may bring the ends of broken bones together and set them, but he cannot fuse the two sections permanently together. The killing of the virus, healing of the wound, and knitting of the bone are processes that only the body can accomplish. Man cannot duplicate or even imitate the body's power to heal, he can only assist in the process.

The body can develop a multitude of degenerative and infectious conditions if it is continually subjected to poisons, much of which enter in the food that is eaten every day. If the body is allowed to detoxify by removing these harmful elements, it will rebuild, replacing diseased tissue with new healthy tissues. Symptoms of degeneration and disease will go away. Fasting has proven beneficial in the treatment of tumors, cysts, arthritis, glaucoma, cataract, asthma, psoriasis, eczema, gastric and duodenal ulcers, colitis, amebic dysentery, bronchitis, neuritis, Bright's disease, Parkinson's disease, sterility, multiple sclerosis, migraine, hay fever, hypertension, appendicitis, pellagra, migraine, epilepsy, kidney stones, and gallstones, to name just a few.

Fasting, however, is *not* a cure. Fasting is a process of detoxification that rids the body of accumulated filth. The body, freed from encumbrances, heals itself.

WHY FASTING WORKS

Why is healing enhanced when fasting? You might wonder that since the body is not consuming nourishment it would get weaker, not stronger. Eating, digesting, and assimilating food takes a great deal of energy. Some foods take more energy to consume and eliminate than they provide. When the body is infected with a virus or other pathogenic invader, it focuses its vital energy toward removing this potentially lethal organism. If it did not stop its growth immediately, the organism would quickly multiply, overpower the body, and cause death. This is why immune deficiency diseases are so serious. When we get sick, our bodies instinctively tell us not to eat and we lose our appetites. Sometimes even the smell or appearance of food will bring on feelings of nausea. The body is telling us not to eat because it needs all the energy it can muster to fight the invading microorganisms.

During a time of sickness, the stomach may grumble because it is empty, but you may not actually feel like eating. An empty stomach is not an indication that the body needs food. It is simply the result of involuntary contractions of the stomach and intestinal muscles. These contractions, known as peristalsis, occur whether or not anything is in the stomach. They have nothing to do with the body's need for nourishment.

When the body is not burdened with the task of digesting and eliminating food, it can focus its energy on pulling out and flushing toxins from the body. Every meal, no matter how clean it is, carries with it bacteria and other harmful debris which the body must deal with. When we eat a meal, the blood circulation to the digestive organs increases. The body does this to fight off harmful substances in the food (by bringing in disease-fighting white blood cells), to absorb nutrients, and to supply oxygen and energy to power all the muscles along the 26 feet of the gastrointestinal tract. Blood volume everywhere else in the body decreases as the body tackles the job of digestion and elimination. This process requires a tremendous amount of internal energy, much more than you may realize. This is the reason why after a big meal, you feel tired and want to take a nap. The body signals to you to take it easy so it can

> The therapeutic effect of fasting is very well documented by the actual clinical experience both in Europe and in the United States. The records of the numerous American and European fasting clinics prove the truthfulness of the statement by Dr. Adolph Mayer, that "fasting is the most efficient means of correcting any disease."
>
> —Paavo Airola, Ph.D.

utilize all available energy to process the meal. Even after a relatively small meal the body channels a great deal of energy to the task of digestion. This is also why it is not good to exercise immediately after eating. Exercise diverts energy away from the process of digestion.

When you fast, you free the body of the burden of digestion and elimination. The organs involved in these processes can rest. Your body can then focus its energy to cleansing toxins which have accumulated in various organs and tissues. The immune system, in essence, gets a boost.

DESIGNED TO SURVIVE

In the newspaper recently a story was carried about an 83-year-old woman who was stranded for eight days without food on the grasslands of Wyoming. Mae Wardell had been visiting her sister at a nursing home in Casper. On her return home she got lost. Her car became stuck in the mud, and her effort to free it wore the car battery down. For the next eight days Wardell lived on a dozen or so cans of juice she had with her and the frost she scraped from the hood of her car. September temperatures in this desolate part of Wyoming dropped down into the 20s. When rescued she was in good health. Even in the cold, surviving on only frost and a little juice, this 83-year-old woman was actually in better health after the ordeal than before.

Such stories are rather common. People who are stranded in air and ship disasters and forced to fast or survive on minimal amounts of food can live for a long time. Although physically weak, as wilderness conditions can be severe, they survive if water is available. Such people have survived and been rescued after as much as two months. On examination by doctors, they are found to be in remarkably good condition. In fact, many of them are probably much healthier as a consequence of their forced fast.

Eating three meals a day is a development of modern civilization. In more primitive societies and in times past, man is and was forced to undergo periods of time without food. The American Indians, for example, typically ate only one meal a day. Many of the primitive tribes in Africa and elsewhere do the same. Interestingly enough, these people do not suffer from degenerative diseases like those in Western countries. For thousands of years they have been able to survive through droughts and famine when getting even one meal a day was difficult.

Famine, drought, floods, and winter cold can all create conditions where food is scarce. These conditions are part of nature. Animals have been endowed with the capability of withstanding these periods, and survive through the hardest of times. Like all other creatures, nature has also designed our bodies with the ability to withstand periods without food.

Animals, like the bear, will hibernate all winter long. During this time all processes of life continue, blood is circulated, respiration continues, and warmth is created. Energy and nutrients are used. Mother bears will give birth to their young and nurse them without eating a thing themselves. Where do they get the nourishment to not only survive themselves but to provide milk for their young?

The bodies of the bear and other animals, including man, store fat. It is the fat tissue which provides the nutrients necessary to carry on life in times of abstinence. Bears eat as much as possible in the summer to build up a thick layer of fat to last throughout the winter. Other animals store fat which can be used in times of drought or cold when food is not available. We also have this survival mechanism built into our bodies.

Our bodies break down carbohydrate, fat, and protein and convert them into energy. From these three nutrients we get all our energy. Any amount that is eaten beyond the body's immediate needs is converted into fat and stored. The body naturally does this to protect itself when food may be scarce. These nutrients, for the most part, are not eliminated from the body no matter how much we eat. When we overeat, the excess nutrients are converted to body fat. That is why overeating leads to weight gain.

By a process called autolysis the body retrieves these stored reserves to be used by vital organs. A healthy body will maintain a reserve of nutrients to supply all its needs for weeks and even months without food. These reserves contain a balanced blend of nutrients to keep the body healthy. Some may worry that fasting will cause malnutrition. They may point out that vitamin C and the B-complex vitamins are water-soluble and that the body isn't supposed to be able to store water-soluble vitamins. We all know that a vitamin C deficiency causes scurvy. But it has been found that even in fasts extending over a month, people do not develop scurvy or beriberi (vitamin B_1 deficiency), pellagra (niacin deficiency), rickets (vitamin D deficiency), goiter (iodine deficiency), or any other deficiency disease. Studies have demonstrated the body's ability to store vitamin C and the B-complex vitamins. Water-soluble vitamins are stored in the liver and other tissues of the body. The body with its innate intelligence has provided a means to store necessary vitamins and minerals so all the body's nutritional needs are met when it is forced to rely on its reserves.

Vitamins and minerals are utilized during the digestive process. When nutrient deficient foods are continually eaten, they are used up and disease develops. A poor diet, which drains stored nutrients, can deplete reserves even more quickly than fasting.

Autolysis is essentially a form of self-cannibalism. As we go without food, tissues are called upon in the reverse order of their importance to the organism. Thus fat (which was stored for this purpose) is the first tissue to be used. As the body consumes its fat reserves, it then begins to dismantle diseased tissues or broken down cells. Once these become depleted, the skeletal muscles are next to go. Organs such as the brain, nerves, heart, and lungs, which are vital to life, are the last to be affected. In fact, even when death is caused by starvation, these vital organs retain all their functional ability and strength until the end.

The tissues of less importance are consumed to provide energy for those necessary to maintain life. Once the body reaches the point where it begins to seriously break down skeletal muscle, the first functional organ to be affected, a state of starvation exists. Fasting, however, never proceeds this far.

When you are fasting, vital organs do not suffer in the least, only unwanted fat and nonfunctional tissues are reabsorbed and consumed. Muscles may look leaner, but that is due primarily to the removal of fat around them and not from removal of the muscle itself. Muscles, as well as other organs, retain their integrity.

Fasting is not simply a withering away of useless tissue. Vital functions of life continue, cells are regenerated, wounds heal, and physical growth continues. In this way the body becomes rejuvenated. In fact, healing is enhanced because the body now has more healing energy than it did when it had to constantly digest food.

During the process of autolysis your vital force (or healing energy, also known as "chi" in Chinese medicine and acupuncture) reaches deep into all areas of the body, into joints, muscles, nerves, bones, marrow, everywhere. Toxins and microbes, buried deep in your tissues and organs are pulled out and discarded. Diseased tissues, which have no functional purpose, are broken apart and consumed. Thus degenerative tissues are removed. The body is at a heightened level of efficiency. Wherever repair is necessary, the body rebuilds. People who have been weakened by deterioration grow stronger as the body builds new cells to replace the old.

One of the benefits of fasting is the reduction of toxins introduced into the body at this time. Since no food is eaten, toxins commonly associated with food do not enter the body. With fewer toxins entering the body our immune systems can focus on cleaning out the garbage that is already there.

If food consumption is reduced, either by fasting or by sensible dieting, the body is able to channel more energy to healing. It is logical to assume that people who eat less (and still get adequate nutrition) are healthier than those who eat more. We are well aware that the reverse is certainly true. Those who are obese suffer from a myriad of health problems brought on by their poor diet.

Studies on animals have shown that underfeeding as opposed to overeating tends to prolong life. Animals that are fed just enough to maintain life outlive those who are fed normal diets. Animals that are allowed to eat as much as they want die earliest. Not only do the animals live longer, but they retain normal body functions longer. Mice that live the equivalent of 90 years of human life are still fertile, long after other mice are not. Their life span extended to 120-140 in terms of human life—nearly twice the normal life expectancy (see *The 120 Year Diet* by Roy Walford, M.D.).

Fasting has a rejuvenating effect, not a detrimental one. Research on animals and insects has demonstrated similar results. In certain species of worm it is found that if given abundant food, they pass through their whole life in three to four weeks, but when the food is greatly reduced or they are forced to fast, they may continue active and young for over three years! Initial studies on diet restriction in humans also shows improved physiological health.

Periodic fasting seems to be what nature has intended for all the creatures of the earth. Our bodies were built to handle periods with little or no food and we actually live longer and healthier lives by doing so. Periods when food is plentiful are always separated by cold, heat, drought, and other conditions when food is scarce. Fasting is nature's cleanser and rejuvenator. It is the simplest and most natural form of bringing about healing.

HOW TO FAST

When is the best time to fast? You can do it any time of year. Chinese medicine recommends fasting at some point during the ten days before and after the equinox. For spring that is between March 10 and April 1. The most natural time to fast is in the spring. In the animal kingdom this is the time when the scanty food forged from winter is nearly depleted and before new shoots have sprung up. Animals go without much food and essentially fast until new growth appears. Likewise with primitive man, by the end of the winter, food stores have been depleted and food is most scarce. At this time he must eat what little is available. In olden times man was compelled by nature to fast just before the new growth of summer appeared. Nature designed it that way. For this reason, extended fasts may be more in harmony with nature if conducted in late spring or early summer. At this time temperatures should be warming up so the decrease in body temperature that accompanies fasting will not be such a discomfort, as it would in colder times of the year.

As expected, fasting involves some degree of discomfort. The stomach groans and growls and may even hurt a bit. This will go away. Thoughts of food may enter your mind. Keep them out. If your stomach rumbles or you are tempted to eat, drink some water instead. This will help to satisfy those urges. Fasting is not easy. But it does become easier with practice.

Fasting can be done any time of the year: spring, summer, winter, or fall. It should be done when you can devote time to it. When you fast, you will feel colder than normal, especially your hands and feet. For this reason, many people prefer to fast during the warmer months. But as long as you can bundle up and keep warm, it doesn't matter when you fast.

No food, whatsoever, is eaten when fasting. Water, however, is absolutely necessary. The faster should drink plenty of fluid to avoid dehydration. Sometimes while fasting, people forget to drink enough fluids. The body needs water to carry on all the processes of metabolism, fluid circulation, and maintenance of chemical balance, as well as the process of cleansing. Therefore, the faster should drink plenty of water, without going overboard. Approximately six glasses a day for an adult is adequate. If you are small in stature, less water is needed. If you larger than average, you may need to drink more water.

Fruit and vegetable juices are not consumed on a water fast. Drink only distilled or filtered water. If the fast extends for more than two or three days, pure water is not usually consumed. For extended fasts, most fasting experts drink a very dilute form of lemonade. The mixture consists of the following ingredients:

2 tablespoons fresh lemon or lime juice

1 tablespoon raw honey or unprocessed maple syrup

8 ounces of filtered or distilled water

A pinch of sea salt

Adding a little lemon and honey to the water is not for nourishment, but simply makes the water taste better and aid in the cleansing process. Lemon juice is a good cleanser and astringent that rids tissues of toxins; it also stimulates liver detoxification. Honey is used to balance the sour taste of the lemon. By far the most important ingredient in this mixture is the salt.

Distilled or filtered water is recommended because it is free from chlorine, fluoride, and other chemicals typically added to tap water. Unfortunately, it also has all naturally occurring salts and minerals removed as well. Water this pure can act as a sponge and leach minerals and salts out of the body causing a mineral deficiency.

If you use filtered or distilled water it is very important to take some sea salt and perhaps liquid mineral supplements every day. If you fail to do this you will increase the discomfort you experience, shorten the time you are able to refrain from eating, and decrease you body's ability to cleanse and heal itself.

You can tell when your body has become salt and mineral depleted when water no longer quenches your thirst and you lose the desire to drink. During a water fast your body is trying to eliminate toxins as efficiently as possible and an adequate amount of water is absolutely necessary for this process. Your natural response should be to have an increase in thirst. If you lose your desire to drink while fasting or the water becomes unpalatable it is a sign that you are becoming minerally deficient; your body is trying to prevent further leaching of salts and minerals by suppressing your desire to drink.

Sea salt is recommend over ordinary table salt because it contains many trace minerals that may also be leached out of the body during the fast. Taking a trace mineral supplement is also a good idea. Be generous with the salt. If you don't want to add it to your water then put it on your tongue and let it dissolve. Do this several times a day. Believe me you will get better results with less discomfit.

In addition to this lemon water mixture you may drink as much pure water as you like. Just keep in mind to get an adequate amount of salt.

Some fasting experts also permit herbal teas (without sweetener) as well. Flavored water is usually permitted only on extended fasts. Short fasts of only a day or two use just pure water and sea salt. Cleansing works better that way.

Medications should be discontinued. They only cause the body to spend energy working to remove them rather than cleaning house. If you must have a prescription drug, check with your doctor before starting a fasting program.

A water fast will cause you to feel less energetic than normal. Part of this is because of the lack of eating stimulating foods and part because the body is utilizing all its energy on internal cleansing. You should avoid strenuous physical activity and get plenty of rest. If you have a physically demanding job or stressful work environment, it may be best not to go to work while you fast; stay at home and take it easy. You might have to take vacation time to do this.

A tendency some might have when fasting is to want

to refrain from all activity and sleep most of the time. Rest is good, but some degree of exercise is necessary to keep muscles in shape and body fluids circulating. Blood and lymph must circulate in order to purge toxins from the tissues and remove them from the body. Cleansing will actually be quicker if you keep physically active. This does not mean jogging ten miles a day or lifting weights, but moderate exercise like walking is highly recommended.

Some people feel, since they are not eating, they should have no energy. So they walk around like a zombie and complain that they don't have the strength to do anything. This is more psychological than physical. Even though you will notice a decrease in energy level as you fast, you will be able to pursue most normal activities. You could continue to go to work and no one would suspect you were fasting unless you told them, which you should not do.

A big factor in the success of your fast is the attitude of the people you are around, especially your family. Most people are ignorant about the process and benefits of fasting. To them, missing a single meal is the onset of starvation. It is wise not to tell anyone you are on a fast. Most people do not understand fasting and will only give you negative comments. Some will argue with or tease and tempt you. To avoid such problems, simply don't tell anyone.

If your family isn't sympathetic to what you are doing, it can make your fast unbearable. They will criticize you. They may even try to tempt you with tasty tidbits of your favorite food. Aromas from cooked foods in the house will be hard to resist. These people work on your senses and mind to break your will. Often, they do it not to be malicious, but more as a form of teasing. Whether they are just teasing you or trying to dissuade you from fasting, you don't need to suffer with it. To make your fast successful, you need to set some ground rules before starting. One is that you should not be required to cook meals or be around when meals are prepared and cooked. They should show you some courtesy and allow you to fast without temptations or criticism. A supportive family can be a big encouragement.

Some people worry that when they fast they do not have bowel movements. Don't worry about it, this will adjust itself after the fast is over. Logically, if you are not eating anything, you should eliminate very little.

Some fasting proponents advocate daily enemas along with the fast. They reason that the body is not having regular bowel movements and material which is in the colon may be sitting there putrefying and releasing toxins into the body. Other experts say enemas are unnecessary. They point out that if the body needs to defecate it will.

Animals need not resort to enemas when they fast, so why should we? Enemas will certainly do no harm, so if you feel you need to have an enema, you may do so, otherwise, don't worry about it.

Almost anyone can fast. Overweight people, since they have more stored fat, can fast a longer time than skinner people. Even thin people carry a reserve of nutrients in their tissues. They too, can benefit from a fast.

For some conditions, however, fasting is not recommended. Obviously those suffering from anorexia or malnutrition should not fast. A pregnant or nursing mother should not fast as she needs nourishment for herself and her baby. Also, unhealthy toxins released during a fast may reach the baby through the placenta or breast milk. People with advanced stages of heart disease, cancer, and diabetes should avoid fasting. If you have a serious health condition, you should first check with you health care provider before attempting a fast.

Except for the conditions mentioned above, most everybody can fast. Even those who are hypoglycemic or diabetic can fast. Most people, however, should not attempt to fast without some preparation first. Most of us eat processed, prepared foods stripped of vital nutrients. Toxins in the environment and packaged foods also leach nutrients from the body. Because of this, many people, particularly teenagers, who generally eat deplorable diets are subclinically malnourished. They are getting just enough essential vitamins and minerals to keep symptoms of advanced nutrient deficiencies from surfacing, but woefully lacking in optimal nutrition to keep them healthy. Fasting for such people would only deprive them further of desperately needed nutrients. Because subclinical nutrient deficiency cannot easily be identified, it is near impossible to identify who or who isn't deficient. A good indicator, however, is diet history. A person who subsists primarily on junk foods is almost assuredly malnourished to some degree. A person who eats plenty of whole grains, fruits and vegetables is most likely getting adequate nutrition.

Since many people live primarily on convenience foods, most people should prepare for fasting by eating a nutritious diet such as the Natural Foods Diet. A nutritious diet such as this should be undertaken for several weeks before fasting. This way the body can build up a store of essential nutrients. Another important reason is to flush out the worst toxins with a clean diet before resorting to the more drastic fasting. Just switching from a typical diet to the Natural Foods Diet will bring about cleansing and rejuvenation. This diet should be continued until the body has had time to cleanse and adjust to the change in diet. Simply cutting out or reducing stimulating foods such as coffee, salt, meat, tea, chocolate, sugar, fat, etc. will affect the body. Eliminating some of these will cause withdrawal symptoms. Such symptoms during a fast can make fasting much more difficult to accomplish. If you eliminate these sometimes uncontrollable cravings from your system before going on a fast, going without food for a few days will be much easier.

HOW LONG SHOULD YOU FAST

Fasts usually last from one to 30 days. They could extend even longer. People have fasted for over 100 days, under supervision. Any extended fast should be supervised by a health care provider who is experienced in conducting fasts. You should limit your first fast to one to three days.

Fasting is not a one-time thing you do to gain instant health. You do not need to jump into a 30- or 40-day fast to purge all your toxins at one time. Most people have so many toxins in their bodies that they couldn't endure an extended fast. Fasting should be broken into smaller periods of time and repeated frequently. Then, as the body becomes cleaner, longer fasts can be attempted.

If you are inexperienced, you should fast no longer than about 14 days. Fasts longer than this should be under supervision by a health professional experienced in fasting. During the fast, huge amounts of toxins are pulled out of tissues and dumped into the bloodstream for elimination. Even if you think you are healthy, a fast can pull out a huge amount of toxins that have been locked deep in your tissues. Dumping these poisons into the bloodstream may bring about symptoms of a healing crisis. The more toxins in the body, the more likely a fast will initiate a healing crisis. Even a short three-day fast can bring on such a crisis. As you have learned in the previous chapter, symptoms can be unpleasant. This is one reason why it is advisable to be under the supervision of an expert if attempting a longer fast.

Short-term fasting means one to three days of taking in nothing but water. Short-term fasting alters both consciousness and physiology. It is a good home remedy for colds, flus, infectious illnesses, and toxic conditions of all kinds. If you combine it with rest and a good mental state, short-term fasting can make you feel like a new person. Many people report that even after one day of fasting their senses are sharper, their heads clearer, their bodies lighter and more energetic. Some like this feeling so much that they fast one day a week.

—Andrew Weil, M.D.

The first three days of the fast are the worst, after that you lose most of your desire and craving for food. The first day of the fast is the hardest. The stomach grumbles and groans. You feel "hunger pangs." You may feel tired. Other symptoms may also surface. The second day is hard too, but easier than the first. The third day is much easier although desires for food are still present. After the third day, desire for food has greatly diminished and fasting no longer is difficult. It gets easier each day. In fact, although it may seem strange, it is easier to lose weight by fasting than by a calorie-restricted diet. When people diet, they must watch what they eat and limit their calories. Food cravings are always present and temptation is fierce. The stomach is always hungry. It is difficult to resist cheating. When fasting, however, after the third day most desire for food and all cravings are gone. There is comparatively little temptation to cheat. So not only is losing weight faster, but actually easier.

The first thing you should do to prepare yourself for a fast is to start on the Natural Foods Diet. Stay on this diet for three weeks before attempting any fast which will last over three days. This isn't a requirement, but it will help to make the fast more bearable. If you have been eating ordinary grocery store and restaurant foods, when you fast you will experience withdrawal symptoms that may be manifested as lack of energy, depression, headaches, and such. Foods that you have become used to eating every day—sugar, meat, dairy, etc.—have a stimulating effect on the body. When you remove these stimulants from your diet, you will feel a let down, which you will interpret as a lack of energy.

If you start on the Natural Foods Diet first, you will experience this lack of energy while you are still eating instead of during your fast. During the fast you battle hunger pangs, which is tough enough at first; you don't need to be troubled with fatigue, headaches, and such as well. If you prepare beforehand by following the Natural Foods Diet, your fast will be easier for you. On the Natural Foods Diet it will take about two weeks for the body to adjust. Then energy will return with renewed strength and vigor.

As a suggestion, you may try one 24- or 36-hour fast a week after you have started your Natural Foods Diet. Then as you feel up to it, try a couple of three-day fasts. Work gradually up to five- and seven-day fasts. Only after you have been on a Natural Foods Diet and gone through several short fasts should you attempt a fast longer than seven days. With this preparation, you may try medium duration fasts of 10-14 days. After each fast, continue with the Natural Foods Diet. The Natural Foods Diet will continue to cleanse the body but at a slower pace, and keep you from adding new toxins to your body.

The shorter fasts give you experience and make the longer fasts easier. Your body becomes accustomed to periods of no food, so it is not so much of a shock for you physically or psychologically. Your body will be cleaner and, therefore, cleansing symptoms less severe. If your body is fairly clean, you may encounter few symptoms even after 10 or 12 days.

A 24-hour fast can last from dinner one day to dinner the next, or breakfast one day to breakfast the next. For example, if you were going to start your fast Friday night, you would eat dinner and then nothing else for the rest of the night. Don't eat a big dinner to tide you over during the fast. Remember, it is the absence of food that brings about cleansing. Saturday morning continue to fast. Skip breakfast and lunch. You will break your fast by eating dinner Saturday evening. Try to make it a full 24 hours. If you want to extend the fast to 36 hours, skip dinner and break the fast when you eat breakfast on Sunday morning.

Fasting may or may not bring about a healing crisis. Whether it does or not, it is still cleansing toxins out of your body. Often a healing crisis will manifest itself a few days after ending a fast. If you experience a healing crisis while fasting, you can continue to fast; often that may be the only thing you can do as you might be nauseous. But if the symptoms become too unbearable, the fast may be broken (if not vomiting) and symptoms will subside as the body channels cleansing energy towards digestion. The toxins that the body was eliminating will still be left in the body if the crisis is aborted. For your health's sake, you should continue with a cleansing program. This can be done slowly with a clean diet and a series of short fasts.

Fasting should be done frequently as the effects are cumulative. If you can't manage a full 14-day fast, several three- or five-days fasts will eventually accomplish the same cleansing. One longer fast is actually easier than several short fasts. The reason is once you have gotten past the first three days, your hunger is so much reduced that the remainder of the fast is relatively easy. With short fasts, you must go through the difficult first three days several times.

The more often you fast, the longer you will be able to fast. Also, fasting becomes easier with experience. The body becomes more accustomed to periods of deprivation. Psychologically you are more familiar with the process and it is not such an ordeal. Attitude has a great deal to do with the success of fasting. Don't get into the mind frame that you are depriving yourself and don't tempt yourself by dreaming of chocolatey desserts, roasted meats, or greasy fried potatoes. Make up your mind from the start to stick to the fast. Think positively! Focus your thoughts on the cleansing your body is doing and on the health you are achieving. Avoid all temptations. Avoid going into stores where there are aromas of foods. Remove yourself from all temptation.

The more toxins your body has, the longer it will take to detoxify. Don't expect psoriasis, colitis, bronchitis, arthritis, or other chronic conditions to mysteriously disappear after fasting for only three days. Although the body will benefit from short fasts, serious degenerative conditions, which have taken years to develop, will take time to correct. Longer fasts will keep the body in a state of detoxification a longer time so more internal cleansing can be accomplished.

You will have toxins stored in your tissues since childhood that will eventually be purged by fasting. Take a person who has been troubled by bronchitis for say the past three years and by chronic psoriasis for 20. The conditions that caused the bronchitis will be cleared up first, since it occurred more recently. It may take several fasts to reach all the way back and cleanse the toxins which cause, the psoriasis. Repeated fasts are necessary to dig deep into tissues and remove all toxins that have been accumulating since childhood.

Fasting should be done on a regular basis. This could be a two-week fast once a year, a seven-day fast every six months, or a two-day fast each month. The idea is to cleanse the body on a regular basis. If the fasts are short, they should be frequent. If longer, than they can be spaced farther apart. Even if your diet is clean, you will still benefit from periodic fasting. You cannot escape completely from environmental pollutants, contaminated foods, or microorganisms. Periodic fasts will purge these toxins from the system.

Fasting expert, Paul Bragg, Ph.D., who lived nearly a century, fasted from 24 to 36 hours every week and seven to ten days four times a year. He felt it was necessary to fast often to clean toxins that constantly accumulate in our bodies, even when we eat right. Bragg ate very healthfully, preferring organically grown produce, but did not have control all the time over the quality of the food he ate, even though it may have appeared healthy. He periodically had analyses of his urine made, and repeatedly they found traces of DDT and other deadly pesticide residues. Although DDT is now illegal in United States and many other Western countries, it still lingers in our environment and it is still used in countries from which produce is imported. We do not know what chemical agents are on the foods we buy.

Fasting should become a regular part of our lives. We need to schedule periods of fasting to clean up debris that finds its way into our bodies each day. Pollutants, foods, mold, skin creams, shampoo, drugs, cigarette smoke, etc.

all contribute to toxic buildup in our bodies. We are exposed to more toxins than we realize and just eating wisely won't keep us clean. Fasting should be done on a regular basis. Short one- to two-day fasts can be done weekly or monthly. Longer fasts may also be done at any time. Every year, try at least one longer fast of 7-21 days. When not fasting, eat according to the Natural Foods Diet plan.

WHEN TO END A FAST

If you don't eat, eventually you will die from starvation. If you fast for too long, you can enter a starvation phase. So how long is it safe to fast and when does fasting turn into starvation?

You don't need to fear, when fasting for a week or two, that you will suffer harm or die from starvation. Most people have enough nutritional reserves to handle periods much longer than this.

When you begin a fast, you will feel hungry for the first few days. But with each day, the hunger diminishes. After about three or four days you will have lost most of your desire for food. The remainder of the fast your desire for food is minimal and there is relatively little discomfort. In fact, you will feel much like your normal self. You can go on for weeks like this.

The body is amazingly intelligent. During a fast, it can tell us when reserves are becoming depleted. As reserves near exhaustion, hunger returns with an intensity that will drive you to seek food. The intensity is much greater than the hunger felt the first few days of the fast. At this time, the fast should be broken no matter how long you have been on it. The time will vary with each individual. Obviously, those with a great deal of stored body fat will be able to fast for much longer than those who have little.

Starvation weakens the body to such a degree that getting around becomes increasingly difficult and eventually you would become bedridden. This is what's expected if the body is cannibalizing functional tissues to maintain life. You would never fast this long.

Never continue fasting after hunger returns. You can make a goal, but don't hold yourself to it if hunger returns. Judge by how you feel. Most anyone can fast seven days without harm (so long as they are free of serious disease). You need three to four days just to get over the initial stages of hunger. After that, hunger diminishes to the point that you don't care about eating. It doesn't bother you unless you allow yourself to become tempted with smells and thoughts. Remove temptation and you will be fine. You may find that some foods you liked before will be unappealing and even nauseating. You will know when it's time to stop, when hunger returns with a passion. It is not likely that you will need to end your fast before twenty-one days has expired. Remember, the longer you can fast, the deeper the cleanse can go. But if you fast longer than ten days, it is advisable to adequately prepare for it with a series of shorter fasts.

WHAT TO EXPECT WHEN YOU FAST

People often complain that fasting doesn't work for them because every time they try it, they get sick, or get a headache, or experience other uncomfortable symptoms. The fact that a person is experiencing these symptoms is a sign that the fast is working and the body is cleansing itself. That's the purpose of fasting—purging the body of filth. Removing this filth will involve an increase in activity of the organs of elimination—lungs, kidneys, bowels, skin. Fasting is a means of detoxification—accelerated detoxification. You should expect some discomfort. You may experience nausea, headaches, diarrhea, skin rashes, coughing, etc. These are the processes of cleansing. Let the body complete its job. Be prepared for it. Welcome it. It is a sign of healing and improving health. You may or may not have a full-blown healing crisis during a fast. This will depend on your health and the length of your fast.

Every ache and pain is likely to be blamed upon the fast whether it was the cause or not. Withdrawal symptoms (fatigue, depression, etc.) will manifest themselves when you stop eating stimulating foods such as sugar and meat. For the most part, this can be avoided if you prepare yourself beforehand by getting on the Natural Foods Diet. It takes two to three weeks on the Natural Foods Diet for the body to adjust. After that, energy returns and discomforts cease. When you enter into a fast, your body will be prepared and will not have to go through the withdrawal symptoms. This makes the first three days of the fast much easier to endure.

Many people can't fast because psychologically they are just too weak. The physical discomfort of the first three days and the temptation of food is too great for them to bear. To be successful, you need to commit yourself. Set a goal of, say, three or five days, and stick to it.

After you start your fast you may find when you wake up in the morning that you have a dry or sore throat. The soreness is usually the result of a lack of fluids. It will go away in a couple of hours after drinking some water. The body requires larger quantities of water than normal as it flushes and carries out toxins. If you don't drink enough during the day, your throat will feel sore in the morning.

It is common during a fast that lasts more than a few days to lose some desire to drink. Not drinking enough water will put an additional strain on the body and you may become dehydrated. So drink plenty of water.

As the body cleanses itself, toxins will be carried out through every orifice and every channel of elimination. You may encounter mucus congestion, runny nose, coughing, slight fever, aches, diarrhea, and discharge from your eyes and ears. At first, you might think you are coming down with a cold or have hay fever. You're not; this is part of the cleansing you are experiencing.

During your fast your body conserves energy. In this process, heat generation is kept at a minimum and focused on vital internal organs. As a consequence, your fingers, toes and other extremities will become cold. In fact, this will make your whole body colder than normal. So you will need to wear extra clothing to keep comfortably warm. If you fast during the summer, this decrease in temperature will be less noticeable to you.

Generally, you will notice that you have less energy and endurance than you normally have. This is to be expected when you fast since you are not consuming energy-producing foods. But you should not be so tired that you drag your body around. If you have prepared yourself by getting on the Natural Foods Diet before the fast, your energy level will remain relatively high and you will be able to do most everything you normally could. Your mind will remain sharp and able to think clearly and you soul be just as alert as normal. It is only if you jump into a fast from a normal diet that you will feel lethargic.

Your tongue can reveal how much toxic material is stored in your cells and vital organs. The tongue is a mirror of the membrane system of your body. While fasting, the tongue will become heavily coated, and your breath will take on a strong offensive odor. You can watch the progress of your internal cleansing by observing the coating on your tongue. As it builds up, the body is removing more and more and breath gets worse and worse. You are likely to also have a strong body odor as toxins are released through your skin and sweat glands. Daily baths will relieve much of this. Do not use deodorants, mouthwash, or perfumes. Wash with mild soap and water. Brush your teeth. If you have to do something about bad breath, rinse your mouth with a three percent solution of hydrogen peroxide. This is a natural disinfectant that is available at most any pharmacy or health food store.

Your urine will take on a dark amber color and it too, will have a strong odor. If you drink plenty of water, the urine color and odor will be less noticeable.

If you continue to fast, you will reach a point where the coating on your tongue starts to get lighter and your breath improves. This continues until the tongue acquires a healthy pink color and the breath smells fresh. Body odor will be gone. Urine will be clear. At this stage, your body has accomplished about all of the detoxification it can at that time, and it is time to end your fast. To reach this state usually takes a few weeks.

Since you are not eating any solid food, you will not have bowel movements. So don't worry about this. And don't take laxatives. Your body will evacuate when it is ready. It doesn't need to be forced. You may, however, experience a bowel evacuation during the fast. You might wonder where this material would came from. You will notice that it will have a foul smell and may be stringy, rubbery, or filled with sticky mucus. This material is feces that has been trapped in the colon. It may have been encrusted on the colon wall for years, putrefying and slowly poisoning your body. Fasting has forced it loose.

Fasting is an intense method of detoxification. Microorganisms, chemicals from foods and cosmetics, environmental pollutants, and old drugs will be loosened up and flushed out. If you have a great deal of this debris dumped into your bloodstream, you will experience a healing crisis as the body removes it. You may experience vomiting, nausea, diarrhea, nasal discharge, aches, pains, fatigue, etc. You can continue with the fast, if you can. Keep in mind that if you are losing a lot of fluid from vomiting and diarrhea you need to drink more to replenish it if you can. If symptoms become too uncomfortable, you can ease them by eating some fruit or mild soup, which

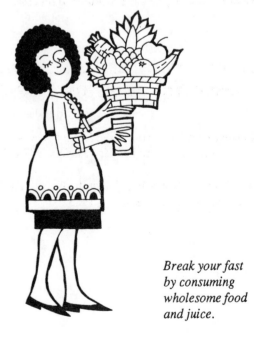

Break your fast by consuming wholesome food and juice.

will be easy on your digestive tract. The toxins you are eliminating need to come out. You may continue with the fast or try again later.

The effects of fasting continue after the fast is over. You may experience only mild discomfort during your fast such as grumbling stomach, bad breath, etc. A few days after ending the fast, however, you may encounter an actual healing crisis. If you start to feel sick three days later you will know that you aren't coming down with the flu, your body is continuing to detoxify. Fasting had loosened up the toxins and the body is now flushing them out.

Detoxing should not be viewed as a period of "sickness." It is a time of cleansing and is a positive experience. You should look with joy in anticipation of having a cleansing crisis and be happy when you feel "sick" as a result of the cleansing process. Cleansing means you are healing, becoming healthier and stronger.

BREAKING THE FAST

If you've been on a fast more than just a few days, you need to break the fast gently. Eating meats, fried foods, packaged convenience foods and other poor-quality foods will cause digestive problems—avoid them. The day you end your fast you should eat only fruits and vegetables in moderation. You may eat fresh fruits and vegetables, salads, vegetable soup, or steamed vegetables, and juices. You may gradually add other wholesome foods in subsequent days. Refrain from meat or greasy foods. Give the gastrointestinal tract time to adjust to processing full meals again before taxing it with meat.

Short fasts may be broken on juices if you wish. But it isn't necessary to restrict yourself to juices. Foods with fiber and bulk are actually preferred because they help stimulate peristalsis—the muscular movement of the gastrointestinal tract.

It is common to be continually hungry for a few days after a prolonged fast. The tendency is to eat too much and undo much of the good you have accomplished. To help control your hunger, drink plenty of vegetable and fruit juices. You should be eating normally again in a couple of days.

One complaint critics give fasting is that even though a fast may help to remove symptoms of degenerative disease, these conditions often reappear sometime later. They then say that fasting only provides temporary improvement and that it is ineffective as a permanent cure.

Keep in mind that fasting is not a cure! It is a process by which the body detoxifies itself, thus allowing healing to take place. The examples the critics cite are of people who, after the fast, return to their previous lifestyle, eating the same types of foods which led to their ill health in the first place. It is important for you to realize that if you are to gain any permanent benefit from fasting, or any other detoxification program, you must change your lifestyle. This involves eating good-quality foods and avoiding all low-quality foods. Ideally, you will follow the Natural Foods Diet plan. In this way, you will get good foods that will continue to allow your body to heal and build strong tissue. Don't undo all the work of a fast by gorging yourself on junk food.

 **ADDITIONAL RESOURCES**

Fasting Can Save Your Life. Shelton, Herbert M. Tampa, FL: American Natural Hygiene Society, 1978.

The Miracle of Fasting. Bragg, Paul C. Desert Hot Springs, CA: Health Science, 1966

Fasting Signs and Symptoms—A Clinical Guide. Salloum, Trevor K. East Palestine, OH: Buckeye Naturopathic Press, 1992.

The 120 Year Diet: How to Double Your Vital Years. Walford, Roy, M.D. New York: Simon & Schuster, 1986.

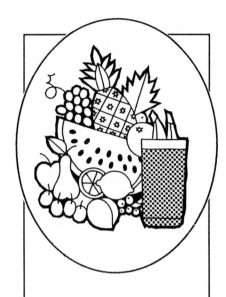

Chapter 7

JUICING

Today, any person not familiar with the nutritional and recuperative value of fresh vegetable and fruit juices is woefully uniformed.
—Norman W. Walker, D.Sc.

The art of medicine consists of amusing the patient while Nature cures the disease.
—Voltaire

THE JUICE FAST

"I was first introduced to juice fasting in 1975," states Elson Haas, M.D., Director of the Marin Clinic of Preventive Medicine and Health Education, "just after I completed my general medicine internship. At the time, I knew nothing about the relationship between nutrition and good health—as evidenced by my own health. I was 40 pounds overweight, had little energy, and suffered daily from terrible allergies.

"After attending a lecture on cleansing through fasting by natural health practitioner Stanley Burroughs, I decided to try a ten-day juice fast under his guidance. By the third day of the fast, I felt healthier. My head was clear, my energy level improved, and I was physically and mentally alert. At the end of the ten days, I felt even better. What's more, the fast inspired me to reconsider my diet. More conscious of how the food I ate affected my health, I began eating better. Within a year, I'd reached a healthy weight, my allergies had disappeared, and I looked younger and felt great. Now, I make a point of fasting every spring to allow my body to heal itself."

In addition to water fasting another type of fasting is the juice fast where fruit and vegetable juices are consumed along with water. This form of detoxification has proven to be highly effective.

In the observation of thousands of patients in clinics around the world, water fasting has proven to be one of the fastest methods of total detoxification and rejuvenation. Water fasting has been used successfully against numerous degenerative diseases as well as infectious illnesses.

A single fast is rarely enough to completely regain health. For some conditions it may take several extended fasts to rebuild health. Benign tumors, for instance, have reduced in size and even been removed. However, cancerous tumors have been harder to treat. Water fasts have halted growth and even reduced the size of malignant tumors, but have not always been successful at completely purging active growths from the body. This does not mean fasting methods are powerless to stop such conditions. Water fasting alone, for such conditions, may not be enough.

THE GRAPE CURE

In the 1920s, Johanna Brandt made a discovery that had a profound influence on fasting treatments. At this time, she was diagnosed with stomach cancer. X-rays clearly showed the cancerous growth overtaking her body. Nothing could be done to help her, and she resigned to the fact that death would soon follow. She was introduced to fasting by a little book called *The Fasting Cure* by the novelist Upton Sinclair. This book gave her new hope for relief from her suffering. She began fasting. Her battle lasted for several years. She would fast four, seven, ten days and even three weeks at a time drinking only water. All this fasting brought about a slight improvement, but not relief. The cancerous tumor persisted. She suffered violent attacks of vomiting and purging with excruciating pain which brought up half-digested blood. Doctors recommended an immediate operation as the only means of prolonging her life. She refused. She fasted another three weeks. It was then that she accidentally discovered a food that destroyed the growth and eliminated the poisons from her body.

She lived in an area in South Africa where there were many vineyards. Grapes were a common part of everyone's diet. After eating grapes exclusively for six weeks, her symptoms and the cancer were gone. X-rays which had clearly shown the cancer before, now showed no trace of the growth. Fasting alone had not been able to dissolve the cancerous mass. Grapes, she reasoned, contained elements that were able to penetrate the cancer, breakup the tissue, and purify the blood. She witnessed that, "abnormal growths, cancers, tumors, abscesses, and fibrous masses seem to be dissolved by the powerful chemical agent in the grape. Diseased tissues and fatty degenerations and every form of morbid matter are apparently broken up into minute particles and thrown into the bloodstream to be carried to the organs of excretion."

As a result of her miraculous healing, she began advocating the grape fast as a cure for cancer and traveled around the world with her message. She supervised many grape fasts which typically lasted one to two months and helped to bring many people to recovery. She was the first person to recognize that grape seeds and skins contained a group of vitamins that had substantial healing properties. The grape seed and skin, it was later discovered, contains bioflavonoids, including proanthocyanidin (also known by the brand name Pycnogenol) an antioxidant that is many times more powerful than Vitamins A or C in neutralizing harmful free radicals. As a result of Johanna Brandt's discovery, fasting clinics began experimenting with grape and other juices. The results have proved quite favorable.

BUT IS IT A FAST?

Purists have claimed that drinking juice is not a true fast. Normally, we think of fasting as refraining from all forms of nourishment, except water. Some people will add a little lemon and honey to the water. This adds a minute amount of nourishment to the fast, but for all practical purposes it is still a water fast. Some will use herbal teas. Again, this is still basically a water fast. Others will go a little farther by adding fruit juice. And still others will take it another step and add both fruit and vegetable juices. These latter two are called juice fasts. Strictly speaking, to fast means to refrain from all forms of nourishment, including juices. Technically, using juice might more appropriately be called a juice diet. However, the results of a juice fast are remarkably similar to water fasts, but with additional benefits. Whether you call it a juice diet or a juice fast makes little difference. What is important is that it works.

As a method of detoxification, the juice fast has shown to be just as good, if not better, than the water fast. In general, it is the preferred detoxification method by most natural health care professionals. The reason is that the juice supplies elements, like Johanna Brandt discovered, that break up and remove toxins and promote cellular rejuvenation better than water alone.

A juice fast has basically the same effect on your body as the water fast. You will get hunger pangs at first, your energy level will decrease somewhat, you will lose weight, toxins will be purged, but cellular growth and rejuvenation will continue. You will also experience depression and fatigue if you don't prepare yourself beforehand. Like the water fast, prepare for the juice fast by following the Natural Foods Diet for at least three weeks. This is not a requirement, you could start a juice fast at any time, but if you don't prepare you will experience withdrawal symptoms from the stimulating meats, sugars, and seasonings you've become accustomed to.

CONCENTRATED NUTRITION

One of the reasons why juicing has been beneficial is because the most nutritional part of the plant is separated from the indigestible fiber. It may take a dozen carrots to get a small glass of carrot juice. In this case, three glasses of carrot juice would be equivalent to eating about 36 carrots. So you consume most of the vitamin and mineral content of 36 carrots without the bulk and without expending energy trying to digest the fiber. (Who could eat 36 carrots a day anyway?) These liquid nutrients are readily digested and absorbed.

Juicing provides concentrated nutrients, including valuable antioxidants that prevent free-radical damage which is a major contributor to cellular degeneration. Free radicals are formed in the body during normal body process, and taken in by the air we breath and food and water we consume. Most people do not get near enough vitamins or minerals in their diet. Juicing produces a mineral and vitamin concentrate that has proven beneficial.

Each plant cell is encased in a tough fibrous shell known as the cell wall. It is the cell wall that gives plants their rigidity and makes up the bulk of the plant's fiber. The fluid part of the plant which is inside the cell provides most of the nutrients. If the cell walls are not broken, the nutrients will not be released. Stomach acids, digestive juices, and enzymes can't penetrate the cell wall, and this fibrous material passes through the intestinal tract intact without releasing its nutrients. The cells in plant foods must be broken in order to make their nutrients available to us. Chewing is essential for the release of the plant's nutrients. This is one reason why health experts tell us to thoroughly chew our food before swallowing. Juicing separates the nutrient-rich juice from the fiber. Without the bulk of the fiber, we are able to consume more of the juice and, consequently, get more vitamins, minerals, and other nutrients.

With a juice fast, even though you are taking nourishment, your normal dietary consumption is drastically reduced. Juice contains no bulk and is digested in a matter of minutes, putting little strain on the digestive organs. Of the three energy-producing nutrients (carbohydrate, protein, and fat), only carbohydrate is supplied in any appreciable quantity and even then the amount is very small. So the body still is able to rest and conserve energy, yet is given just enough carbohydrate to supply the energy it needs. Cleansing of toxins and removal of fat and dysfunctional tissue continue as it does with a water fast.

When no energy-yielding nutrients are consumed, as in a water fast, there is a general feeling of lethargy. Heavy physical activity is discouraged, for the body needs all its energy for detoxifying and healing. Consequently, normal activities like housework, job, school, etc. may be tiring.

The juice fast provides the body with enough nutrients to keep the energy level up close to normal. With juice, you are still able to carry on daily activities, go to work, and study without being hampered by excess fatigue. In fact, you can keep up an exercise program with a juice fast. Exercise is important because it stimulates blood and lymph circulation which removes toxins and distributes nutrients to the cells. Exercise is an important aspect of healthy living and you are encouraged to get some physical activity while fasting. Brisk walks provide an excellent form of exercise which is not too strenuous, yet stimulating.

The nutrients in the juice also give energy to the immune system which is doing the bulk of the job of detoxification. In addition to providing more energy, juice supplies vitamins and minerals that help all the bodily functions which, in turn, enhances cleansing and promotes cellular rejuvenation.

During a juice fast you are also encouraged to drink pure water. Your body needs the liquids to remove toxins. Like with a water fast, if you drink distilled or filtered water you may need to add a little sea salt to your liquid diet. The way to tell if your body is becoming minerally depleted is if the water you drink has an unusually bland or stale taste and doesn't seem to quench your thirst.

Keep in mind that juice fasting is only a temporary method of detoxification and is not supposed to be a long-term diet. Juices do not give you fiber which is necessary for healthy bowel function. For a few days or weeks, juicing can have great health benefits and the temporary decrease of fiber intake is well tolerated. But a prolonged diet devoid of fiber can lead to digestive problems. (See pages 147-149 for additional information regarding fiber.)

FRUIT AND VEGETABLE JUICES

Juices can be made from a variety of fruits and vegetables. You can drink the juice from a single source or mix them as you please. Fruits are considered the best detoxifiers and vegetables the best cellular rebuilders.

Use fresh juice rather than canned or frozen drinks. V-8 juice may taste great, but processing destroys many of the nutrients, and chemical or incidental additives are almost always present. Use clean, unadulterated produce free of pesticides, herbicides, mold, and other contaminants. The quality of the ingredients in prepared juices is also in question. When apples, for example, are sold, where do the big, unbruised, appetizing ones go? They end up in the

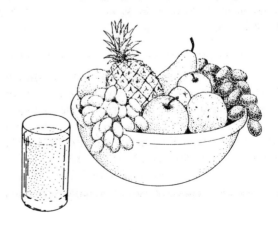

supermarket. What happens to all the small, underripe, overripe, bruised, and partly moldy ones? They get made into juice. Do they wash off the pesticides and dirt? Several incidents have occurred where people have gotten food poisoning from E. coli bacterium by drinking apple juice that was made from unwashed apples. E. coli is a bacteria that normally grows in the lower digestive tract of animals. It can cause food poisoning and even death when food contaminated with fecal matter is eaten raw or undercooked. It is not unusual for meat to be contaminated with E. coli since the organism is associated with animals. Occasionally it is found in unpasteurized juices. Processed juices are often made from fruits that are not produce quality and may have mold, pesticide residue, and even bird droppings. For these reasons, you should use only fresh, washed organic fruits and vegetables.

Vegetables which make the best juice include: cucumber, celery, lettuce, tomato, spinach, beets (including the tops), cabbage, carrot, bell pepper, parsley, potato, onion, garlic, kale, turnip greens, asparagus, Swiss chard, broccoli, brussels sprouts, cauliflower, dandelion greens, eggplant, kohlrabi, turnip and turnip greens, parsnips, zucchini, radish, watercress, and alfalfa sprouts.

The best fruits for juicing include: apple, peach, pear, pineapple, grapes, berries (all types), cherries, apricots, melons (all types), plums, oranges, lemons, grapefruit, and limes. Some fruits and vegetables don't juice well, like bananas and avocados. They just turn into mush and clog the juicer.

Vegetable juice can be consumed cool or hot. Although heating destroys some of the nutrients, hot vegetable juice makes a tasty broth and adds variety to a juice fast. Onion and garlic gives vegetable juices a soup-like flavor. Carrots add sweetness.

You can mix any of the vegetable juices together. You can mix any of the fruit juices together. But mixing fruit and vegetable juices does not generally produce the best flavors. Apples and carrots are the exceptions—they can be used in both fruit or vegetable juices. Carrots make a nice complement to fruit drinks and apples sweeten up vegetable juices.

> I am not the only doctor who realizes this, but I'll tell you, it's taken 65 years of sanitarium practice to confirm that when we replenish the chemical elements in a person through vegetable juices, fruit juices and through liquids and supplements, along with a balanced diet, good health is restored.
> —Bernard Jensen, D.C., Ph.D.

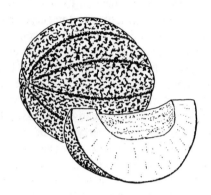

Make just enough juice for one serving. Never store fresh juice over 12 hours as it will begin to oxidize immediately and decompose, losing nutritional value. Many vegetables and fruits taste good without combining with other produce—apple juice, grape juice, carrot juice, etc. Combining juices adds some variety and fun to the drinks. Be creative. Some fruits produce very sweet juices and it is best to dilute them with distilled or filtered water. Pure carrot juice, for instance, is very sweet and should be diluted.

Green vegetables are rich in chlorophyll. Chlorophyll is the pigment which makes plants green and is considered the life-blood of the plant. Chemically it is almost identical to hemoglobin found in human blood. The basic difference is that the hemoglobin (which gives blood its red color) is built around an iron atom while chlorophyll is built around a magnesium atom. Because of its similarity to blood, chlorophyll is considered a natural remedy for blood-related disorders. It is also known to have a soothing, cleansing, healing influence on the bowel and the entire digestive tract.

Many health resorts such as Ann Wigmore's Hippocrates Health Institute serve their guests chlorophyll-rich drinks to help them overcome degenerative illnesses. Ann Wigmore made the use of raw wheat grass juice famous. She showed that the nutritional effects of fresh chlorophyll-rich juices are often accompanied by a powerful reversal of disease.

Juices have been used therapeutically for decades. In the 1930s H.E. Kirschner, M.D., demonstrated the effectiveness of raw chlorophyll drinks. He was in charge of 200 tuberculosis patients at the Olive View Sanitarium near Los Angeles. Each of his patients was give a green drink daily containing a variety of chlorophyll-rich vegetables along with a healthy diet. Many of the emaciated patients gained weight, improved digestion and bowel function, and showed an increase in hemoglobin. Patients considered hopeless were out of bed in six to eight months. Even cancer patients improved when put on a healthy diet which included a green drink. Wheat grass, barley grass, and alfalfa are all rich in chlorophyll. Juices made purely from these grasses have a strong disagreeable flavor. You may dilute them with distilled or filtered water. Combining grass juices with more mild green vegetables such as fresh parsley, mint, spinach, or celery or adding flavor with carrot, pineapple, or apple juice will make the drink more palatable.

There are special slow-grinding juicers called wheat grass juicers which press the juice from delicate wheat, barley, and other grasses. You can also juice grasses and other soft leafy green vegetables in ordinary juicers if you juice them together with hard vegetables. Wheat grass, barley grass, alfalfa, and other grasses can be purchased at health food stores and even some supermarkets. You can also grow your own by simply buying seeds and sprouting them. After they have sprouted, make sure to expose them to the sun so that they can manufacture the green chlorophyll. Juice the sprouts after they have grown a couple of inches and are a nice green color. Health food stores sell packages of seeds for sprouting complete with instructions on how to do it.

Vegetables in the cabbage family which include broccoli, brussels sprouts, kale, cauliflower, collard greens, and kohlrabi are known for their remarkable healing qualities. These vegetables are rich in antioxidants, vitamin C, calcium, potassium, sulfur, and other minerals. Juice from these vegetables accelerates healing, especially within the digestive tract. Dr. Garnett Cheny, clinical professor at the University of California, found that raw cabbage juice helps in the healing of stomach ulcers. He discovered that after his ulcer patients drank raw cabbage juice over a period of 4-5 days, most of their symptoms disappeared.

Vegetables in the cabbage family are also good in helping to overcome constipation, improve liver function, clear up skin problems, and destroy infectious organisms in the blood. Studies have found that people who eat more of these types of vegetables have lower colon and stomach cancers.

Juices must be made with a machine designed specifically for juicing. Blenders do not make juice. There is a big difference between juicers and blenders. Juicers extract the juice, separating the liquid from the bulk. Blenders chop the fiber into pulp and mix it with the juice. Blenders are good in their own right, but should not be used if you are going on a juice fast.

There are many good books on juicing which contain a wide variety of juice recipes. You really don't need recipes, just combine the fruits you like and the results will usually be satisfying. The following are a few sample recipes. You can adjust the ingredients to suit your taste and the amount of juice you want.

Vegetable Green Drink
3-4 cups consisting of two or three green vegetables (parsley, spinach, beet greens, watercress, broccoli, kale, chard, alfalfa sprouts, etc.)
4-6 carrots

Cabbage Power Drink
1-2 cups cabbage
1 kale leaf
4 carrots
1 cup pineapple (or 1 large apple)

Carrot-Celery Juice
6-8 carrots
2-4 stalks celery
6 sprigs parsley

Melon Cocktail
1 cup watermelon
1 cup cantaloupe
1 cup casaba
Other melons can also be added. Include the seeds and inside rind of the melons as they contain many nutrients.

Apple-Berry Delight
2 large apples
1 cup raspberries (or blackberries)

Carrot-Pineapple Delight
6-8 carrots
1-2 stalks celery
1 cup sliced pineapple

Vegetable Cocktail
3 tomatoes
1 stalk celery
2-3 sprigs of parsley
2 slices lemon
1/4 green pepper
1 slice onion
A dash of vegetable broth seasoning can be added if desired.

Vegetable Broth
3 carrots
3 celery stalks
1 small beet
1/8 small onion (or 3 scallions)
This drink can be consumed either hot or cold.

Spicy Broth
3 carrots
3 celery stalks
1 tomato
1/8 small onion (or 3 scallions)
jalapeno (to taste)
May also use a clove of garlic. Fresh garlic is hot so go lightly.

MONOFOOD DIET

In a monofood diet you eat only one type of food. The food, usually a fruit but may also be a vegetable, can be eaten in any form. It may be juiced, eaten whole, or dried (unsulfured). Usually, fruit of some type is used because they are good cleansers. Grapes are the most popular fruit used and are one of the most effective detoxifiers and cellular rejuvenators. Grapes can be eaten whole, juiced, or as raisins. Apples, watermelon, and carrots are other foods commonly eaten on a monofood diet. You can eat them juiced, fresh, or dried as you like throughout the fast so long as you eat only one kind of fruit. Johanna Brandt's grape diet was, in fact, a monofood diet. She believed that a diet of raw fruits and vegetables can correct abnormal conditions of the blood, but that the grape diet produces the quickest results.

This diet is sometimes called a juice fast or juice diet because juices are often the primary food consumed. Sometimes it is called a grape fast, or apple fast, etc. Although not a true fast, it still provides many of the benefits that water and juice fasts offer.

When eating only one type of food, your total food intake is greatly reduced. Thus your body must rely on stored reserves for a complete range of nutrients and for energy. As a result, you lose fat and weight, and toxins are drawn out of the tissues and discarded. Since you only eat healthy produce, you avoid most food contaminants (chemical additives, mold, waxes, solvents, etc.) that sneak into our everyday diets. You also get a healthy dose of vitamins and minerals, especially if you drink a lot of juice.

With a monofood diet, you experience much of the same detoxification reactions characteristic with water or juice fasting. The one major advantage with the monofood diet is that you can eat solid food. This allows your stomach and intestines to digest a small portion of food and continue normal processes. Even though this uses up energy that could go into detoxification, it keeps material flowing through the bowels and helps relieve feelings of hunger.

If you find fasting too difficult, a monofood diet can give similar health benefits without the severe hunger pangs. Try a monofood diet a couple of times. Then as your body becomes healthier and more accustomed to going without the foods you normally eat, try juice fasting.

On prolonged fasts some people find that they can handle a juice fast easier if they start it with a three-day monofood diet. The first three days are the hardest when you go on a fast. Eating a little fruit helps to relieve the hunger and satisfy the appetite.

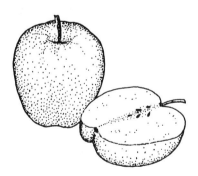

 ## ADDITIONAL RESOURCES

The Complete Book of Juicing. Murray, Michael, N.D. Rocklin CA: Prima Publishing, 1992.

Juicing for Good Health. Keane, Mauree B. New York: Pocket Books, 1992

Juicing for Life. Calborn, Cherie and Keane, Maureen B. Garden City Park, NY: Avery Publishing Group, 1992.

Juicing Therapy. Jensen, Bernard, Ph.D. Escondido, CA: Bernard Jensen, 1992.

Chapter 8

OXYGEN THERAPY

Oxygen, the great invisible food, stimulant and purifier, builds our resistance to infections and strengthens our weak points. It's Nature's most vital aid in helping the body to heal itself and to stay healthy.
— *Paul C. Bragg, Ph.D.*

NATURE'S MIRACLE CLEANSER

Imagine for a moment, a time in the distant future. After centuries of scientific medical advancements, a new powerful wonder drug is developed. This drug is like no other that has been available before. It is just as useful inside the body as out. It can be applied externally to kill disease-causing fungi, bacteria, and viruses—such as athlete's foot and ringworm—and to disinfect cuts and infections. It can be taken internally to destroy infectious organisms that cause such diseases as candidiasis, pneumonia, and AIDS. It can be used to purify drinking water, killing disease-causing organisms like *Guardia lamblia* and neutralizing chemicals such as chlorine, insecticides, and industrial solvents. Taken internally, it stimulates the immune system, encourages cell rejuvenation, and detoxification. Metabolism is invigorated and the body is cleansed of harmful toxins, removing arterial plaque, thus reversing cardiovascular disease, and killing cancer cells. It can be used for practically any and all forms of degenerative or infectious disease known to mankind. People suffering from arthritis, asthma, cancer and any number of other conditions could find relief.

Although this new wonder drug is a powerful disease killer and toxin neutralizer, it is completely harmless to healthy cells with no undesirable side effects. Unlike most drugs, it is inexpensive and safe enough that it is available to anyone without a prescription. This substance would make most other drugs obsolete. It would be hailed as the most important medical advancement of all time!

Such a drug, you may say, is impossible, especially within our lifetime. Not so! In fact, we already have it available today. What is this wonder drug? It is not really a drug, it is a natural substance freely available to all. That substance is oxygen. Yes, ordinary oxygen, the type you breathe every day.

Oxygen has more healing power than all drugs or therapies ever invented. It is nature's miracle cleanser. It gives life, blocks disease, and stimulates the growth of healthy cells. In fact, it is the lack of adequate oxygen that is the root cause of many diseases in nature.

Oxygen is the most widely distributed element in nature. It is a colorless, tasteless, odorless gas, constituting one-fifth of the atmosphere, eight-ninths of water, and about one-half of the crust of the earth. About 65 percent of the human body is composed of oxygen. Chemically it is very reactive, having the property of combining with almost all other elements (making it a good cleanser and detoxifier). Oxygen forms oxides by direct combination with nearly all other elements. It is this property that allows the body to use it to produce energy and

106

which destroys pathogenic organisms. It is utilized in essential chemical reactions in nature and in living organisms.

THE BREATH OF LIFE

Every living thing breathes. Fish remove oxygen from water through their gills. Insects, worms, and other invertebrates breathe through pores in their skin. Vertebrates, including humans, extract oxygen through their lungs. Plants, too, must breathe, exchanging gases through pores in their leaves. Plants, however, absorb carbon dioxide and give off oxygen while animals inhale oxygen and exhale carbon dioxide. The exchange of gases between plants and animals provides the balance in nature where both can thrive. Abundant clean, unpolluted oxygen is necessary for good health.

Oxygen is inhaled into the lungs where it diffuses into the bloodstream and is carried by arteries and capillaries to every cell in the body. Respiration, which is the exchange of gases in living organisms, must occur in every active, living cell if life is to be maintained. Every one of the 40 trillion cells in our bodies demands a continuous supply of life-giving oxygen in order to live. Hundreds, probably thousands of diverse chemical reactions are constantly proceeding in every active living cell. The sum total of these chemical changes are referred to as metabolism. Oxygen is the fuel each cell uses to power metabolism. Without oxygen, metabolism would be impossible. Without oxygen there would be no life! It is absolutely essential to life.

Oxygen is necessary in order to generate many processes within the body. It is necessary for regulation of tissue repair, cellular respiration, growth, immune functions, hormone synthesis, and the production of cytokines (chemical messengers that are involved in the regulation of almost every system in the body). So the body functions better when oxygen is readily available.

Of all the elements that the body needs, only oxygen is in such constant demand that its absence brings death in minutes. When oxygen is restricted, even in the smallest degree, disease and death result. The importance of oxygen to good health has long been recognized. It is used in many medical applications from treating periodontal disease to severe burns. Oxygen is so vital to good health that hospitals have it installed in patients' rooms. All rescue units, ambulances, and life support systems are equipped with it. Although oxygen can be used for numerous purposes, it has received little attention because pharmaceutical companies, the ones who manufacture our drugs and medical supplies, cannot make a significant profit from it. So oxygen therapies in medical use are generally limited to those requiring extensive medical training or expensive equipment such as hyperbaric chambers and oxygen tents. However, the healing and detoxifying power of oxygen is available to everyone at little expense.

When cells are deprived of oxygen, they weaken and die. Cells are continually dying and being replaced throughout the body. As long as cells can get adequate oxygen and other nutrients, they can continue to multiply and replace dead cells. But if circulation is chronically restricted to any particular organ, the cells die faster than they can be replaced and the entire organ begins to deteriorate and eventually malfunction. At times, when dead and degenerative cells and other toxins cannot be removed, they poison surrounding cells, causing them to mutate forming abnormal growths. Oxygen-starved tissues gradually deteriorate and die, often causing noticeable symptoms and increased susceptibility to infectious disease. These symptoms are typically blamed on aging or genetics.

The buildup of plaque in the arteries restricts the transport of oxygen through the body and is a major cause of circulation problems. Breathing polluted air and smoking not only cuts down on the amount of oxygen getting into the body but also adds dangerous toxins, putting even a greater strain on an oxygen-starved body. The lack of oxygen can lead to the development of numerous degenerative conditions, lower resistance to infection, as well as promote abnormal and potentially fatal growths. A lack of circulation in joint tissues may lead to arthritic-like pain. In the kidneys it may lead to kidney disease. In the heart it may cause heart disease.

The heart gets its oxygen from the coronary artery. If this artery becomes blocked, the cells of the heart begin to die. As plaque builds up, choking off oxygen, more and more cells die and the organ slowly deteriorates. The heart reaches a point where it cannot continue normal function and stops. This is a heart attack.

Strokes which can affect mental and physical ability are very similar. An artery feeding the brain becomes clogged, preventing the delivery of oxygen, which causes brain cells to die, producing a stroke.

Bed sores are yet another example of what happens when tissues and cells are deprived of life-sustaining oxygen. People who lie in one position for too long restrict circulation in certain areas of their bodies, thus depriving cells of oxygenated blood. These cells die and literally begin to decay. This forms a breeding ground for disease-causing microorganisms. This is what a bed sore is.

Any place in the body that is deprived of adequate oxygen will begin to deteriorate. Such places are prime collecting sites for metabolic waste, environmental toxins, and pathogenic organisms which further aggravate surrounding tissues leading to a number of degenerative conditions. This is one reason why disease-causing bacteria and other parasites are often found in degenerative tissues. In an oxygen-starved environment, normal cells can easily mutate and become cancerous. Cancer cells live in an oxygen-restricted environment deriving their nourishment from the fermentation of sugar rather than oxygen. These cells grow rapidly, but since they are mutated, do not function normally.

Oxygen is required for respiration by all organisms except for anaerobic organisms, which are the cause of many diseases in both humans and animals. Most disease-causing organisms reproduce with more vigor in the absence of oxygen or are able to survive and grow in living cells whose ability to ward off infection is weakened by a low-oxygen environment. Fungi (which include the yeast *Candida albicans*), viruses (which are neither plant nor animal and not even considered living organisms), and anaerobic bacteria (such as type A Streptococcus) flourish in an oxygen deprived environment.

One of the best, determinations of physiological age is the measurement of lung function called vital capacity (VC). This represents the amount of air that can be taken in and breathed out rapidly in one very deep breath. The vital capacity reflects the integrity of the entire respiratory system and the body's ability to absorb and distribute oxygen. Studies have shown that VC is the most significant single predictor of human life span. One notable ongoing study involving nearly the entire population of Framingham, Massachusetts, has clearly demonstrated this fact. The Framingham population has been closely monitored for over forty years, to see how obesity, cholesterol levels, diet, exercise, and other factors affect the incidence of degenerative disease and life span. Results have shown that individuals with a low VC (indicating poor oxygen delivery throughout the body) for their age do not live as long on average as people with high VCs (good oxygen delivery). The ability of the body to utilize oxygen has a direct impact on health.

As you can see, getting adequate amounts of oxygen plays a vital role in our health. People who get the oxygen they need age slower, have less illness, and experience fewer degenerative conditions than those who don't. Their physiological age, in essence, is much younger than their biological or actual age. A 75-year-old who is free from degenerative disease, mentally alert, and physically active is physiologically much younger than a 50-year-old who has numerous physical ailments, failing memory, and is wasting away.

OXYGEN DEPLETION

Some people have theorized that the reason degenerative diseases have increased so drastically over the past century is due to the decrease in oxygen in the atmosphere and the increase of pollution. It is no secret that the air we breathe is far more polluted now than it was a few decades ago. Industrialization has poured billions of tons of pollutants into the atmosphere, decreasing the amount of oxygen available to us. We are not even safe in our own homes. Harmful chemical residues continually disperse into the air from drapes, carpets, wood finishes, paint, and such for years. Polluted air displaces healing oxygen with harmful gases and chemicals. The body requires an increased amount of clean oxygen to neutralize and offset pollutants in the air. Yet, we are breathing in less clean oxygen.

The oxygen level in the atmosphere is slowly decreasing due, in part, from pollution and the destruction of forests, aquatic algae, and other plants which provide our oxygen. Scientists have analyzed air bubbles trapped in ice formed hundreds and even thousands of years ago and the bubbles in amber (i.e. fossilized tree resin) that are millions of years old. These tiny air bubbles provide samples of the earth's air at the time they were formed. The oxygen content of these ancient air pockets is much greater than it is now. According to the U.S. Geological Survey, 75 million years ago, when dinosaurs roamed the earth, the atmosphere contained 50 percent oxygen. Over time, the oxygen level dropped to 38 percent. Geologists attribute this to a decrease in volcanic activity which reduced the escape of oxygen from igneous rock (igneous rock consists of 464,000 parts per million of oxygen, some of which is released into the atmosphere when the rock is exposed to or comes near the earth's surface). Some paleontologists speculate that this 12 percent drop in oxygen was one of the factors which contributed to the extinction of the dinosaurs.

The earth's atmosphere contained 38 percent oxygen as recently as the mid 19th century. With the advent of the industrial revolution in the late 1800s which brought the burning of fossil fuels, industrial pollution, and eventually car exhaust, by the 1950's the percentage of oxygen in our atmosphere dropped to 21 percent. This is a drop of 17 percent in less than one hundred years! More than the 12 percent that occurred over the previous 75 million years. Although 21 percent is normally quoted as our current level, recent tests indicate that the oxygen level may now be at only 19 percent.

It has been suggested that one of the reasons why degenerative and infectious diseases have been steadily increasing over the past century is due to the decrease in oxygen. This may also explain why so many pathogenic microorganisms like HIV (AIDS virus), Epstein-Barr virus (chronic fatigue syndrome), Hanta virus, Type A Streptococcus (flesh-eating Strep), and others, which were previously unknown, are now becoming modern-day epidemics.

OXYGEN AND HEALTH

Increasing the amount of oxygen in our bodies can and does reverse degeneration, stimulate the immune system, and promote healing. Probably the most natural method of increasing the oxygen level in the body is through deep breathing exercises. By increasing the amount of air taken into the lungs we increase our oxygen consumption. Other ways to increase oxygen include exercise and heat therapy, both of which increases respiration and are discussed in more detail in following chapters. In medical settings oxygen masks, hyperbaric chambers, and other devices are routinely used. Oxygen, however, does not have to enter the body solely through the lungs. It can also be absorbed into the bloodsteam through our skin or through the mucous membranes in our digestive tract. This can be done using oxygen compounds such as ozone or hydrogen peroxide.

There are numerous different types of therapies utilizing oxygen in various forms to promote healing. Some are very simple and can be self-administered such as the use of hydrogen peroxide taken orally, through inhalation, rectally, vaginally, or by absorption through the skin. Other methods require qualified health care professionals where an oxygen solution is given by injection or where blood is drawn out of the patient, mixed with ozone or oxygen and recirculated back into the bloodsteam (autohemotherapy).

Although many people are unfamiliar with oxygen therapy, it is not new. Medical literature contains thousands of studies on the use of oxygen to treat illness. Doctors and scientists began treating diseases and other conditions with oxygen well over a hundred years ago. From 1880 to 1904 Charles Marchand, a chemist, published eighteen book editions on the oral ingestion and topical use of hydrogen peroxide, ozone, and glycerin to treat typhoid fever, cholera, gastric ulcer, asthma, bronchitis, catarrh, hay fever, whooping cough, and tuberculosis. A. L. Cortelyou of Marietta, Georgia, treated diphtheria with a peroxide nasal spray in 1898. Ozone was used successfully during World War I to combat battlefield infections.

In 1918 and 1919 the flu epidemic that swept around the world killed nearly 21 million people. In the *Lancet*, a prestigious British medical journal, the success of oxygen therapy was reported in combating this flu. In a hospital in India, 80 percent of the people were dying from influenzal pneumonia. Nothing worked. Knowing of the use of oxygen therapy during the war, Drs. T.H. Oliver and D.U. Murphay decided to use it as a last resort. They selected the hospital patient who was in the worst condition, one who had been delirious for two days and which they felt had no chance of recovery. They probably figured that if the treatment didn't work, or was even harmful, that he would die anyway. The patient was so delirious that he had to be tied down on his bed. They took two ounces of three percent hydrogen peroxide, mixed it in eight ounces of saline solution and injected him with it. The man recovered. In just six hours he was sitting up asking for food. They administered oxygen therapy to the other flu patients resulting in significantly reduced mortality rates.

As early as 1924, Frederick Koch, M.D., advocated oral hydrogen peroxide for the treatment of cancer. In the 1950s Dr. Reginal Holeman at the St. Thomas Laboratory in Cardiff, Wales, demonstrated the use of hydrogen peroxide in cancer treatment. He put hydrogen peroxide in the drinking water of cancerous mice. Within 60 days the tumors completely disappeared. Following the positive results with mice, four human subjects with very advanced inoperable tumors were then treated with oral administration of hydrogen peroxide. Two of them showed marked clinical improvement and a decrease in the size of their tumors.

Even in the 1950s, the use of oxygen to fight cancer was not new. Two-time winner of the Noble Prize, Dr. Otto Warburg, a biochemist and Director of the Max Planck Institute for Cell Physiology in Germany, demonstrated in 1931 that oxygen deficiency causes cancer. He showed that oxygen deficiency and cell formation are part of the cancer process. According to Dr. Warburg, when cells are deprived of 60 percent of their oxygen, they regress or mutate into "primitive" forms and enter into glucose reactions, deriving energy, not from oxygen, as normal cells do, but from the fermentation of sugar. This primitive mode of survival is thought to be the way organisms first existed on earth, before they began using oxygen. It is a much less efficient method, as the rapid reproduction of cancer cells uses up large amounts of glucose, breaking it down into lactic acid, a waste product, which puts a severe strain on the body. This also causes a distortion in the body's acid-base balance. As the acidity of the body rises, it becomes even more difficult for the cells to use oxygen normally. It has been shown that cancerous tumors contain as much as ten times more lactic acid than healthy tissues.

Dr. Warburg further demonstrated that cancerous cells will die when exposed to oxygen. Oxygen stops the fermentation process and normal oxygen respiration returns. He proposed that a lack of oxygen at the cellular level may be the prime cause of cancer, and that oxygen therapy could be an effective treatment for it.

Dr. Warburg said, "Cancer, above all other diseases, has countless secondary causes, but there is only one prime cause. Summary: the prime cause of cancer is the replacement of the normal oxygen respiration of body cells by an anaerobic cell respiration."

Because of Dr. Warburg's work, scientists now can control the development, rate of growth, and regression of cancerous cells. In laboratory experiments when scientists want cells to mutate, they reduce oxygen levels. To stop, they give them more oxygen.

Many pathogenic microorganisms also proliferate in an environment that has less oxygen and is slightly more acidic than normal body pH. When such a condition exists, disease-causing organisms grow abundantly. Friendly organisms such as acidophilus bacteria that inhabit the intestinal tract do not thrive in this type of environment and are overcome by the rapid growth of unfriendly bacteria, yeast, and other pathogenic organisms. Candida, a fungus, that is present in all of us to some extent, is kept in check by friendly organisms, the acid level in the internal environment, and the immune system. When the environment in the body changes, this organism reproduces faster and overcomes more friendly organisms and causes the condition known as candidiasis which produces numerous symptoms.

Oxygen therapy stimulates the immune system, helps neutralize toxins, and kills invading viral, fungal, parasitic, and bacterial organisms. It deactivates toxic substances. Oxygen stimulates cleansing and healing of human tissues and the growth of good microorganisms. Oxygen therapy has proven beneficial in cleansing toxins, killing infections, improving circulation, alleviating allergies, and treating cancer, multiple sclerosis, and numerous other degenerative conditions.

Oxygen therapy has been utilized in Europe for decades with great success. In North America it is still controversial and although used to some extent in hospitals and medical clinics, the self-administered forms of oxygen therapy (using hydrogen peroxide and ozone) are not yet fully accepted by the traditional medical establishment. The reasons for this are discussed later in this chapter.

FORMS OF OXYGEN

There are basically three forms of oxygen available to individuals that can be used for cleansing and healing. They are: free oxygen in the air (O_2), ozone (O_3), and hydrogen peroxide (H_2O_2).

Free Oxygen

Free oxygen is the oxygen in the air we breathe. It consists of two oxygen atoms. This is the form of oxygen that the body needs for respiration and metabolism. We can increase our oxygen intake by simply breathing clean fresh air and by practicing deep breathing exercises.

In Asian cultures the breath is the source of strength and energy. Holy men, yogis, martial artists, and others practice deep, slow breathing as a form of health enhancement, spiritual enlightenment, and mental stimulation. They believe that deep breathing increases the body's vital force or chi, as it is called in China.

Paul Bragg, one of the foremost authorities on natural health and longevity, traveled throughout the world studying cultures where people were particularly healthy. He met with the holy men of India who spent hours devoted to building physically and mentally powerful bodies as an instrument for high spiritual advancement. Some of these people are known to live 120 years or more. One holy man he met in the foothills of the Himalayan Mountains told him that he was, at that time, 126 years old. This man had no reason to lie, because his whole life was spent seeking truth and spiritual enlightenment. This holy man had perfect vision and a beautiful head of hair. He had all his teeth and the endurance and stamina of an athlete. He spoke five languages. Bragg stated that this holy man was one of the most amazing men that he had ever met. When asked to what he owed his great strength and mentality, he answered, "I have made a long life practice of breathing deeply and practicing faithfully all of my breathing meditations daily." Deep breathing exercise increases our vital capacity (VC) and brings more healing oxygen into our bodies.

The main drawback with breathing exercise is finding a place which is free from air pollution. Industrial exhaust and household fumes pollute the air both outside and inside. Unless you live in the country and have access to fresh clean air, the air you breathe is probably filthy. Breathing this type of air can actually make you sick. The only way to practice deep breathing in metropolitan areas is to use an ionizer or ozone generator to clear pollutants out of the air.

Ozone

Free oxygen gas is comprised of two atoms of oxygen (O_2). Ozone, another form of oxygen gas, contains three oxygen atoms (O_3) and is less stable. Ozone is a product of nature. It is formed in the upper atmosphere when ultraviolet light from the sun bombards oxygen (O_2) splitting it into two separate oxygen atoms. The single oxygen atoms are chemically highly reactive and quickly hooks onto other oxygen molecules forming O_3 (ozone).

Ozone forms a thick protective coat around the earth, shielding us from the damaging rays of ultraviolet light from the sun. It is necessary for our survival.

Because ozone is less stable than free oxygen, it readily reacts with other chemicals producing a normal O_2 molecule and one free oxygen atom. This atom oxidizes compounds it attaches to. If this substance is a chemical pollutant in the atmosphere or a bacteria or virus, the oxidative reaction will chemically render them harmless. For this reason ozone is often used as a disinfectant.

It is up to 5000 times more effective as a disinfectant than chlorine and, unlike chlorine, is nontoxic. Many cities in Europe and some in North America use ozone to disinfect their swimming pools and drinking water.

When taken into the body, ozone increases the oxygen content of the blood and tissues. For this reason, ozone therapy has been successfully used to oxygenate the body and bring about improvements in health.

Ozone is found in country air to a much greater extent than in cities and towns, and on mountain tops to a greater extent than in deep valleys. The reason for this is probably because ozone readily reacts with chemicals in the air and is consequently destroyed. In cities and near the surface of the earth where pollution and airborne debris is more concentrated, the ozone is depleted by chemical reaction.

It is a surprise to some people to learn that ozone is a beneficial gas and not a dangerous environmental pollutant as we are often told. Since ozone can be and is made artificially, it is often considered a pollutant and spoken of in the same context as industrial byproducts like sulfur dioxide or carbon monoxide which are very poisonous. Ozone is a natural form of oxygen gas, and to label it as a dangerous pollutant is ridiculous. Ozone can be generated in the air by certain types of electrical equipment and has a distinct chlorine-like smell. The smell has made people suspect it to be a harmful pollutant and some tests seem to indicate the possibility that it can be harmful. According to Ed McCabe, author of the book *Oxygen Therapies*, any adverse effects on health are attributed to contaminants such as nitrogen oxide (a deadly poison) that can be associated with it when generated by man. In the laboratory, nitrogen oxide is formed when ozone is electrically produced. Nitrogen oxide can then react with oxygen and water vapor to form nitrogen dioxide and nitric acid which are nasty pollutants. So, it's not the ozone that is dangerous, but the contaminants sometimes associated with it.

Opponents to the medical use of ozone, such as the FDA, claim that ozone irritates the mucosa of the lungs. They have studies which seem to indicate this, but they fail to recognize what happens when someone breathes ozone.

It starts to oxidize all the pollutants, tar, ash, chemical contaminants, microbes, and dead cells in the lung tissues, causing coughing and mucous discharge. This is the body's natural means of cleansing toxins out of the respiratory system and is not a disease in itself. Because the body is discharging oxidized toxins, the FDA says ozone is an irritant. However, it's the toxins that are the irritants, not the ozone.

Initial studies with ozone were performed on animals to observe the detrimental effects this "pollutant" would have on living cells. The results, interestingly enough, proved just the opposite. Instead of causing ill health, the ozone improved health. The test animals became healthier. Veterinarians have used oxygen therapy to treat animals for decades, so these results were nothing new to them.

Later, in order to create adverse symptoms in test animals, researchers began using extremely high levels of ozone. They actually created a form of oxygen poisoning. Anything, even oxygen, can be toxic at extremely high levels. Rats forced to breathe massive quantities of ozone developed bleeding in their lung tissue. This "proved" the danger of ozone in the atmosphere. But such levels are never encountered outside the laboratory. The idea that ozone is a dangerous gas is unfounded and inaccurate. The level of exposure you get in nature and even from ozone generators is well below any degree of potential hazard. Ozone is, in fact, one of the best things we can pump out into the environment, not just to help build up the ozone layer which shields us from harmful ultraviolet radiation, but to neutralize harmful pollutants that are continually dumped into our atmosphere.

Ozone is nature's natural disinfectant. It is produced by both sunlight and by lightning. You can faintly smell it in the air after an electrical storm. People with asthma, bronchitis, and other respiratory problems typically report a gradual decrease in symptoms after a thunderstorm.

Although ozone has received a bum rap, many researchers and health care providers are using it. Ozone kills disease-causing microorganisms and so is used to disinfect swimming pools, hot tubs, and drinking water. It is also used as a disinfectant during surgery and dentistry. It has been shown to be effective against most all viruses including HIV. Ozone is known to damage viruses which have a high amount of fat in their membranes. HIV membranes have a high fat content so it has been effective. Healthy cells are not damaged, they have antioxidant enzymes to break down ozone, viruses do not.

Ozonated water is used to treat periodontal disease, swallowed for treatment of gastric cancer, and applied as a wash in intestinal or bladder inflammation. Even cancer has been successfully treated by injecting an ozone solution directly into tumors. Material cost of using ozone is only a few cents. Ozone therapy has shown to be of benefit for these and numerous other health conditions in both animals and humans. It is widely used and practiced in Europe, but since the FDA has not approved it, its use in the United States is primarily limited to veterinary medicine.

Ozone generators that oxygenate water (such as in a swimming pool) or air (like an air filter) are available. Pool and spa suppliers would be the best source for ozone generators for use in water. Some of these companies produce household water purification systems that remove contaminants such as heavy metals as well as ozonate the water. To find a generator for the air, inquire at your local health food store, some carry ozone generators or know how you can get hold of one. Health oriented magazines also, occasionally, carry advertisements where you can order one. There are many different brands and styles. One of the best for home use is the Living Air purifier. If you have difficulty locating a source, write to The Family News, 9845 N.E. 2nd Ave., Miami Shores, Florida 33138. This health periodical routinely publishes information about oxygen therapy and ozone generators.

Hydrogen Peroxide

Hydrogen peroxide (H_2O_2) is water with an extra oxygen atom attached (H_2O+O). It is the most commonly used form of oxygen for therapeutic purposes. The reason for its popularity is because it is readily available, inexpensive, and very powerful.

Some people mistakenly assume it is poisonous, perhaps because the name sounds like a man-made chemical. Hydrogen peroxide is simply oxygenated water and is found naturally in lakes, streams, rainwater, and snow. It is also manufactured in our bodies. It is a product of nature and without it we could not exist.

We get hydrogen peroxide in the environment from ozone. Ozone formed in the upper atmosphere is heavier than oxygen and as a consequence migrates downward. As ozone intermingles with water vapor (clouds) it turns into hydrogen peroxide. If it is not destroyed by pollution in the atmosphere, hydrogen peroxide reaches the ground in rain and snow, oxygenating surface waters.

Plants do better with rain water than with well water or city water because there are trace amounts of hydrogen peroxide in it. Have you ever noticed how green and healthy your lawn looks after a heavy rain? Not only does the grass get water but it is gets natural hydrogen peroxide. The lawn doesn't look nearly as vibrant and healthy after watering from a sprinkler, which delivers water that is devoid of hydrogen peroxide. Even house plants flourish when a few drops of hydrogen peroxide are routinely added to watering. Oxygen is life-giving to both plants and animals. It is the way nature intended.

Hydrogen peroxide is a liquid at room temperature and looks just like water. Because it is less stable than water, hydrogen peroxide reacts chemically, becoming simply oxygen and water. So, it is completely nontoxic. Like ozone, it readily frees its extra oxygen atom initiating an oxidizing reaction which can neutralize harmful chemicals and destroy microorganisms. It is commonly used in many pharmaceutical preparations, mouthwashes, dentifrices (substances used to clean teeth) and as a topical disinfectant. It is widely used throughout the world for sterilizing soft drink and milk containers and is totally environmentally friendly.

Hydrogen peroxide can be self-administered topically, orally, rectally, or vaginally. Topically it is used as a disinfectant for cuts, open sores, and acne. It speeds the healing of wounds and burns, and it kills parasitic fungi. Used as a mouthwash, it can kill harmful bacteria that cause gum disease, plaque, and dental carries (cavities). Taken internally it has been effectively used to treat ulcers, atherosclerosis, vascular headaches, gangrene, strokes, allergies, asthma, lung infections, diabetes mellitus, candida, and viral infections. In fact, most any degenerative or infectious disease can be treated with hydrogen peroxide.

Atherosclerosis is a cause of high blood pressure, heart disease, stroke, memory loss, and many other health problems. Arthritis patients characteristically suffer severely from atherosclerosis, and their blood cholesterol levels tend to be higher than normal. There is evidence that the plaque which accumulates in the blood vessels prevents the normal transfer of oxygen to joint tissues. Joint tissues which are thus deprived of oxygen become inflamed and arthritic. Studies at Baylor University Medical Center have demonstrated that fatty deposits in arterial walls that lead to atherosclerosis are dissolved by hydrogen peroxide.

In testing natural spring waters, it was found that the water at Lourdes, France, which is famed for its healing properties, contains one of the highest concentrations of natural hydrogen peroxide.

Many people are skeptical about the uses of oxygen for so wide a variety of conditions. But oxygen acts as a cleanser. When toxins are neutralized and removed from the body by oxidative reactions, circulation improves and the body heals regardless of the symptoms that may have been present.

"I used to get the flu and colds constantly," says Ed McCabe author of the book *Oxygen Therapies*. "I started by ingesting a few drops of diluted 35 percent solution of food-grade hydrogen peroxide in juice two or three times a day. Ignoring the bleachy taste and uneasy feeling, I knew it was breaking down into water and oxygen in my system. I did this for four months. The first thing that happened was that my intestines emptied accumulated waste-matter heavily for three days. A few weeks went by as I slowly increased the dosage, and then I came down with a fever for two weeks. A week went by and then I started coughing and expectorating. This lasted for about two months."

After these healing crises McCabe notice a marked improvement in health. After initiating self-administered oxygen therapy, he said, "So far, I have not had a cold or flu in over two years . . . I haven't had to go to a chiropractor in two years. Before, my old spine, neck, and pelvic conditions were increasingly going out and requiring constant treatment. These increasingly frequent and painful events were probably due to the aging process of arthritic spurs growing on my joints. I saw them on x-rays. I don't know exactly why this is, but I assume metabolic waste toxins and microbes in my joints are being oxidized and eliminated, and my connective tissues are regaining flexibility. Any microbes that were living in my cells and creating waste product buildup, are also being oxidized and eliminated. I also have fewer and lesser allergic reactions now, my hay fever has stopped, and my normal ear wax has increased, after being dried up for years."

Walter Grotz, one of the pioneers of self-administered hydrogen peroxide therapy, published the ECHO Newsletter for several years. His newsletter contained many testimonials on the use of hydrogen peroxide. For instance, a lady from Alaska wrote that she started taking hydrogen peroxide for her asthma, but after taking it three times a day for a month, her hemorrhoids disappeared and her eyesight and complexion also improved. She now takes 23 drops a day and notices that this is detoxifying her considerably.

A man from Arizona wrote that he suffered with asthma and emphysema for several years and was always under medication. He was introduced to 35 percent food grade hydrogen peroxide after being released from the hospital as an emergency asthma case. He started taking three drops three times a day and followed through to 25 drops three times a day. He is now on 15 drops per week. "I'm going on my fourth month and I must say, it's a new life for me. I'm feeling so good I just had to write and thank you." He wrote again later to say he is very happy with his program, over six months now and he hasn't had to take any kind of medication.

A woman from Illinois said that her son developed a severe case of folliculitis (inflammation of the hair follicles) over his buttocks and down his legs. It was caused from wearing skin tight jeans. She spent $50 on a dermatologist visit, plus another $60 on a prescription salve. The condition took three weeks to clear up. After learning about hydrogen peroxide and buying some food grade, her daughter developed a severe case of folliculitis from shaving her legs with a dull razor. She mixed up a three percent solution of hydrogen peroxide, and applied it with a cotton ball, and it cleared up in three days.

Another man says that at first he was skeptical about using hydrogen peroxide, but decided to try it on his pet collie who had arthritis. The vet said nothing could be done to improve her health; they could only give a prescription to ease the pain. Within a week after using hydrogen peroxide, she was showing signs of recovery and began to be more active. After about a month, the arthritis disappeared completely.

This amazed him, so he added it to his own drinking water and within a month's time the arthritis in his right foot went away. The same arthritis he had for over 15 years due to an auto accident that left him with a hairline fracture and calcium build-up around the bone.

He also wrote that he had hemorrhoids which plagued him for four years, off and on, and they were partially controlled by larger than normal amounts of prune juice. After a month of being on 10 drops of 35 percent food grade hydrogen peroxide, three times a day, the problem disappeared and has been gone since.

His son's allergies flared up one day so he doubled his hydrogen peroxide solution and the next day it was gone except for some nasal congestion. He then mixed one drop of 35 percent hydrogen peroxide with five ounces of distilled water for him and he used it as a nasal spray. It worked great and there were no side effects.

"I firmly believe we are on our way to being a happy and healthy family," he says. "My wife and I are not doctors, but we don't need to have a doctor's degree to tell us we feel great."

Hydrogen peroxide is available in different strengths and purity. Pure hydrogen peroxide, like pure oxygen, is extremely flammable; in fact, a solution consisting of 90 percent hydrogen peroxide and 10 percent water is used as rocket fuel. The hydrogen peroxide available in stores is always diluted with water. The most common type found is typically sold in drug stores. It is nearly 97 percent water and only three percent hydrogen peroxide. At this strength it is completely safe and can even be taken orally, yet still strong enough to kill germs on contact. You can tell when it is reacting chemically with germs or toxins because it will bubble and foam. The cost is only about $2 a quart. This type, however, is *not* recommended. The reason is because it contains chemical stabilizers.

Different strengths are available for different uses—

six percent, 30 percent, 35 percent, etc. Most contain stabilizers. The only type you should use is 17 or 35 percent *food grade* hydrogen peroxide. A solution of 35 percent hydrogen peroxide contains 65 percent water—without any additives. Diluted it can be safely taken internally. Never use 35 percent hydrogen peroxide without diluting it first. It is much too strong. If you spill some on your fingers it will temporarily turn them white and produce a burning sensation. If you get some on your hand, quickly rinse it under running water. Before using 35 percent solution you should dilute it to three percent or less. At this concentration there is no harm in contact with skin, including sensitive mucous membranes of mouth, throat, and nose.

To dilute 35 percent solution to three percent, mix 11 parts distilled water with one part hydrogen peroxide. For example, to get 12 ounces of three percent solution, mix 11 ounces of water with one ounce of food grade hydrogen peroxide. Always use distilled water. Tap water contains contaminants that will partially use up and decrease the strength of the final solution.

Use these measurements as a guide for mixing up a three percent solution:

1 oz = $\frac{1}{8}$ cup
2 oz = $\frac{1}{4}$ cup
4 oz = $\frac{1}{2}$ cup
8 oz = 1 cup
32 oz = 4 cups = 1 quart

A convenient amount of solution to keep on hand is three cups (24 oz). This can be kept in a quart-sized container with room to spare. In an empty container, mix $2\frac{3}{4}$ cups (22 oz) of distilled water with $\frac{1}{4}$ cup (2 oz) 35 percent food grade solution. Hydrogen peroxide does not need to be refrigerated, but keep it in a cool place away from sunlight. If you use it every day as a mouthwash, it will last a month or so. If kept too long, however, it may lose some potency.

OXYGEN DELIVERY

Basically, there are three ways to get oxygen into the body—(1) through the lungs, (2) through the skin, and (3) through the mucous membranes of the digestive tract. Other means which require professional assistance, are also available, such as by injection, but they are beyond the scope of this book.

Oxygen Delivery: Lungs

The lungs are the primary system of oxygen delivery to the body. Increasing the amount of oxygen in the air we breathe is perhaps the most obvious way to accomplish this. The oldest and simplest method in which to do this is with deep breathing exercises.

There is a system of breathing the Asian masters have perfected that not only increases oxygen delivery, but stimulates and exercises the internal organs. It is a form of internal exercise and is basic to all Oriental forms of physical exercise and meditation.

You can do this while standing, sitting, or lying flat on your back. Since it involves using muscles in the chest and abdomen, you should do it on an empty stomach, either before meals or at least two hours after.

Begin by lying on your back, arms to your sides, eyes closed. Now, exhale slowly and at the same time tighten the abdominal muscles slightly to form a depression below your ribcage. This forces air from the bottom of the lungs up and out. Most people breathe too shallowly, using only the top portion of their lungs, thus not bringing in as much air as they should (decreasing vital capacity). This exercise will help circulate air throughout the entire length of the lungs increasing oxygen-carbon dioxide exchange and increasing your vital capacity. The abdominal movements will also exercise and stimulate circulation of internal organs and improve digestion.

Continue to exhale until all air is out and the abdomen is tight. Don't tighten the abdominal muscles to the point of straining, just enough so the muscles are slightly firm and air is expelled. While doing this, imagine that every bit of air is leaving the lungs.

After you exhale completely, stop momentarily, relax your abdominal muscles and begin to inhale slowly. As you inhale, extend the abdomen outward so that it swells up like a balloon. This will pull the incoming air into the bottom of the lungs. Try not to allow the chest to expand until the abdomen is fully extended; you want to use only the muscles in the lower abdomen while doing this.

It is not necessary to force either the inhale or the exhale. With continued practice, you will be able to extend and empty the abdomen quite easily while breathing very slowly. Try to center your entire concentration on the area surrounding the navel and imagine that you are only using the lower part of your lungs to breathe.

You should breathe through the nose. Nature has designed our air passageways with several functions. Besides serving as channels for air transfer, they also clean and regulate temperature. The hairs in the nose and moist mucus lining filter out dust and other debris. The sinuses warm or cool the air, as needed, before it enters the lungs.

In normal breathing you should inhale and exhale through the nose. During vigorous physical exertion, the mouth can act as a secondary air entrance to get greater amounts of oxygen in a shorter amount of time. But breathing exercises do not use up body oxygen so quickly as to require air to be quickly pumped in and out of the lungs. So when you are doing deep breathing exercises, breathe naturally—through the nose. This will keep the air that enters as clean as possible and the temperature suitable. You may, if you like, open the mouth slightly when exhaling, and this is frequently done, but keep the mouth closed when inhaling.

One complete exhale followed by an inhale comprises one round of breathing. Continue in this fashion for several minutes. Do not strain your abdominal muscles; use them to aid in the breathing without overtaxing them. This breathing exercise will stimulate and energize you. It is good to do in the morning before starting the day.

You can do this breathing exercise while sitting. Sit comfortably in a chair with your back gently against the back of the chair and both feet flat on the floor, legs uncrossed. The breathing motions are exactly the same as when lying down. Use the abdominal muscles to fill and empty the lungs entirely. In the sitting position you can practice deep breathing exercises at work without being conspicuous. It helps to oxygenate the brain and stimulate circulation, providing a boost of refreshing energy during the middle of the day.

Deep breathing exercise is not the only way to increase oxygen delivery to the lungs. You can attend to your normal activities and still increase your oxygen intake by breathing oxygenated air from an ozone generator. The added advantage of a generator is that ozone also detoxifies the air. A drawback to deep breathing exercises is that the air you breathe may be polluted and you could do yourself harm inhaling these toxins. Using an ozone generator to remove toxins and oxygenate the air is the best way to breathe clean, oxygen-rich air.

Another way to get a concentration of oxygen is by using a solution of oxygenated water. You can put it in an empty nasal spray bottle, vaporizer, or humidifier. This is particularly useful in combating sinus infections and allergies. Using a vaporizer every night will help those with emphysema, lung cancer, and other respiratory problems. Put one-eighth cup (1 oz) of 35 percent hydrogen peroxide solution per gallon of water in the vaporizer. Or mix 1 pint of three percent hydrogen peroxide to one gallon of water.

Ozone generators look much like ordinary portable air filters. You can set them on the floor or desk, turn them on, and have a room or whole house flowing with clean, oxygenated air. With one of these devices, the quality of the air in your house can be far superior to the mixture of gases often found outside.

Exercising in an environment with polluted air can be dangerous to your health. Running along side of a busy street is a poor idea. During exercise the body demands more oxygen, and respiration increases accordingly. When we breathe air contaminated with carbon monoxide, we not only starve the body from getting the amount of oxygen it needs, but we poison the system, killing vital cells throughout the body including those in the brain, heart, and lungs. People who run, or even walk alongside busy streets are inhaling dangerous amounts of carbon monoxide and may be doing themselves more harm than good.

If polluted air is a problem in your area, a portable ozone generator can provide you with fresh clean oxygenated air. Set it up at home and exercise in the same room. There are many excellent forms of exercise you can do within the confines of your own home. Work out while listening to an aerobics tape or use a stationary bicycle, a Nordic Trac, or other exercise equipment. Rebound exercise can take the place of jogging or running and provide much better results (see Chapter 9).

Take the generator to work and set it up in your office. This is particularly advantageous in a work environment where coworkers smoke or where you may be exposed to other air pollutants. Besides providing oxygen for your body, ozone produced by these generators will also neutralize toxins in the air. Poisonous fumes, such as formaldehyde, slowly released by carpets, drapes, paint, varnish, etc. which are a part of all homes and offices, are rendered harmless when in contact with ozone. Thus, the harmful effects of these deadly, yet invisible, gases are neutralized. If you are in a room with someone who is coughing or sneezing due to a cold or flu, ozone will kill the germs before they can infect you. There are no adverse side effects from breathing ozonated air.

Pulmonary (lungs and associated organs) problems like hay fever, asthma, bronchitis, tuberculosis, smokers lungs, etc. decrease the lung's ability to absorb oxygen. This, in turn, lowers the body's oxygen content and hampers the immune system, decreasing cleansing and allowing anaerobic pathogens and cancerous cells to grow with little restriction.

Oxygen therapies oxygenate the body and clean out the lungs and bronchial tubes. Coughing, sneezing, and sinus drainage are natural functions the body uses to clean the respiratory system. During a cleansing reaction, coughing may be intense, sinus drainage may be copious, and mucus thick. Bacteria, dead cells, and environmental toxins (such as tar from tobacco smoke) that have been trapped in the lungs for years may be dislodged and expelled. But once the offending material has been removed, breathing is more efficient, and vital capacity (VC) is increased. Utilization of oxygen by your respiratory system improves. Not only do breathing problems subside, but the whole body gets more oxygen so other seemingly unrelated symptoms improve. Infections decrease, as do diarrhea; arthritis; wound healing; and energy levels increase; the mind is clearer and memory better; blood pressure drops; blood fat decreases; asthmatic attacks stop; allergies disappear; ulcers clear up; and back pain subsides.

Oxygen Delivery: Skin

Normally we think of the lungs as the only way by which we get oxygen, but the skin also is a living, breathing organ. Through its 96 million pores, oxygen is absorbed into our tissues. For this reason, the skin is sometimes referred to as our third lung.

Oxygen can be increased in our bodies by means of bathing in a tub of oxygenated water. You can oxygenate water with either ozone or hydrogen peroxide. If you use ozone you need an ozone generator. When ozone is produced in water it converts to hydrogen peroxide. So you can get the same results by mixing a hydrogen peroxide solution in the water. If you have a swimming pool or hot tub, it is cheaper to buy an ozone generator than to use hydrogen peroxide. For a smaller volume of water used in a bath tub, hydrogen peroxide is more convenient.

For detoxification of the body, put 1 1/2 cups (12 oz) of 35 percent food grade hydrogen peroxide in your bath water and soak in it for 30 minutes. Or use about 2 quarts three percent hydrogen peroxide to a tub of warm water. Because hydrogen peroxide is so soluble, oxygen is absorbed by your body tissues. Absorption is enhanced by the water temperature. Hot water dilates pores and blood vessels facilitating oxygen absorption. Keep the water as hot as you can comfortably stand by adding more hot water as necessary. This treatment can energize your body, and some people claim it keeps them from sleeping for a couple of hours after taking the bath. You may not want to do this too soon before going to bed.

Some people express concern because tap water often contains chlorine and other chemicals which may also be absorbed by the body. To prevent this, some people use filtered bath water. This isn't really necessary. The hydrogen peroxide in the water will neutralize chlorine and other chemicals.

If you like, you can enhance the oxygen absorbed into your body by doing deep breathing exercises while you soak. Don't overdue this. Ten minutes or less is usually enough, then just soak the rest of the time. If you become light-headed you're getting too much oxygen. Breathing normally again should clear your mind.

For a foot problem, such as athlete's foot, you could soak the feet in a small tub of water containing hydrogen peroxide. Feet can be soaked for 15-30 minutes every day until the condition is improved.

A three percent hydrogen peroxide solution can be applied topically to disinfect skin or treat eczema, acne, fungal infections, skin ulcers, eczema, etc. But keep it out of direct contact with the eyes. Commercial ointments or gels are also available that combine healing qualities of hydrogen peroxide and other substances such as aloe vera.

External use of oxygen therapy is effective not only for skin problems and wounds but internal symptoms as well. Oxygen is absorbed into the bloodstream and circulates throughout the body. Arthritis is effectively treated this way. "I have seen an arthritic knee, locked up tight," says Dr. Kurt Donsbach, "get approximately 80 percent motion in less than two weeks after external use of hydrogen peroxide."

Oxygen Delivery: Mucous Membranes

The third way to get oxygen into your system is by taking it internally where it is absorbed through the mucous membranes. Taken this way, the oxygen starts from the inside of the body and filters out, just the opposite of oxygenated baths. It has an added benefit in that it can come directly in contact with disease-causing organisms in the digestive tract. A healthy digestive tract is vital to our overall health. If the environment there is overrun with pathogenic organisms and putrefying toxins, the body can suffer from any number of symptoms. Taken internally, hydrogen peroxide is an effective gastrointestinal cleanser.

Orally administered hydrogen peroxide will clean the upper digestive tract (stomach and small intestine) and be absorbed into the blood. Applied rectally, during an enema, it will clean the lower digestive tract (colon), which is the most disease-prone segment of the entire body. In the colon it kills harmful anaerobic bacteria that thrive in an oxygen-starved environment, but will not harm the beneficial aerobic bacteria such as acidophilus that require oxygen. Applied vaginally, in a douche, it can clean out yeast and bacterial infections.

You can use a three percent solution as a daily mouthwash and breath freshener. It kills bacteria that cause cavities and gum disease. Dentists often comment to those using hydrogen peroxide how clean and healthy their patients' teeth and gums are. Hydrogen peroxide is a secret to making teeth whiter.

As a mouthwash, take half a mouthful and swish for about five minutes, then spit it out. Do not use too much because as it kills germs in the mouth, it becomes foamy and expands. Leave enough room in your mouth for the expansion.

When taking it orally you do not need to worry about mixing any particular solution strength. You are only concerned with the total amount of hydrogen peroxide that is ingested and not with the solution strength. This means that, so long as you get a certain amount of hydrogen peroxide, it doesn't matter much how dilute the solution is. So you do not need to prepare a mixture in advance like you would for a topical application or a mouthwash. All you do is add a few drops of 35 percent solution to a glass of distilled water. The size of the glass is inconsequential. It is the number of drops of 35 percent solution that is important. So go according to drops rather than worrying about percentages.

Tolerance levels vary from person to person, and taking too much can cause nausea and unpleasant cleansing reactions. Start slowly as the body is not accustomed to so much oxygen. As your body gets used to it, you can gradually increase the dose. The amount normally taken varies from 2-30 drops, 1-3 times a day. For some, a few drops per glass is all they can tolerate; others can handle 30 drops. Twenty-five drops in 8-12 ounces of water is substantial.

You don't need to purge the toxins out of your system all at once. Oxygen is a powerful cleanser. Give it time to clean out the system and prevent too drastic a cleansing reaction. Normally, you will start off with low concentrations, gradually building up to a maximum as you purge toxins, then taper off to a maintenance dosage.

Drink the mixture on an empty stomach (to avoid nausea). Take it at least two hours after eating or 30 minutes before. A few drops in a glass of water is pretty much tasteless, but when you start adding several more drops, the hydrogen peroxide solution takes on a somewhat bleachy taste. This does not bother some, but others can't stand it. About 12 to 16 drops of 35 percent solution in eight ounces of water is the level at which most people detect an unpleasant taste.

Hydrogen peroxide shouldn't be combined with most types of juice because certain compounds in the drink, such as beta-carotene, react with the hydrogen peroxide, releasing oxygen before it has a chance of getting into your system. Adding aloe vera juice has been suggested as a way to maintain potency and make it a little more palatable. Putting hydrogen peroxide in five ounces of fresh watermelon juice has also been suggested as another way to mask the taste.

In 1985, Dr. Kurt Donsbach began to test various oral hydrogen peroxide formulations to make the taste of hydrogen peroxide more palatable for patients at his hospital in Mexico. Dr. Donsbach also adopted the IV use of hydrogen peroxide and uses both oral and IV extensively at his clinic. Dr. Donsbach developed a product he calls Superoxy Plus. It comes in five different flavors: lemon lime, herbal tea, cherry berry, orange, and plain. It's made with a special blending process that inhibits aftertaste. It's good enough that you can take it by the spoonful rather than mixing it with water. Each tablespoon contains the equivalent of about 12 drops of 35 percent food grade hydrogen peroxide. He suggests taking one ounce (two tablespoons) of his solution morning and evening. This is the equivalent of 48 drops per day, of 35 percent hydrogen peroxide. A few other companies also have hydrogen peroxide solutions available that do not have the bleachy aftertaste. You should be able to find food grade hydrogen peroxide or one of these preparations at your local health food store.

To start off, you can use two drops of 35 percent hydrogen peroxide solution in a glass of distilled water three times a day. Good times are a half hour before breakfast, lunch, or dinner, and just before going to bed at night. Increase this amount by two drops for each serving every day until you reach about 20 drops per glass *or* as much as your taste can tolerate.

Twenty drops taken three times makes a total of 60 drops a day. If 20 or more drops in a glass of water is too much for you to handle (tastewise), cut down on the number of drops you use but increase the number of glasses you drink. So, instead of taking 20 drops three times a day, take 15 drops four times a day. Either way, you still get a total of 60 drops.

Maintain your maximum dose for at least a week. You can then back off on the amount until you are at a comfortable level. Then stay at that level until you get the results you are looking for. One thing to remember is that persistence pays off. For chronic conditions you can stay on 20 drops three times a day as long as you think it is necessary.

The suggested program is as follows:

• 2 drops 3 times a day on 1st day
• 4 drops 3 times a day on 2nd day
• 6 drops 3 times a day on 3rd day
• 8 drops 3 times a day on 4th day
• 10 drops 3 times a day on 5th day
• 12 drops 3 times a day on 6th day
• 14 drops 3 times a day on 7th day
• Continue to add two drops a day until you reach 20 drops or as much as you can stand.
• Remain at 20 drops 3 times a day for 7 days.

Finally, back off to a comfortable level, adjusting the dosage and frequency to suit your tolerance level.

Dr. Donsbach recommends working up to a dosage of 25 drops of 35 percent food grade hydrogen peroxide twice a day (a total of 50 drops). However, many people do very well on 10 or 15 drops 2-3 times a day. Dr. Donsbach says that he only goes higher for his active cancer patients, maintaining them on 75 drops, twice a day.

In an enema or colonic, oxygen breaks up impactions and kills harmful fungi and bacteria, without destroying the good bacteria. Use one drop of pure 35 percent food grade hydrogen peroxide for every six ounces of water. That's pretty dilute, far less than the three percent used as a disinfectant and mouthwash. See Chapter 11 for specific information regarding colon cleansing.

For a douche, add 6 tablespoons of three percent solution to a quart of warm distilled water.

PRECAUTIONS

Although oxygen is natural and the body requires it to live, too much can be detrimental. There is little to worry about in getting too much oxygen from breathing exercises or ozone generators. But there is a possibility of using too much hydrogen peroxide. Strong solutions can be irritating to living tissue, so caution should be taken. As mentioned before, a 35 percent solution of hydrogen peroxide can burn the skin if not diluted. In an enema, if too strong a dose is used it may cause inflammation. Consuming too much will also have adverse reactions. Basically, problems only occur with the use of too much or too strong of a concentration. At the levels described in this book, hydrogen peroxide is completely safe.

Oral use of hydrogen peroxide has been documented since at least 1884. There are, however, a few side effects with hydrogen peroxide therapy even at low levels. Since it bubbles when it reacts, taken orally it will create some bubbling in the stomach. If too much is taken, this could cause nausea and even vomiting. You can avoid this reaction by starting off with small doses and gradually building up. This way the stomach has time to get used to it. Making sure to take it on an empty stomach will also help.

Since hydrogen peroxide is a clear liquid, it can be mistaken for water. So keep concentrated solutions (especially those over three percent) out of the reach of children. Never transfer the concentrated solution into an unlabeled or improperly labeled container.

If concentrated hydrogen peroxide is accidentally ingested, drink large amounts of water to dilute. Stay upright and contact your doctor.

If you spill the solution, flush the spill area with water. Do not return spilled material to the container.

Many people have criticized oxygen therapies as dangerous because treatment is often followed by cleansing reactions. Those people who do not understand the healing process or the healing crisis see symptoms of healing as signs of distress or illness. Consequently, they label oxygen therapy as dangerous or questionable. The worst "side effect" you may experience is a cleansing crisis as your body removes toxins.

Hydrogen peroxide is just a water molecule with an extra oxygen atom attached. When the H_2O_2 comes in contact with harmful microorganisms and toxins, it liberates the singlet oxygen (O_1) killing the germs and neutralizing toxins by oxidation. White blood cells scurry around gathering up this debris, dumping it into the body's channels of elimination. This increase in activity and elimination creates the symptoms of a healing crisis. Therefore, you may experience skin eruptions, nausea, sleepiness, fatigue, diarrhea, nasal discharge, and the like.

Symptoms of cleansing can be made manifest in many ways. One woman, after starting oxygen therapy, suddenly developed severe bleeding in her nose and eliminated two large blood clots from her right nostril. When the crisis was over, she reported that she could breathe through the nostril for the first time in years! Another person had bleeding from the mouth and spit up huge amounts of mucus. Another had rectal bleeding as his hemorrhoids were reduced. These are signs of natural cleansing and although they may cause discomfort, they will be of short duration. After the toxins are removed, the body will be healthier and more vital.

Perhaps the biggest criticism to oxygen therapy is in regard to free-radical generation. Free radicals are highly reactive atoms or molecules that quickly pull electrons from surrounding molecules. When the molecule loses its outer electron, it too becomes a free radical and attacks another nearby molecule, creating a chain reaction that may affect hundreds and perhaps thousands of molecules. The problem here is that once an electron is removed from the molecule, its electrical charge is changed which affects its chemical properties. Thus the normal function of the molecule is disrupted. This can cause death, destruction, and even mutation to living cells. Singlet oxygen (O_1) and especially the hydroxyl ion (OH) can function as powerful free radicals. Free-radical damage has been linked to numerous degenerative diseases. Antioxidants are substances that stop the free-radical chain reaction. They are often sold as food supplements. Their use has brought about significant improvements in health in some people.

Critics to oxygen therapy say ozone and hydrogen peroxide generate free radicals and therefore are dangerous. Free radicals are a necessary part of life and you can never be free from them. Every breath of air we take creates free radicals (especially if the air is polluted or the person is exposed to tobacco smoke). Normal metabolic processes in our cells create free radicals. Chemical reactions with the food we eat (particularly from food additives and chemical contaminates) create free radicals. Some nutrients in our foods such as vitamin C, vitamin E, and beta-carotene function as antioxidants and stop free-radical chain reactions. This is one reason why we should eat plenty of grains, fruits, and vegetables which are our primary sources of natural antioxidants.

The body also manufactures its own antioxidants such as catalase, superoxide dismutase (SOD), co-enzyme Q10, glutathione reductase, and others. If the body is given adequate nourishment and if exposure to environmental toxins is minimized, it can manufacture all the antioxidants it needs. People who eat a poor-quality diet and live in polluted cities develop conditions that are aggravated and maybe even initiated by free-radical reactions.

So what about oxygen therapy, is it dangerous? Will it cause even more free-radical damage? If oxygen therapy did cause serious free-radical damage, it would not be used. Both traditional and alternative health care practitioners use it. Oxygen therapy has been successfully used to treat numerous health conditions. It has proven to be beneficial. If it caused massive free-radical damage, you would expect these conditions to get worse, not better!

When hydrogen peroxide is absorbed into the bloodstream, it is broken down into water and singlet oxygen. The free electron of the singlet oxygen either combines with a free electron of a molecule, such as in a cancer cell, or with the free electron of another singlet oxygen, becoming O2, the form necessary for respiration.

When singlet oxygen, from a source such as hydrogen peroxide, comes into direct contact with tissue cells outside of the circulatory system such as in a cell culture or test tube, the cells die. This is viewed by some as evidence that oxygen therapies are harmful. However, in *living organisms*, free-radical damage does not occur.

The reason ozone and hydrogen peroxide do not pose a threat via free radical formation is that these substances are natural to the environment and to our bodies. Hydrogen peroxide is, in fact, manufactured by many of our own cells. Neurophils, for example, are one type of white blood cell. They attack foreign substances in our bodies by squirting them with hydrogen peroxide. Whether it be an invading microorganism, chemical toxin, or renegade cell from our own body (such as cancer), the hydrogen peroxide oxidizes it, killing it or making it harmless. In this process, hydrogen peroxide is spilled into the bloodstream. Our body manufactures enzymes specifically for the purpose of breaking down hydrogen peroxide. These antioxidant enzymes float abundantly throughout the bloodstream, the excess is quickly taken care of. Hydrogen peroxide is a vital component of our immune system; it is the main weapon our body uses to defend itself from foreign substances.

If a person is in ill health due to poor nutrition and toxic overload, their natural production of antioxidant enzymes may be low. Enzyme synthesis requires an abundant supply of vitamins and minerals that are often lacking in modern diets consisting of processed foods. Oxygen therapy requires antioxidant enzymes for optimal health benefits. Some people may not experience noticeable improvement in health simply because they are enzyme deficient. The benefits they receive from getting more oxygen may be offset by unchecked free-radical reactions.

Before beginning any oxygen therapy program, it is recommended that a person first improve the diet. This is necessary to build up the nutrient reserves needed to produce the enzymes required to remove excess free radicals. A full month on the Natural Foods Diet described in Chapter 4 is recommended before trying oxygen therapy. Taking antioxidant supplements can help, but should not be a substitute for proper nutrition. If used, supplements should be taken *with* meals. Antioxidants and hydrogen peroxide should not be taken at the same time as the benefits of each will be depleted.

 ## ADDITIONAL RESOURCES

Dressed to Kill: The Link Between Breast Cancer and Bras. Singer, Sydney Ross and Grismaijer, Soma. Garden City Park, NY: Avery Publishing Group, 1995.

Hatha Yoga: Manual 1, 2nd Edition. Samskrti and Veda. Honesdale, PA: The Himalayan International Institute, 1985.

Hydrogen Peroxide Medical Miracle. Douglass, William Campbell. Atlanta, GA: Second Opinion Publishing, 1992.

Oxygen Therapies. McCabe, Ed. Morrisville, NY: Energy Publications, 1988.

The Use of Ozone in Medicine, First English Edition. Rilling, Siegfried and Viebahn, Renate. Heidelberg, Germany: Haug Publishers 1987.

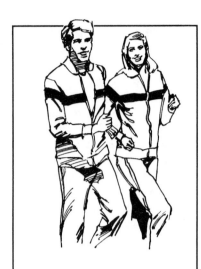

To rest is to rust and rust means decay and destruction. In other words, activity is life, stagnation is death. If we do not use our muscles, we lose them. In order to keep muscles firm, strong, vigorous, and youthful, they must be continually used. Activity is the Law of Life!
—Paul C. Bragg, Ph.D.

Chapter 9

EXERCISE DETOXIFICATION

THE MIRACLE OF EXERCISE

Louis raced toward the tennis net for a return shot. As he extended his racket to scoop up the ball, he felt a burning, knifelike pain suddenly shoot into both his calves. It spread up to his thighs, then his legs went numb.

The cramping pain persisted days later. At 72, Louis thought he was physically fit; he still swam and played tennis occasionally. "I thought I was immune to the gradual physical decline that age seemed to inflict on others," he said. Then came the incident on the tennis court. In the days that followed, he discovered he could walk only two city blocks before his feet tingled and grew numb and his legs cramped up with the same excruciating pain.

He underwent a CAT scan, MRI, and other tests. The diagnosis: excessive buildup of plaque in the arteries of both legs that extended all the way up to the heart. "This often happens in older people who are prone to atherosclerosis," the doctor said. "I spend most days operating on people who cannot be treated any other way. They waited too long." He said an operation would be dangerous and expensive, but offered Louis another option.

"You know," he said, "you're in pretty good shape for your age. If you'll walk at least a mile every day, I think your body will cure the clogged-artery problem by itself."

Louis, surprised at the doctor's recommendation, complained, "I can't walk two blocks, much less a mile."

"You can stop every two blocks, wait a couple of minutes and start again when your muscles have recovered," the doctor replied. "Just so you get a mile in every day. It may take you a year to get results, but you can do it."

At first it was a struggle, walking two-block increments. It took a full hour. "Going up a modest incline felt like climbing the Himalayas," Louis says. "Still, I kept to my promise, no matter how many times I had to stop."

When winter weather came, every step seemed harder. Louis seriously considered giving up and just having the operation.

His son, a physician, urged him to stop eating fatty foods. "I virtually gave up red meat for fish and poultry. I ate raw vegetables and fresh fruit at breakfast, lunch, and dinner. I cut way back on sodium and drank 12 bottles of water a day. Within six months, I'd shed ten pounds."

As time progressed, walking became easier for Louis, even enjoyable. His one mile walks increased to three and four miles every day. His body became stronger and healthier. Atherosclerosis no longer was a threat. "I have been celebrating my new life, " Louis says. "I allow nothing to get in the way of my daily walk. My endurance and quickness on the tennis court have returned."

He continues to walk even after his return to health because the doctor warned him that if he stopped exercising, his body would again deteriorate.

"I have found a new purpose in life," says Louis. "I tell others who are in the predicament I was in to walk. They should ask their doctor whether they, too, could avoid invasive surgery by doing something as simple as walking. The healing powers of our bodies are there, just waiting to be used."

Exercise has long been known as a revitalizer. Research has verified this. Look at people around you. The ones who look the oldest, sickest, and have the most health problems, are the ones who are the least physically active. Look at people who exercise regularly—especially older people. They walk with a spring in their step, they stand straight and tall, their skin is healthy and elastic, they are full of energy, and they are generally happy.

They look and act years younger than their chronological age—why? Because they exercise. A person who exercises regularly will have a means of internal cleansing that will remove a great deal of debris from the body. Regular exercise will cleanse the body more so than probably most other methods of detoxification.

There are two common denominators in cultures where people are particularly long-lived and degenerative disease is rare. Diets of these people vary greatly from one culture to the next, even among those people who are extraordinarily healthy. One similarity is the absence of toxins in their food and environment. The second, is exercise. These people remain physically active throughout life and even into old age. The Hunzas of Pakistan, for example, who have more people per capita over a hundred years of age than any other culture engage in manual labor until the day they die.

The health-enhancing benefits of exercise have been known for many years. In the 1930s researchers were able to decrease the incidence of tumors in a strain of cancer-prone mice from 88 to 16 percent merely by raising some on calorie-restricted diets and abundant physical activity as compared to others who had unlimited food and little exercise. In 1960, scientists discovered that an extract of exercised muscle, when injected into mice with cancer, slowed the growth of tumors and sometimes eliminated them entirely. An extract of nonexercised muscle had no effect.

Exercise has been successfully used to treat depression and is a potent defense against all degenerative diseases. The health benefits of exercise have been well established.

Studies have shown exercise to:

- Increase detoxification (flush out metabolic waste, environmental poisons, and other toxins)
- Decrease risk of degenerative diseases such as heart disease, atherosclerosis, arthritis, cancer, and diabetes.
- Increase energy
- Improve joint mobility
- Combat depression
- Relieve stress
- Improve blood and lymph circulation
- Improve flexibility
- Enhance immune system function
- Improve brain and nerve function
- Enhance healing
- Improve digestion and bowel function
- Remove excess fat
- Lower cholesterol level
- Prevent insomnia
- Improve strength and endurance
- Normalize hormone secretion
- Prevent osteoporosis

DETOXIFICATION THROUGH EXERCISE

Most people don't ordinarily think of exercise as a form of detoxification, but it is one of the best natural detoxifiers available. Exercise is just as important to detoxification as a good diet. It can also enhance the cleansing effects of any detoxification program.

Exercise should become a regular part of your life. In past generations physical labor was common. Nowadays, with all of our modern conveniences, modes of transportation, and automation, most people do not get the exercise they need. Combine that with the enormous amount of pollutants we are exposed to daily, and our bodies become over toxic and slowly degenerate. Regular

Cancer
    Physically fit men die four times less often from cancer, and physically fit women die 16 times less often from cancer than unfit men and women.
    —Dr. Steven Blair, et al., Physical Fitness and All-Cause Mortality, *Journal of the American Medical Association*, November 1989

Body Mass Index

A standard derived from height and weight measures, which is useful for estimating the risk to health associated with obesity, is the body mass index (BMI).

The extent to which weight reflects fatness depends partly on a person's frame size. The larger the frame, the heavier a person is expected to be, due to the density of bones and muscles.

$$BMI = weight\ (kg)/height^2\ (m)$$

Or using the conversion factor (707.61) you can plug pounds and inches into the following formula.

$$BMI = \frac{weight\ (lb)\ x\ 707.61}{height^2\ (inches)}$$

A BMI greater than 27.7 for men or 27.2 for women indicates overweight. Ideal weight 20.7 to 24, for men and 19.1 to 23.5 for women.

	Men	Women
Underweight	< 20.7	< 19.1
Acceptable weight	20.7 to 27.7	19.1 to 27.2
Overweight	>27.7	>27.2
Severe overweight	>31.0	>32.2
Morbid obesity	>45.3	>44.7

exercise can overcome and remove a great deal of the toxins we are subjected to.

Removal of Fatty Tissues

One of the biggest deterrents to good health is the accumulation of excess body fat. Fatty tissues clog the arteries, increase blood pressure, strain the heart, hamper circulation, and slow down metabolism, among other things, all of which lead to aches, pains, fatigue, and degeneration and dysfunction of body tissues and organs. Weight problems have been identified as a major contributing factor to numerous health problems, ranging from coronary artery disease to cancer and numerous gastrointestinal disorders.

Many of the toxins that find their way into our bodies are stored in the fatty tissues. As you recall from Chapter 5, when fat is dissolved these toxins are dumped into the bloodsteam and if the load is heavy, it will initiate the symptoms of a healing crisis. Excess fat also hampers circulation, preventing adequate removal of toxins. Toxic accumulation in the tissues encourages cellular deterioration which increases the toxicity of the body. An overweight body is, therefore, a toxic body.

When we lose weight, we reduce our fat and thereby our toxic load. By so doing we remove a great deal of strain on the body. Losing excess weight greatly reduces our chances of developing disease.

There are many theories of how and why people gain excess weight. Some say it's caused by slow metabolism or emotional or social problems or even genetics. These factors may all contribute, but the fundamental reason people gain weight is consuming more calories than they use. In other words, overeating. When we eat more than the body requires for its daily functions, the excess calories are stored as fat. The only way to remove excess fat is to eat less or increase physical activity to burn more calories.

Dieting alone does not work well. Most diets (as well as diet pills, sauna baths, and fad diets) primarily remove water, not fat, and water will be reabsorbed as soon as liquids are consumed in adequate quantities. Losing too much water can be dangerous as it may lead to dehydration.

To get rid of fat, a healthy diet, such as the Natural Foods Diet, needs to be combined with exercise.

Some people who want to lose weight hate the idea of exercise. Obese people particularly do not enjoy moving their bodies. They feel heavy, clumsy, and intimidated. They choose to lose weight by a means other than exercise. Studies have shown that obese women put on a calorie-restricted diet without exercise lost the same amount of weight as obese women who exercised and dieted—with one noticeable difference. The exercise group lost more fat. The dieting group lost more water.

Weight will come off easier and will more likely stay off when exercise and sensible eating are combined. Part of the reason is that the body's metabolism will adjust to the increased energy output and consume more calories even when not exercising.

The conditioned body tends to use fat, rather than glucose, as fuel, therefore more body fat is burned during exercise. Regular vigorous exercise will also increase metabolism for as long as two days, so more calories are consumed even after exercising.

Losing excess weight is only one of the benefits of exercise detoxification. Skinny people can also benefit from exercise and weight management. Although a thin person may have less fat, the fat he has may be loaded with toxins. Exercise and proper eating will help him remove these toxins and rebuild with clean healthy tissues. We all need some body fat, but the fat should be clean. With detoxification exercise, people who are underweight will lose a little weight at first as their bodies detoxify. After removing toxin laden fat and deteriorating cells, the body will rebuild with strong healthy tissues and weight will be gained. Weight will adjust naturally to a trim, but more ideal, norm.

Many people believe that exercise increases appetite and, therefore, you'll tend to eat more if you exercise and negate any weight loss. This is not true. Most people who work out moderately (up to an hour a day) actually eat less than sedentary people. A lean person may eat more following increased activity, but the exercise will burn up the extra calories. If you have extra fat, you will react differently to exercise than those who are lean. Unless you exercise to excess, your appetite will generally not increase from the exercise, because when the body has excess stores of fat, the appetite is not stimulated by moderate exercise.

Increase Circulation and Bodily Function

Exercise stimulates blood and lymph circulation throughout the body. These fluids distribute essential nutrients to the cells and remove metabolic wastes and other toxic substances. If circulation slows down, the cells starve and choke on their own metabolic waste.

Our cells are individual living units. Just as we need oxygen to live, so do the cells. Without oxygen we would die in a matter of minutes. The same is true for each cell in our bodies. Denied oxygen for just a short time, they die. A heart attack results when an artery which feeds oxygen to the heart becomes clogged. A stroke is caused when a blood vessel in the brain is blocked. When oxygen cannot get to these and other organs in sufficient quantities, they immediately began to deteriorate and die.

Restricting the free flow of body fluids limits the delivery of oxygen and other vital nutrients. Lack of nutrition to the cells will cause the cells to deteriorate and mutate. Metabolic waste, dead and deteriorating cells, and other toxins accumulate and poison surrounding tissues, increasing toxic load in the body and causing disease-like conditions to develop.

Exercise detoxification increases circulation of nutrients and flushes out harmful toxins. Metabolism increases both during and after exercise. This speeds up body processes, thus enhancing kidney and liver function—two of the body's primary detoxifying organs.

The production of white blood cells increases with exercise. This is important because white blood cells are an essential part of our immune system and vital in the body's detoxification process. Among other things, they neutralize and destroy microorganisms and other harmful substances and remove them from the body. After vigorous exercise the white blood cell count will remain elevated for as much as two hours. During this time they are busy cleaning and detoxifying the body.

Building up a sweat is also an important part of exercise detoxification. One of the functions of the skin is that of elimination. Uric acid, a waste product which is also removed in the urine, is excreted when we perspire. Along with this come heavy metals and other harmful toxins. Sweating is important for the removal of toxins from the body.

Exercise stimulates the growth of new blood vessels, thus enhancing oxygenation and delivery of nutrients to all body tissues. Many pathogenic microorganisms are anaerobic in nature. That is, they do not like oxygen. Exercise oxygenates the blood and tissues and thus inhibits the growth of harmful microorganisms.

Getting the Most from Exercise

Exercise should be a regular part of your life. It is one of the best methods of cleansing. Most other detoxification methods are used only for a short time. Exercise can and should be done regularly.

As amazing as exercise is, it can be undermined by other factors such as poor diet, drugs, alcohol, smoking, etc., as well as heavy exposure to environmental contaminants. Combined with a proper diet and lifestyle habits, regular exercise can have a marvelous rejuvenating effect on the body.

Athletes and others who exercise regularly have extraordinarily strong, healthy bodies. However, occasionally you read in the news where an athlete dies or comes down with one of the typical degenerative diseases of our society. People may ask, why didn't exercise help him? Heredity may be a factor in some cases. The fact is, many athletes have horrible diets and lifestyle habits. They eat far too much meat, dairy, sugar, fat, and convenience foods and generally overeat, often gorging themselves, reasoning that they will burn off the excess calories. Some, aware that exercise cleans the body, eat whatever they want. Others eat lots of high-protein foods like meats and protein powders, believing it is necessary to build muscle. Some use steroids and other drugs (pharmaceutical and recreational). As a result, many athletes destroy much of the health benefits of exercise and in time succumb to disease.

Exercise alone will not save you if you continually subject yourself to poisons. The two most important things you can do for your health is exercise regularly and eat a good diet.

MOTION IS LIFE

When you look at a corpse, what do you see? A lifeless, motionless mass that is deteriorating. Let's come up one step on the scale of life. If a person is in a coma, what do you see? Is the person moving, getting stronger, improving mental capacity? No. The basic functions of life are working at only a minimal level; most of the body is atrophying—wasting away. It is slowly deteriorating.

Let's come up farther to someone who can consciously move but is limited—say wheelchair-bound. Is this person's legs getting stronger? Is he getting healthier by sitting all day? No. Why is that? Because there is no appreciable movement.

Now take a person who is capable of free movement but is physically inactive, the typical couch potato who sits down all day at work then comes home and sits all evening in front of the television set. Is this person getting stronger and healthier with time or is he deteriorating?

Our bodies adjust to the level of physical activity we put upon them. Without movement the body atrophies. With movement body functions improve. A body builder becomes strong and flexible because he moves. A runner develops cardiovascular and pulmonary efficiency because he moves. We become stronger and healthier with movement. Every cell in the body requires movement to get nourishment, remove metabolic waste, and to fulfill its function. If the cells did not have movement they would be dead or dying. If we do not move, a similar situation occurs.

Effects of aging can be retarded. Look at seniors who are physically active and healthy. Exercise will bring life back into your body and keep life there. Even people who have physical disabilities can improve their health. Being wheelchair-bound, for example, does not prevent a person from exercising.

Some people avoid exercise by trying to convince themselves that diet alone will make them healthy. You can eat all the best foods you can, but if you don't exercise, your body cannot use the nutrients optimally. Dr. Bernard Jensen, renowned nutritionist and naturopath, stated that "Food alone is not the cure" to poor health. Dr. Paavo Airola, also a world-renowned authority on nutrition, stated in a radio interview that exercise is the most important thing we can do for our health, even more important that diet. That is quite a statement to be coming from a nutritionist.

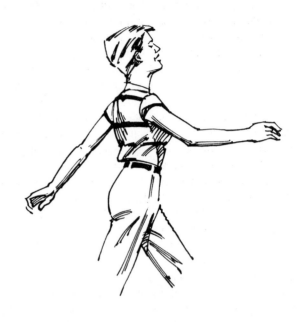

Motion is life. Stagnation is death. Without movement we deteriorate and head toward disease and death. Physical activity is the closest thing we have to the fountain of youth.

CIRCULATION: THE KEY TO GOOD HEALTH

Blood and other body fluids transport nutrients from the digestive organs and lungs throughout the body. Blood carries oxygen from the lungs to essentially every cell in the body. It carries vitamins, minerals, proteins, and other nutrients to the cells which need them to carry on the process of life.

Not only does blood deliver nutrients to the cells, but it also collects and removes metabolic waste. Each cell is a living unit and, like our entire body, consumes nutrients and produces waste. This waste is toxic and must be removed. Along with metabolic waste, the blood removes other debris such as dietary poisons, environmental toxins, microorganisms, and dead cells.

Blood is pumped by the heart through the arteries, which branch out into smaller and smaller arteries until they form capillaries—tiny channels with walls only one cell thick. Here plasma, the blood water, filters through small pore spaces in the capillary walls. Red blood cells and other large blood proteins are too big to fit through these openings and continue to circulate through the capillaries, returning to the heart by way of the veins.

Once the blood plasma penetrates the capillary walls it is called interstitial fluid. With it comes the oxygen and other nutrients transported by the blood. Lymphocytes (a type of white blood cell), which are larger than red blood cells, are flexible and therefore able to squeeze through the capillary openings. They too, circulate in the interstitial fluid.

Interstitial fluid bathes all the cells in the body. When you scrape or cut yourself, but not deep enough to bleed, the watery yellowish fluid that you see on the injury is this fluid. It is the medium which actually transports nutrients to each cell. By osmosis, the cells absorb the oxygen and other nutrients and expel metabolic waste. The interstitial fluid picks up this waste as well as other toxins and removes them from the cells. Interstitial fluid is a sea of both nutrients and toxins. Much of the toxic debris, such a carbon dioxide which is produced as oxygen is metabolized, is filtered back into the blood stream where it is expelled through the lungs. Other toxins are transported by the lymphatic system and eventually flushed out of the body by way of the kidneys, colon, and skin.

Interstitial fluid flows around the cells until it is sucked up into a lymph vessel and enters the lymphatic system. Here the interstitial fluid is known as lymph fluid. The lymphatic system is completely different from, although similar to, the circulatory system which carries the blood. Lymph vessels branch throughout the body sucking in interstitial fluid and the debris floating in it. Lymph nodes spaced along these vessels serve as filtration plants that neutralize most of the toxins as they pass by. These vessels merge into larger and larger vessels and eventually drain back into the bloodstream near the heart. In the bloodstream lymph fluid is again referred to as plasma. Interstitial fluid, lymph, and plasma are all basically the same thing—water carrying nutrients and waste materials. Because their function is similar, for simplicity, I will refer to both interstitial and lymph fluids as lymph or lymph fluid.

Our hearts supply the force necessary to pump blood through the circulatory system. The lymphatic system, however, does not have a pump as such. The pumping force in the lymphatic system is supplied primarily by muscular contraction. The milking action of muscles squeezing the lymph vessels pushes the lymph along its pathway. Intermittent one-way valves prevent the lymph, once it enters a lymph vessel, from moving backwards.

The rate of lymph flow is governed primarily by muscular movement although pressure from massage or gravity may also move lymph to some extent. If you don't move your body, the lymph cannot circulate. In fact, the blood can continue to release plasma through the capillary walls, but if it is not sucked into the lymph vessels, it builds up causing edema (swelling) which can cause numerous other symptoms.

The body must move to circulate the lymph fluid throughout the body and around the cells. A person who sits all day at work, drives home, and sits all evening watching television, then goes to bed and repeats this cycle day after day, gets no exercise. Lymph circulation is, consequently, sluggish and even stagnates in certain areas of the body.

One of the vital functions of lymph fluid is to transport lymphocytes and antibodies. It is the lymph that brings these vital elements of our immune system into contact with invading microorganisms. They neutralize or destroy pathogenic bacteria, viruses, and fungi, and remove harmful toxins, such as heavy metals and chemical contaminants. A lack of lymph circulation hinders the transport and function of the immune system.

A person who does not exercise has a sluggish lymph system, which means his immune system will be less effective, and toxins (microbiologic or chemical), metabolic waste, and dead cells will collect in areas of stagnation. Toxins collect and build up in the slowest areas of circulation, such as in scar tissues, inherently weak or diseased organs, or areas continually restricted from circulation like the feet and hips. As this debris collects, it agitates surrounding tissues and causes further cellular destruction and provides an ideal breeding ground for microorganisms. These areas become the focus of disease and infection.

Cells need vitamins, minerals, proteins and other nutrients to live and function properly. When these materials are not provided—due to lack of motion—cells become sick, die, or mutate. Cancer cells are in us all, but our immune system destroys them. When circulation (motion) is restricted, removal becomes inefficient and cancer cells can gain a foothold and multiply.

A person who is confined to bed due to an injury, such as a broken leg, will start to feel terrible after a few days. The reason is because lack of circulation has caused a buildup of toxins in the body.

A person who lies in one position for too long a time decreases circulation to parts of the body. As a result, these nutrient starved areas begin to deteriorate and literally rot. This is what a bed sore is. Hospital patients must be moved regularly to avoid bed sores. But a similar thing happens inside the body when circulation is hampered. The tissues begin to deteriorate and mutate which leads to abnormal growths and disease.

The pelvic area is of major concern because so many people sit all day. Sitting creates pressure in this area, restricting circulation. Organs in this region become starved for oxygen and other nutrients and become clogged by their own metabolic waste and toxic accumulation. Is it any wonder why prostate, uterus, and ovary dysfunction is so widespread? These organs are struggling in a sea of toxins. They cannot function properly in such an environment and consequently they deteriorate and malfunction. The kidneys, bladder, colon, and rectum—all vital organs of elimination—are affected, hampering their ability to detoxify the body. The reproductive organs that produce estrogen, progesterone, and testosterone affect the entire body. When hormones are out of balance, numerous other body processes are affected. PMS, headaches, impotence, cancer, prostate enlargement, endometriosis, irregular menstrual cycles, and other related abnormalities may be caused, in part, by a simple lack of circulation in the pelvic area.

Circulation can be restricted by wearing tight-fitting clothing as well. Studies have shown a correlation between the wearing of bras and breast cancer. Any restrictive clothing will hamper lymph circulation.

Recent studies have given conclusive proof that cancer can and does develop as a result of restricting lymph movement. A century ago it was popular for women to wear corsets to improve their figures. These tight-fitting undergarments extended from the bust to the hips. Lacing along the back allowed them to be bound tightly around the body, enhancing a woman's figure and making her look more slender. The corset eventually gave way to the girdle, a similar garment made of tough elastic which was squeezed and wiggled into, often with great effort. It was noticed that women who frequently wore these confining garments often developed a number of adverse physical conditions. The bra, which was much less restricting, yet could add support or padding to enhance the figure, came into popular use. Most women in North America and in other Western countries wear bras. It has become a standard piece of clothing. The bra, however, like its relative, the corset, is terribly confining and blocks the free flow of lymph to the bust. The pressure exerted by the straps on the bra is not strong enough to cut off blood circulation, but it is tight enough to prevent lymph from flowing to lymph nodes near the breast and around cells. This creates a pooling of toxins which irritate surrounding tissue. The result is breast cancer.

Breast cancer is of major concern in America and other civilized countries. However, it is almost unheard of in Third World countries. In the United States and Canada, one out of every eight women will get breast cancer sometime in her life. Why is it so high in Western countries and relatively rare elsewhere? In a study conducted by Sydney Ross Singer, a medical anthropologist, and Soma Grismaijer, and outlined in their book *Dressed to Kill,* the connection between tight clothing and cancer was made. In this study, 4,500 women, half of which had breast cancer and half of which did not, the effects of wearing a bra were determined. Of the women who did not wear bras, only one out of 168 got breast cancer (a dramatic improvement over the national average). For women who wore their bra at least 12 hours a day, but not to bed at night, one out of seven developed breast cancer (close to the national average of one out of eight). For women who wore their bra at least 12 hours and slept with them on at night, the rate of breast cancer was three out of four!

This supports the observation that in Third World countries where women don't wear bras, breast cancer is rare. Women who have developed lumps in their breast have had the lumps disappear within a couple of months after they stopped wearing their bras. The evidence of breast cancer being directly related to wearing bras is clearly evident. Keep in mind, however, that the bra is not the only factor involved. Exercise and diet are also important. Environmental pollutants, food additives, as well as microorganisms provide the source for the toxins which accumulate in the breast tissue. A lack of exercise allows circulation to be sluggish. Combine that with a restrictive garment, like a bra, and you end up with trouble. Any tight fitting clothing can have a similar effect, as will sitting on your rear end all day.

Movement or exercise is the only way to adequately circulate lymph through the body. Without exercise, your body becomes a stagnant toxic dump. Movement is life.

YOUR EXERCISE PROGRAM

What type of exercise should you do to detox? Any type of exercise that gets your whole body moving and your body fluids circulating will be beneficial. You don't need to follow any one particular exercise program. The important thing is that you exercise regularly.

However, you should avoid stressful exercise that may cause injury or discouragement. You should choose an activity that you enjoy. This way you will be more apt to make it a regular part of your life. It should be convenient so that you can do it easily rain or shine. And it should fit your budget.

Many people lack the motivation to exercise or they get discouraged easily. To make your exercise program successful, you need to make it a habit. Even if you've always avoided exercise, once you have made up your mind to do it and make it a habit, the psychological barriers vanish and you will actually come to enjoy it. Here

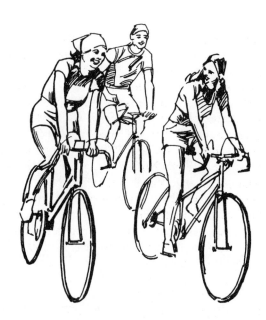

are some guidelines to help you set up and maintain a successful exercise program:

Commitment. The first step is to make a commitment to yourself. Set a goal to exercise regularly. You should exercise a minimum of three times a week. Five to six days a week would be better.

Duration. Exercise at least 20 minutes at each session. Thirty minutes or more is even better. The more time you can spend, the more benefit you will receive.

Activity. Choose an activity you enjoy doing. The more you enjoy your workout, the more likely you are to make it a habit.

Convenience. An ideal exercise will be one that you can do at most any time. Joining a health spa is fine, although, it is not the most convenient, nor is it normally cheap. But if you like that sort of thing and it encourages you to exercise regularly, then do it.

Schedule. You need to set a specific time to exercise and stick strictly to it. This is very important! If you do not set aside a specific time for exercise, you will not keep it up. Other things always have a way of popping up and, before you know it, there is no time to exercise. Scheduling is a most important step in developing a successful exercise program. When you set a time to exercise, you adjust all other activities around your exercise schedule so nothing else interferes. Having a set time will also psychologically prepare you for the workout. Before the habit is formed, you may argue with yourself after a hard day at work: "I'm too tired; I've got to make dinner; I've got to do this or that." But if you have a schedule, it will encourage you to exercise regardless of the excuses.

Place. Choose a place to exercise and do it in the same place each time, a room in the house, the garage, a health club, or even outdoors. Your mind associates this place with exercise, mentally you feel more prepared, and your desire to exercise is increased. One reason some people prefer to exercise at health spas or clubs is that the atmosphere there helps get them into the mood.

Clothes. Some people can get into the mood of exercising better by changing into an exercise outfit. If this helps encourage you, then do it. Special clothes are also recommended if your exercise is vigorous enough to cause you to perspire, which it should.

Set goals. Set goals for yourself and focus on accomplishing those goals. You should have at least two goals, one long-range and one short-range. The long-range goal would be to gain better health. This is your primary purpose in initiating an exercise detox program. Short-range goals will be based on performance such as time or distance. The short-range goals will make your workouts more enjoyable and give you feelings of accomplishment and progress. Make the goals realistic, not too easy, yet achievable in a matter of months. Once you have achieved one goal, set a new goal and go for it. Continue to set new goals as you accomplish old ones. Setting goals will give your workout more purpose and allow you to see the improvement you are making.

Don't overdo it. Avoid stressful exercises or overextending yourself. Tiring yourself out may lead to injury and may make you so exhausted that all you want to do afterwards is rest. Exercise should be vigorous enough to give you a good workout, yet not so demanding as to sap all your strength and make you exhausted for the rest of the day. If you injure yourself, then you will need to take time off to recuperate. Also, stressful exercise may make you dread working out. The right amount of exercise

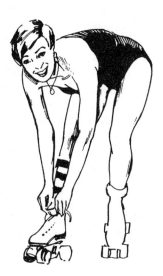

Exercise for Headaches

Just about everyone has suffered from headaches. Some people experience them more often than others. Women are two to four times more likely to get them than men. Approximately 10 percent of the population experience headaches four or more times a month.

Some chronic headache sufferers find relief by walking or other aerobic exercise. They get fewer headaches, their headaches are less severe, and they have less of a need for medications, say researchers who study and treat headache patients. "People who regularly walk briskly or jog have reported dramatic relief from their headaches," say Fred D. Sheftell, M.D., and Alan M. Rapoport, M.D., founders and directors of The New England Center for Headache in Stamford, Conn. "By making changes in your diet, your exercise patterns, and your ways of dealing with stress, you can substantially reduce and prevent headache pain."

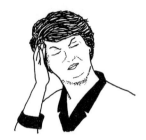

The majority of all headaches is caused by tension, which can be relieved by exercise. "An exercise schedule that involves some aerobic activity—walking, running, swimming, and so on, four or five times a week—does seem to make an appreciable difference in reducing headaches and promoting a general sense of well-being," they say.

Aerobic exercise brings about a number of changes in the body that can prevent headaches. It:

Improves circulation. When you exercise regularly, your body responds to increased blood flow by developing extra capillaries. As a result, your tissues receive more blood and thus more oxygen, which removes nerve-irritating wastes from tissues more efficiently.

Detoxifies. The liver neutralizes and removes toxins from the blood that irritate nerves and muscles and cause pain. Aerobic exercise increases the volume of blood that is pumped into the liver. The liver can then remove more toxins that cause headaches.

Releases pain-relieving chemicals. Vigorous exercise causes the body to produce pain-relieving substances such as endorphins, chemicals that are more powerful than morphine. Endorphins block the effects of pain and thereby raise the headache sufferer's pain threshold.

Reduces stress. Stress and depression trigger some headaches. Exercise can relieve both stress and depression and thus ease headaches caused by these factors.

Improves posture. Poor posture can strain muscles in the back and neck, causing headaches. Exercise improves posture by relaxing and strengthening the muscles in the spine.

will tire you temporarily, but you will shortly gain renewed vigor and alertness. You should be able to carry on a conversation while you are exercising. If you are too out of breath to do that, ease up. Warning signals of pain or excessive fatigue must be heeded, but they're signs to ease up, not to stop entirely.

Bathe. Take a hot soothing shower or bath after you exercise. This is part of your reward for exercising. The bath will soothe tired muscles and wash off toxins excreted in perspiration. It can also refresh you. Although you may not feel like you perspired much, you may have more than you know. In dry climates perspiration can evaporate almost instantly. If perspiration is not washed off, it becomes a breeding ground for microorganisms. Toxins in the sweat may also be reabsorbed into the body.

Make it a part of your life. Don't limit your physical activity to just your regular exercise program. Take an opportunity to exercise whenever you can. Go bowling, take tennis lessons, play baseball, or get involved in other activities. Since exercise will make you more physically fit, take advantage of it. Instead of driving to a friend's house, walk or ride a bicycle. When you go to work, park your car at the far end of the lot and walk the rest of the way. Instead of taking the elevator, use the stairs. Take spontaneous walks outside. Go to the park and eat your lunch. Avoid sitting for extended periods. Get up and move about and get the blood and lymph circulating. Remember, motion is life.

DETOXIFICATION EXERCISE
Choosing the Best Exercise

The type of exercise you choose is very important. It must be convenient, economical, enjoyable, not too strenuous, and yet effective. What works for someone else may not be the best for you.

Most people think of jogging when exercise is mentioned. The jogging craze hit in the 1970s and still remains popular. It's an excellent form of exercise if you wear the right shoes, are young, and in good physical condition. If not, it is very strenuous on the body. The pounding the skeletal system receives with each step is extraordinarily stressful. Shinsplints, fallen arches, blisters, pulled muscles as well numerous foot, ankle, knee, and hip problems are common. Experienced joggers know that if you are serious about jogging, you *will* suffer injury. Running and injury seem to go hand-in-hand. The constant pounding on a hard surface saps the energy and speeds the onset of fatigue. Most injuries occur when the body is fatigued. When the body tires, it loses its ability to handle stress. An awkward step, which would ordinarily result in relatively minor discomfort, turns into a sprained ankle or torn muscle.

Any aerobic exercise like jogging, dance aerobics, or basketball has the potential for such injuries. For people who are just starting an exercise program, these types of activities may be too strenuous.

Nonaerobic exercises focus on strength training. Weight lifting is a nonaerobic exercise. Much of the exercise equipment in health spas is of this type. Strength-building exercise focuses on working certain muscles or muscle groups while the rest of the body remains relatively inactive. Such exercises are good for building strength and toning up, but are not the best for encouraging blood and lymph circulation. For a detoxification program, you need an exercise that involves the entire body.

Swimming is one of the best exercises. It is fun. It works the entire body. Anyone at any fitness level can benefit from it. And it does not subject the body to the pounding that jogging and other aerobic exercises do. Swimming, however, has some drawbacks. Public swimming pools are shared by thousands of people. As a consequence, the water becomes polluted with an assortment of pathogenic viruses, bacteria, and fungi. These microorganisms can remain in the water and infect anyone who swims in it. It only takes one infected person to contaminate an entire pool.

These organisms are controlled to some extent by dumping chlorine into the water. Chlorine is highly poisonous to both microorganisms and humans. Our skin is not an impenetrable barrier; it excretes sweat, hormones, and oil as well as absorbs chemicals and toxins from the environment, including chlorine. When you swim in a chlorinated pool, your body absorbs the chlorine which increases the toxic load inside the body.

Chlorine quickly evaporates, so it must be added to swimming pools on a regular basis. When it is first dumped into the pool, it is strongest and can even burn your skin. At this stage, most microorganisms are killed. After a time, most of the chlorine has evaporated and the microorganisms have begun to return en masse both from the environment and from swimmers. So depending on when you go swimming, you are either poisoned by the chlorine or subjected to a barrage of biological organisms which may be highly pathogenic. Unless you can find a pool that is kept clean by an ozone generator, which kills microorganisms with oxygen and is harmless to humans, you should think seriously about going swimming.

Cycling machines, Nordic Trac, and other such exercise equipment can provide good resistance exercise as well as an aerobic workout. Any form of exercise will be beneficial so long as it works the entire body and you enjoy it. There are two forms of exercise, however, that deserve special mention. They are walking and rebound exercise.

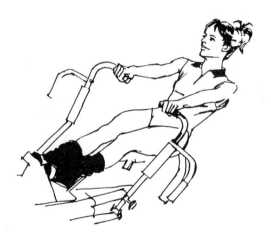

Walking

In the last few years, walking has become the most popular form of exercise in America. It is the most convenient and economical exercise there is and definitely the easiest. You can do it anywhere, and with the proper attire, anytime. Regardless of age or fitness level, most people can walk. Even if it is difficult, like Louis in the story recounted at the beginning of this chapter, you can build up strength and overcome discomfort caused by a sedentary lifestyle.

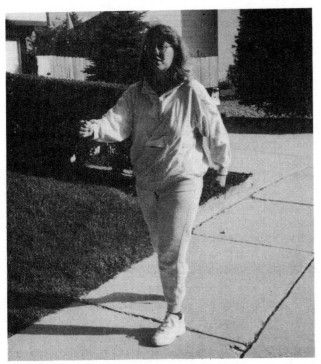

Walking is one of the best forms of exercise.

Although walking is a mild form of exercise, it provides enough physical activity to detoxify the body and enhance bodily functions. You don't need to run or indulge in strenuous activities to benefit from exercise. The adage "No pain, no gain" is a myth. Engaging in even moderate activity can counteract the effects of a sedentary lifestyle. Recent studies performed at Harvard University Medical School demonstrated that a couple of hours of brisk walking each week can decrease colon cancer risk by 30 percent. The more hours spent exercising, the lower the cancer risk. The risk for numerous other diseases also declines with regular walking.

Unlike many other forms of exercise, you can easily find a time and place to walk. If you need to, you can even split up your walking time into shorter segments and spread them out over the day. If your goal is to walk 30 minutes a day, you can take a 15-minute walk at lunch time, five-minute walk instead of a coffee break, and park your car far enough away to walk five minutes coming and leaving work. By the time you get home you've also finished your exercise. Walking during the day like this will invigorate you and actually make you more productive. Some companies recognize this and even provide exercise facilities for their employees.

With the abundance of shopping malls, mall walking has become a popular activity, especially with older people. Malls are relatively safe and weatherproof. The shops and people give the walk an added dimension of interest.

If you are just beginning an exercise program, start off at an easy pace. Walk a minimum of 20 minutes a day, preferably five to six times a week, but no less then three. Work up to 30 minutes or more a day with a brisk walk. Swing your arms. You may even hold hand weights to help tone your upper body. After each workout your heart rate should be elevated, blood freely flowing, and breathing heavier.

Set goals for yourself either in time or distance. Walk faster and farther for a longer amount of time. Don't overtax yourself. Keep in mind that you should be able to carry on a conversation while walking. If you can't, you're working too hard. You should feel tired after a walk, but not exhausted. Energy should return after a few minutes of rest.

The Institute for Aerobics Research recommends the following:

Minimum Dose For Moderate Fitness
Women: Walk 2 miles in 30 minutes or less 3 days a week or walk 2 miles in 30-40 minutes 5-6 days a week.
Men: Walk 2 miles in 27 minutes or less at least 3 days a week or walk 2 miles in 30-40 minutes 6-7 days a week.

Minimum Dose For High Fitness
Women: Walk 2 miles in 30 minutes 5-6 days a week
Men: Walk 2.5 miles in 38 minutes 6-7 days a week

Rebound Exercise

The most amazing detoxification exercise is without a doubt rebound exercise. Rebound exercise or rebounding, as it is sometimes called, consists of jumping on a cushioned surface. Trampolining is rebound exercise. The trampoline was originally created as a form of recreation. Smaller versions known as mini-traps or indoor joggers were created. The portable type used for most rebound exercise nowadays is called a rebounder.

Rebound exercise is almost as convenient as walking. You can do it anywhere at anytime. One advantage it has over walking is that you can do it in the comfort of your home when it is scorching hot or blustery cold outside. However, you do not get the change of scenery that many walkers enjoy.

Rebounders are cheap. You can get an inexpensive model for about $30. Heavy-duty models cost as much as $300, but are worth the price. The better models are built to absorb the shock of impact and have more spring. They also last many times longer than ordinary rebounders. One model can even fold up to the size of a large briefcase and fits a nylon case that can be carried over the shoulder.

Rebound exercise has been described as the most efficient, most effective, form of exercise yet devised by man. Rebound exercise provides all the benefits of ordinary exercise plus many others unique to rebounding. As a form of detoxification no other exercise comes close. The reason rebound exercise is so good is because it works the entire body, not just the arms or leg muscles.

The secret behind the efficiency of rebound exercise is gravity. All exercise, no matter what it is, has one common element—opposition to gravity. When we do pushups we are working against gravity. When we lift weights, the force we work against is gravity. Even with walking and running we work against gravity as we take each step.

With most forms of exercise, some muscles always get disproportionally more exercise than others and some get almost none at all. When lifting weights with the arms, for example, the muscles moving the weight are getting by far most of the exercise. There is little if any benefit to the neck, jaw, hips, legs, feet, etc. Also, circulation of lymph is focused primarily in the moving muscles. A similar analogy can be made to most any other exercise.

With rebounding you also work against gravity, but the gravitational force is not limited to just one part of the body as it is with other exercises. As the body bounces, the gravitational force changes. This force varies from zero Gs (one G is the earth's normal gravitational pull) at the top of the bounce, where the body is momentarily weightless, to as much as four Gs at the bottom of the bounce. With a force of four Gs at the bottom of the bounce you literally weigh four times more than normal. A 150-pound man would weight 600 pounds at each bounce!

You experience a similar change in forces acting on the body every time you get on an elevator. When you go up it feels like your body is being pushed down. When you are coming down, you feel lighter. The force of gravity increases or decreases over the entire body when riding on an elevator. Likewise, when rebounding, the force of gravity oscillates up and down.

A gentle bounce, where the feet barely leave the mat, can produce a force of two Gs. A 150-pound person would weigh 300 pounds with each bounce. This weight is evenly distributed over the entire body. And the entire body responds. This response is what makes rebounding an amazing form of exercise.

The body adapts to the increase in weight and builds stronger tissues. As gravity on the body increases, each cell in the body senses increased pressure. In essence, the cells work to compensate for the pressure by becoming stronger. In theory, rebounding at a force of two Gs (a relatively easy bounce) will double the strength of all body tissues. This includes all of the muscles, both skeletal and non-skeletal or involuntary muscles.

If your heart (which is a muscle) were twice as strong as it is now, wouldn't your chances of suffering a heart attack decrease? If the muscles around your blood vessels were twice as strong, wouldn't your chances of having an aneurysm, varicose veins, or hemorrhoids be lessened? If the muscles surrounding your intestines were twice as strong, wouldn't your chances of constipation and colitis be lessened? And wouldn't your digestion and elimination be improved? Yes they would.

Rebound exercise does not just strengthen the muscles, but it strengthens every single cell of the body, both muscle and nonmuscle. It strengthens the bones, cartilage, joints, and every organ of the body. The liver, pancreas, kidneys, brain, etc. all are subjected to the increased gravitational force of rebounding and will respond by growing stronger. In so doing, they build up increased resistance to disease. As a result, all of the systems and organs of the body function more efficiently. If the organs work better, they can also remove toxins better.

As a method of detoxification, rebound exercise is an excellent internal cleanser. The up-and-down motion compresses and decompresses the body tissues and fluids. Toxins are squeezed out of cells and tissues as lymph fluid is pushed throughout the body. Rebound exercise is the best lymph-pumping exercise known. As a result of this pumping action, toxins are washed out of tissues throughout the entire body and flushed out. Rebound exercise is such an effective detoxifier that it can initiate a healing crisis in a matter of days.

Rebound exercise also stimulates the peristaltic muscular contractions of the colon, accelerating the elimination of body waste. It helps to relieve constipation thus prevent reabsorption of toxins from a slow-moving bowel. Some people complain when they first start jumping that it causes them to have diarrhea. It isn't

Osteoporosis and Exercise

Weight-bearing exercise such as walking, rebounding, and the use of light free-weights helps protect against osteoporosis. A study at the U.S. Department of Agriculture's Human Nutrition Research Center on Aging found that women who walked at least 1 mile a day (7.5 miles/week) had greater bone density than those who walked less or not at all. Exercise also helps increase muscle mass, which in turn helps strengthen bones.

actually diarrhea; their bowels, which have probably been sluggish for years, are finally beginning to function normally again.

Rebounding can be done by people of any age and almost any physical condition. With assistance, even wheelchair-bound people can benefit. In fact, rebounding has been used to reverse the effects of severe arthritis where people have lost all mobility of their legs. After detoxification therapy using a rebounder, they have regained the use of their legs and can get around without aid of any sort.

The intensity of rebound exercise can vary to fit your level of fitness. It can be gentle enough for those who are physically handicapped or have severe degenerative conditions, or it can be as intense as running a record-breaking mile. Either way brings physical benefits.

When starting a rebound exercise detoxification program, it is best to begin slowly. Too much, too soon or too vigorously can initiate unpleasant effects from cleansing. You will feel worse while it is making you healthier. Rebounding can unload more toxins into your bloodstream

Aerobic Exercise

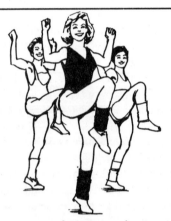

Based on the studies of Kenneth Cooper, M.D., there are five basic principles of aerobic exercise.

(1) Frequency. Exercise at least three times a week.

(2) Intensity. Exercise within 65-75 percent of your maximum work capacity, known as your *target zone*.

(3) Duration. Exercise within your target zone for 20-30 minutes each time.

(4) Type of exercise. Exercises should be rhythmic and continuous, and should utilize the large muscles of the legs and hips. Such exercises include walking, rebounding, jogging, bicycling, swimming, cross-country skiing, and aerobic dance.

(5) Warm up and cool down. Do 10 minutes of slow, smooth stretching before exercising and five minutes of walking and some stretching after exercising.

The target zone is the level of activity you need to maintain to get the most benefit from aerobic exercise. The target zone is based on age and contains an upper and a lower limit.

To determine your target zone, first measure your resting heart rate by feeling your pulse and counting the beats for one minute. Since this is your *resting* heart rate, you must do this when your body is at rest and at least 30 minutes after any strenuous physical activity. The best way to find your pulse is to touch the fingertips to the side of your neck just below the jawbone. Move your fingertips around until you can feel a good strong pulse. Record the number of beats per minute. This is your resting heart rate.

Subtract your age from 220. Then, subtract your resting heart rate from this number. Multiply the result by 0.65 and then multiply the same number again by 0.75. Add your resting heart rate to the results to get the lower and upper heart rates of your target zone.

The formula is as follows: A = age, B = resting heart rate

$$[(220 - A - B) \times .65] + B = \text{lower limit}$$
$$[(220 - A - B) \times .75] + B = \text{upper limit}$$

Example: A 30-year-old with a resting heart rate 70 beats/minute.

$$[(220 - 30 - 70) \times .65] + 70 = \text{lower limit}$$
$$[(120) \times .65] + 70 = \text{lower limit}$$
$$[78] + 70 = 148 = \text{lower limit}$$

$$[(220 - 30 - 70) \times .75] + 70 = \text{upper limit}$$
$$[(120) \times .75] + 70 = \text{upper limit}$$
$$[90] + 70 = 160 = \text{upper limit}$$

As you warm up, your resting heart rate increases until it is in your target zone. Maintain a level of activity to keep your heart rate within your target zone. Check your pulse from time to time during your workout. Count the number of beats your heart makes in 15 seconds and mutitply that by four to get the rate per minute. Do not sit down or rest; continue to walk or lightly exercise as you take this count. If your heart rate is low, increase the speed or intensity of your exercise. If your heart rate is high, slow down.

At first, you will need to check your heart rate frequently, but as you become more familiar with your exercise routine and how your body functions, you will be able to "feel" the pace you need to keep.

than you're used to. In the beginning you can actually feel lethargic, fatigued, and even sick as toxins are released.

You don't need to detox this quickly. Take it easy and detox gradually. Start by limiting yourself to only ten minutes a day. That is all you need to do at first. Exercise five to six times a week. Each week add an additional three to five minutes to your workout time until you spend at least 30 minutes a day rebounding.

One of the beautiful aspects of rebounding is that effects are cumulative. You don't have to do your full workout all at one time. You can break it up into increments spread throughout the day. In fact, it is actually more beneficial to do it this way. If your total workout time is ten minutes, you can split it up into three sessions, two three-minute sessions and one four-minute session. Add a minute or so to each session each week until you are doing three ten-minutes sessions. You may also do four or five sessions if you like. A good time to exercise is just before breakfast, lunch, and dinner because the exercise will decrease your appetite.

A problem with rebounding is that it looks too easy. People think that exercise has to be hard or hurt to be effective. Or that you need expensive hi-tech equipment. That is not so. Walking as well as rebounding are excellent forms of exercise and both are simple and inexpensive.

Rebounding has been studied by NASA scientists and universities over the past several years. Their conclusions all collaborate the many health benefits of this form of exercise. The merits, theory, and evidence for rebound exercise as described here is aptly presented in the book *The New Miracles of Rebound Exercise* by Albert E. Carter.

Thousands of people have discovered the healing benefits of rebound exercise simply by doing it. Dorothy had arthritis in her right knee and both ankles; bursitis in her right shoulder and both hips; suffered constant back aches; and was chronically fatigued. Headaches, high-blood pressure, ringing in her ears, and poor balance plagued her as well.

"All this had been going on for years on end. I was constantly under a doctor's care. He told me I was just getting old and had to expect this sort of thing."

Her husband Walt had severe problems too. He suffered a heart attack, was diabetic, and had four cancer surgeries.

This all changed. Dorothy explains that one day, "Walt brought home a rebounder. He was excited, but I was skeptical. For three days I watched him bounce for 30 seconds at a time. Each day he seemed brighter and had more energy. His disposition turned happy and sunny and he literally began to whistle while he worked, something I hadn't heard for a long time.

"Following his example, I tried to use the rebounder but couldn't keep my balance. Walt held my hands to steady me morning and evening for three days. Sure enough, I began to feel better too! In two weeks my blood pressure dropped 30 points! I had more stamina, and I lost 8 pounds. I began to sing while I worked—literally sing! Life took on a whole new outlook. I had hurt and been tired for so long, I had actually forgotten how it felt to feel really good—no, really great!

"After just two and a half months, my back aches and headaches were gone. No more arthritis or bursitis pain. The leg and foot cramps that woke me up every night disappeared. I went from a size 24 to a size 18!

"And listen to what rebounding has done for Walt! His stamina and recuperative powers have reached phenomenal dimensions. He lost 18 pounds. His cholesterol level is 10 points below normal. His heart rate dropped 8 beats per minute. His eyesight has cleared. He watches television and drives without glasses. The doctor says that he is now in better physical condition than any time since he has known him!"

Much more can be said about the health benefits of rebound exercise, but there is not space enough in this volume. For more information on rebound exercise, see Carter's book.

 ADDITIONAL RESOURCES

Aerobics: The Aerobics Program for Total Well-Being. Cooper, Kenneth, M.D. New York: Bantam Books, 1980.

Rebound to Better Health. Fife, Bruce, N.D. Colorado Springs, CO: HealthWise Publications, 2000.

Getting in Shape: Workout Programs for Men and Women. Anderson, Bob; Burke, Ed; Pearl, Bill. Bolinas, CA: Shelter Publications, 1994.

The New Miracles of Rebound Exercise. Carter, Albert E. Orem, UT: American Institute of Reboundology, 1988.

Walking for the Health of it. Ralston, Jeannie. Glenview, IL: Scott Foresman & Co., 1986.

Walking Medicine. Yanker, Gary and Burton, Kathy. New York: McGraw-Hill, 1990.

Chapter 10

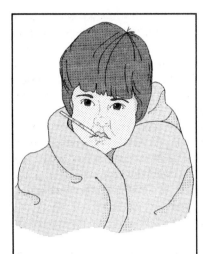

Give me the power to create a fever, and I shall cure any disease.

—Parmenides (500 B.C.)

HEAT THERAPY

Heat therapy, technically referred to as hyperthermia, is also known as sweat therapy, because it generates perspiration; or fever therapy, because it induces an "artificial" fever. Heat therapy is one of the most powerful natural cleansing methods known. Heat draws out toxins, helps clean out clogged pores, kills harmful microbes, increases circulation and oxygenation of tissues, stimulates glands and organs, enhances the immune system, gives a cardiovascular workout similar to aerobic exercise, and invigorates and refreshes the mind. Hyperthermia is, in a sense, a natural all-purpose body cleanser.

Hyperthermia is one of the oldest forms of therapy. For thousands of years people have known of its powerful health-enhancing effects. The early Romans built elaborate baths which included saunas, cold-plunge pools, and swimming areas. Before them the Egyptians, Greeks, and other Mediterranean cultures all practiced some form of heat therapy. In the Middle East and northern Africa, the people have their bathhouses which are still a part of Muslim life. The Turkish bath has been popular in Europe for centuries. Native American cultures used sweat lodges as a part of their cleansing practices. Japan, India, Russia, Finland, and many other countries have long traditions of using steam baths and saunas for purification and healing. The benefits of heat, in one form or another, have been recognized in many cultures around the world. Even now, health clubs and spas include therapeutic baths and saunas.

The Greek physician Parmenides is credited with saying, "Give me the power to create a fever, and I shall cure any disease." Heat therapy which incorporates steam baths and saunas is a way in which we can produce an "artificial" fever.

Over the years, physicians have observed that people suffering from many diverse ailments have been cured following a high fever from another illness. A treatment for cancer was derived this way. People with cancer, when afflicted by malaria with its accompanying high fever, if they survived the infection the cancer also disappeared. This began the treatment of cancer using benign forms of malaria to induce a cancer-killing fever. Before the advent of antibiotics, people suffering with syphilis and other contagious diseases were often infected with malaria to control their illness—a risky practice since the malaria itself could be fatal.

Modern research has found heat therapy to be effective against a wide range of conditions, ranging from the common cold to influenza, hemorrhoids, acne, arthritis, prostatitis, and chronic fatigue syndrome, as well as life-threatening illnesses like cancer.

With all the historical evidence, recent research, and facilities available, it is surprising to find that the majority of people are unaware of the marvelous healing and cleansing benefits of steam baths and sweat therapy.

THERAPEUTIC BENEFITS OF HEAT
Fever

In the past, an artificial fever was almost always induced to treat a person suffering from an infectious illness. It was common knowledge back then that increasing the patient's temperature to the point of inducing profuse perspiration would "sweat the infection out." And it worked great for many viral and bacterial infections as well as other conditions.

Nowadays, fever is often mistakenly thought of as an undesirable symptom of illness because it increases our discomfort during this time. People will often take medication to reduce their fever. This stifles the natural healing process and prolongs the illness. Elevating internal temperature is one of the body's major defense mechanisms against invading organisms. It is vital to the healing process for many illnesses.

Bacteria and viruses, which cause most infectious illnesses, are heat sensitive. At 104 degrees F, for example, the growth rate of the polio virus is reduced by a factor of 250; the growth rate for pneumococcus, a bacterium responsible for pneumonia, also is retarded and dies at 106 degrees. The body ordinarily does not need to raise temperatures this high to fight off most infections. Raising the temperature just a few degrees above normal is effective in combating rhinovirus which causes the common cold and is responsible for one-half of all respiratory infections. Heat also can effectively control influenza, including all the new strains that appear from time to time for which there is no vaccine. Other infectious conditions that respond to fever include upper and lower respiratory tract infections, bladder problems, urinary tract infections and a diverse number of diseases such as chickenpox, shingles, herpes, syphilis, gonorrhea, and even AIDS. Virtually every known disease-causing virus and bacteria is vulnerable to heat within the range of human tissue tolerance. Medical literature is filled with references to the use of heat therapy in conventional medicine as an aid in the treatment of numerous illnesses.

A fever exists when the body's temperature rises above its normal level of 98.6 degrees F. Some fevers are mild, raising body temperature only a degree or two while others can be severe—over 104 degrees F. Microorganisms can usually tolerate only a narrow range of temperature. This range is generally much narrower than what human tissue can endure without injury. Disease-causing organisms which thrive at normal body temperature, when subjected to temperatures just a few degrees higher, will either die or slow down their growth rate, giving the immune system time to mobilize its defense forces which purge the invaders from the body.

Heat therapy is a process that raises the body's internal temperature just like a fever. This artificial fever has the same healing effect as the body's own heat generating mechanism. An artificial fever can be induced when the body's natural healing mechanisms are weakened by toxic accumulations, prolonged illness, or injury and cannot effectively fight off infections or generate an adequate fever.

Inducing a fever when an infection is just starting and before the body has had time to respond, is the quickest and easiest way to cleanse troublesome microorganisms from our system. Symptoms of infection, particularly low-grade infections, can go nearly unnoticed until the organism has thoroughly overrun the body and a full-blown disease crisis exists. Periodically inducing a fever with heat therapy, even when no symptoms are present, will kill offending organisms before they can establish a foothold. This also relieves the immune system from a frantic mobilization, thus reserving vital energy and nutrients needed for normal metabolic functions.

Not only does fever or heat kill harmful microorganisms but it stimulates body systems to increase metabolism, immune function, and circulation, which greatly enhances the body's cleansing and healing processes.

Increased Metabolism

Heat stimulates cellular activity, increasing metabolism. According to A.C. Guyton, M.D., an authority in the field of medical physiology, the metabolic rate increases 25 percent with a rise in temperature of five degrees F (from 98.6 to 103.6 degrees measured orally). As temperature increases, bodily functions are supercharged, working at an increased level of efficiency. This is very important because the cleansing and healing processes are enhanced.

Glandular functions, circulation, healing and tissue rebuilding, and other processes are all stimulated into vigorous activity. Injuries heal faster, toxins and metabolic wastes are removed faster, and hormones and enzymes are produced quicker. Heat stimulates all bodily functions.

Many people are frequently sick and slow to heal because their metabolism is slowed by toxic encumbrance and tissue degeneration. Because of slow metabolic rate, weight problems are common for such people. They may eat little but still gain weight. When metabolism is slow, calorie consumption by the body decreases and excess dietary calories are converted to fat. Excess fat hampers all body systems, increasing blood pressure and adding strain to the heart and numerous other organs. Being overweight is a risk factor associated with many degenerative diseases.

Heat therapy helps to burn calories and reduce weight. Using heat to lose weight is not a new idea. Saunas and sweat baths have been used for this purpose for years. The weight-reduction principle associated with sweat therapy is not based on the loss of water (sweat), as many believe, but on the stimulation of the metabolic rate which causes an increase in calorie consumption. Combined with a calorie-restricted diet, heat therapy can help burn off excess body fat, cleansing the body of needless and harmful tissues.

Increased Circulation

Much of the therapeutic effect of heat comes as a result of improved circulation of body fluids. The importance of blood and lymph fluid circulation is extensively covered in Chapter 9 on exercise. Heat gives you much of the same benefits as exercise. Like exercise, it increases oxygen intake, increases the heart rate, dilates blood vessels, and stimulates blood and lymph flow throughout the body, which in turn, distributes healing nutrients, oxygen, antibodies, hormones, leukocytes (disease-fighting white blood cells), and removes harmful wastes and toxins.

Pulse rate increases from about 75 beats per minute to between 100-150 beats per minute in 15-20 minutes. This greatly increases blood circulation, but *not* blood pressure, because heat also causes the blood vessels and capillaries to dilate, allowing an increased flow of blood.

Fluids reach deeper in greater quantities, penetrating throughout the body, even where circulation is normally sluggish. Delivery of oxygen is increased throughout the body. Oxygen neutralizes toxins (see Chapter 8), and kills pathogenic microorganisms and malignant cells like cancer. Widening of the capillaries enables the blood to carry great amounts of nutrients to the skin, enhancing the health and appearance of the skin. It also allows toxins deep in the body to be carried to the surface and excreted in the sweat. All organ systems benefit from the cleansing action of improved circulation.

Heat gives the heart and blood vessels a cardiovascular workout much like you would get from aerobic exercise. In a sense, heat therapy could be considered the lazy person's exercise. You can get much of the same benefits of exercise, such as increased metabolism, burning up calories, and improved circulation without physical exertion.

You wouldn't, however, get the muscular toning which is also an important aspect of exercise.

Detoxifier

Inducing a fever stimulates all organs and glands, including the immune system which has the job of neutralizing and cleansing toxins and pathogenic organisms from the body. Heat stimulates the production rate of white blood cells which increases the generation of antibodies and interferon (a group of proteins that attack viruses and which also has powerful cancer-fighting properties). White blood cells in the bloodstream increase by an average of 58% during artificially induced fever. The increased number of white blood cells boosts the immune systems capability to combat invading microorganisms and remove metabolic waste and toxic debris.

The body stores many toxins in fatty tissues. Heat therapy is one way to pull these toxins out of the cells and eliminate them from the body. Toxins are removed through the organs of elimination—skin, bowels, and kidneys, all of which are stimulated into feverish activity.

Studies show that heat can remove calcium deposits from the blood vessels and break down scar tissue from their walls. It has been determined the heat can remove harmful chemicals such as DDE (a metabolite of DDT), PCBs (polychlorinated biphenyls from plastic), and dioxin which have accumulated in fat cells.

Sweat therapy cleans clogged pores, and removes uric acid, heavy metals, and metabolic waste. Heat causes pores in the skin to open up, allowing millions of tiny sweat glands to excrete sweat which consists primarily of water and uric acid (the major component of urine). Because sweat contains almost the same elements as urine, the skin is often referred to as the third kidney. It is estimated that as much as 30 percent of body wastes are eliminated through perspiration.

People who have heavy toxic accumulations, such as heavy smokers, can leave a thick yellow residue on towels after a sauna. It has been observed that when sauna benches from public baths are replaced, the floors under the benches are covered with a thick, black layer of tar from accumulated perspiration.

HEAT TREATMENT

You can induce an artificial fever by soaking in a tub of hot water, sitting in a sauna or steam bath, wrapping yourself in blankets with a hot water bottle, or in any number of other ways. Choose a method that works best for you. Electric heating sources such as electric blankets, pads, or heaters should not be used. They emit electromagnetic radiation that disrupts the healing process.

The idea is to get hot enough to raise your body temperature to about 101-104 degrees F for 15-30 minutes. You can raise it as high as 105 degrees, but only maintain this temperature for about 15 minutes. The hotter you get and the longer you maintain the heat, the more relaxed you become. Heat may cause you to feel exhausted, just as if you had a vigorous workout, because the cells and tissues of the body have in effect, been working at an accelerated rate.

After a sweat bath your body will be totally relaxed and you will sleep very comfortably. For this reason, it is recommended that you do heat therapy in the evening and preferably just before retiring for the night. Otherwise, you may find yourself dozing off in the middle of the day or becoming too tired to focus on regular activities. If you don't feel tired after receiving heat therapy, you probably didn't stay in long enough or the temperature was not hot enough. Sometimes if you overdo it, you will feel fatigued and even become dizzy or light-headed. The body is drained of energy and the brain is essentially over oxygenated by the increased oxygen-rich blood flow. This will not hurt you, but it makes walking or driving uncomfortable. Take a nap and you will be okay.

One thing you should do before and after any heat treatment is to drink a full glass of water or fresh juice. You lose a lot of water through sweat and need to keep fluid levels up to prevent dehydration. Do not drink coffee, black tea, soda, milk, or any powdered sugary drinks. Drink only water, pure fruit or vegetable juice, or herbal tea.

Profuse sweating removes heavy metals, minerals, sodium chloride, and other metabolites. If you are on a salt restricted diet, you should increase your salt intake before engaging in heat therapy. You would do well to add a mineral supplement to your diet as well to replace essential trace minerals excreted during the purging process. There are many brands of liquid minerals available that will supply a wide range of trace minerals. If you have subclinical mineral deficiencies, sweat therapy can compound the problem. Eating the foods in the Natural Foods Diet on a regular basis and taking a mineral supplement will prevent mineral depletion during heat treatments.

Drink a full glass of liquid immediately after the therapy and more within the next 30 minutes if you do not go immediately to bed. Juice will restore some of the energy consumed by the heat-induced metabolic workout.

Since heat therapy stimulates most all body processes into vigorous activity, a great amount of energy is expended. Drinking juice will help replenish some of the lost energy-producing nutrients and help you recover your

strength quicker. Do not eat anything for at least an hour after treatment. Just like when you exercise, your blood is channeled away from the digestive organs and pumped into the skeletal muscles and skin tissues. The body does this to move heat to surface tissues and stimulate perspiration in its attempt to regulate temperature. Consequently, the digestive organs, lacking blood, become sluggish. Food eaten at this time is not digested or assimilated well. Ordinarily, after a heat treatment you will not be hungry anyway. The body is saying it doesn't need or want food at this time.

HEATING METHODS

Heat treatments can be accomplished in a number of ways. Perhaps the best heat sources are saunas and steam baths offered at spas and health clubs. The heat of a sauna is generally considered a dry heat; the heat of a steam room is wet or humid. This distinction is only partially correct. Although the heat in a sauna is generally dry, humidity is elevated to as much as 40 percent. Without some moisture, the hot dry sauna air can irritate the mucous membranes. The heat in steam baths is, as the name implies, from hot steam and is very humid. Regardless of the humidity, your temperature increases in either one, so it makes no difference which method you choose.

If you have the money, you can buy a portable sauna or steam unit designed for home use. These can hold one to two people and work very well. Most require no plumbing or attachments. You simply fill a small tank with water and turn on the heating device.

You can induce an artificial fever at home in numerous other ways with little or no expense. You do not need water. Lying under several warm blankets was the method utilized most often in the past to induce a fever to help fight off infections. Hot herbal teas that created internal heat were also consumed to enhance the effects of the blankets. You need to sleep through the night with the blankets on. This method works, but is not particularly enjoyable. You will sweat and if you have a lot of toxins in your body, these toxins will permanently stain the sheets.

The most convenient heat source is a bathtub full of hot water. A hot bath can work just as well as any sauna. Simply sitting in a tub of hot water or taking a hot shower does not work! You need to be completely submerged, except for the head, in water that is hot enough to raise your own body temperature.

Turn on the water as hot as you can stand it. Sit in the tub as it is filling up, keeping the water as hot as you can tolerate. Filling the tub in this way will help your body adjust to the temperature. After the tub is filled to capacity, turn off the water and submerge your entire body, keeping only your head above water. Relax and rest your head on a towel or a plastic air-filled pillow. While you soak and as the water cools, you can drain some out and add fresh hot water to keep the temperature as hot as possible. Usually as your body adjusts to the heat, you can withstand a little more hot water. Even though you are covered with water, your body will sweat profusely. Remain in the bath for 20-30 minutes.

The major problem with bathtubs is that most of them are too small. In order to make heat therapy effective, the entire body, except for the head, needs to be submerged. Most bathtubs are not big enough to do this. One solution to this problem is to buy a plastic sheet, available in various lengths at garden supply stores, and drape it over the tub, water, and yourself like a blanket. You do not wrap it around your body and it is not put in the water with you. It covers the top of the tub to seal in heat even though your knees or toes may stick out of the water.

Keep the plastic off your face. The head in any heat treatment should be left exposed to cool air. This will allow you to remain in the water longer, gaining full benefit. Covering the head is too draining on the body. It also helps to prevent headaches or dizziness that sometimes accompanies heat treatments. If you get headaches, try applying a cold compress to your forehead as you soak.

If you are concerned with exposure to chemicals, such as chlorine in the water, or if you don't have a bathtub, you have other options that will work just as well. Pouring a cup of 35 percent hydrogen peroxide in the bath water will neutralize these toxins. Another option is to use the heat from the sun. This can be done during summer months or anytime if you live a warm climate. The healing warming rays of the sun can be used to get a wonderful "sunbath."

Buy a piece of clear plastic that is at least 7 x 4 feet in size and 6 millimeters thick. You can use the thinner 4 millimeter size but 6 millimeters is better. The thicker size is important because it holds the heat in better and is more durable. You want a sheet of plastic large enough to cover your entire body with room to spare. Plastic sheets are inexpensive. You can get them wherever they sell garden or building supplies. These sheets are normally used to cover floors when painting or on gardens to keep weeds under control. Plastic sheeting is available in black or clear. Get the clear variety. If you use a black sheet outside, it can get extremely hot in the sun and even burn your skin.

The only things you need are a sheet of plastic, a towel, wash cloth or sunglasses, and a place to lie down. A reclining lawn chair works fine. You can also lie on the lawn or a mattress. If you have a trampoline that makes an ideal spot.

For the sweat-induced sunbath, lay the plastic down flat. Lie on top of one half and fold the other half across your body. Tuck the ends of the sheet under your feet to prevent draft from wind. Use a rolled up hand towel and put it under your neck for comfort. Tuck the edge of the plastic sheet under your body to keep out any cooling draft. Some people have described this as being wrapped up like a burrito. While lying on your back, wear sunglasses or put a washcloth over your eyes to protect them from the sun. Lie in this position for 10-15 minutes, then turn over onto your stomach for another 10-15 minutes. Keep your head out of the plastic.

If you are fair-skinned and sensitive to the sun, you may need to gradually increase your time of exposure, working up to about 30 minutes. Most people do not have to worry about exposure to ultraviolet light for this small amount of time. If the sun in your area is very intense, you can sunbathe at cooler times of the day, such as before noon or in the early evening. Full sunlight is actually healing and beneficial,

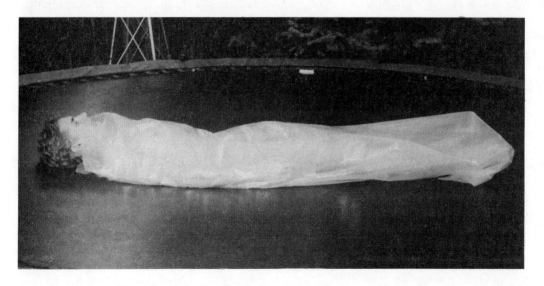

The warm rays of the sun can be used to create an effective steam blanket.

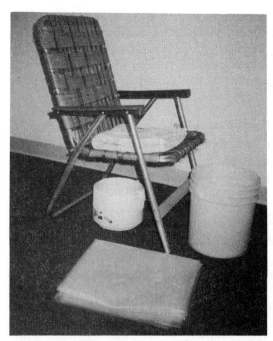

Items needed to create your own portable steam bath.

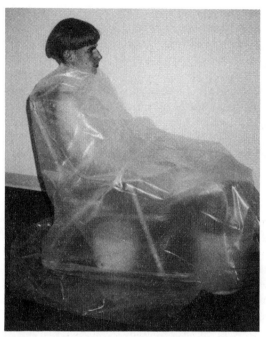

The portable steam bath in operation.

so long as you don't overdo it. If you are eating nutritious foods and you gradually increase your time in the sun, 30 minutes a day is therapeutic! Eating poor-quality foods encourages the growth of skin cancer and the deterioration of skin health which is associated with prolonged exposure to sunlight.

Another option, and one of the best, is to make your own portable steam bath. This portable steam bath can be used any time of year and in almost any location.

What you need is a lawn chair, towel, large plastic sheet, bucket, and steam-producing appliance. Basically what you do is sit in the chair wrapped in the sheet as steam fills the tent-like structure enclosing your body.

The steam-producing appliance can be an electric vegetable steamer, vaporizer, or electric fry pan. The vegetable steamer or vaporizer are the best choices. The steam source of your choice is placed under the lawn chair. Put a folded towel on the seat to protect your bottom from the hot steam. The plastic sheet needs to be big enough to drape around both you and the chair. You want the sheet to be large enough to go all the way to the floor to keep cool outside air out. Fill the bucket with very warm water.

Put the steamer directly under the chair and turn it on. Wait until steam begins to rise. Now sit in the chair on top of the towel, put your feet in the warm bucket of water, and drape the sheet around both the chair and you. Wrap the sheet around your neck. Keep your head exposed to the outside. Cover the bucket and your legs. You've created a

steam tent. The heat will build slowly. Keep the sheet tight so that too much steam is not lost. You may stay in the tent for up to 30-45 minutes.

Drink a glass of water before any heat treatment. To enhance the effects of the heat therapy, you can drink very warm water. This will speed the onset of an induced fever. Traditionally, teas have been used to generate internal heat. Herbs, classified as diaphoretics, heat the body and induce sweating. When combined with heat treatment, teas cause the cleansing results to be quicker and deeper. Diaphoretic herbs include: yarrow, ginger, sassafras, chamomile, blessed thistle, thyme, hyssop, catnip, spearmint, and cayenne. They work best taken in the form of tea. Even hot water by itself is diaphoretic.

Do not add sugar. Sugar depresses the immune system. If you can't drink the tea without some sweetener, use a half teaspoon of raw honey or preferably, molasses. You do not need to drink tea, but you should at least drink a glass of water before and after treatment.

End the treatment by taking a shower to wash off toxins and to refreshen yourself. Finishing the shower with cool water will help to invigorate you.

If you are coming down with an infection, such as a cold, you can fight it by continuing the heat treatment throughout the night. Immediately after the steam bath, get out of the tub or tent and dry yourself off. Immediately get into bed under a stack of warm blankets. You need to keep sweating throughout the night. Drink some diaphoretic tea to keep the cleansing process going. Go to sleep. Have water or tea ready if you become thirsty during the night. Use sheets that are old as they will be stained by your perspiration. In the morning, shower and drink plenty of liquids.

If you initiate heat treatment at the very first signs of a cold, you can drastically shorten the duration and severity of the illness. This is particularly true if you take care of yourself by avoiding stress and eating properly. Heat treatment will have little effect on a cold if you abuse your body by stuffing yourself with sugary donuts and greasy hamburgers, and wear down the body with work or other stress-causing activities.

HOT AND COLD TREATMENT

The effects of sweat therapy can be enhanced if you end the session with a cold shower. Heat causes blood vessels and capillaries to dilate, filling with blood. Cold causes tissues to constrict, forcing fluids deep into tissues and squeezing toxins out. Heat followed by cold generates increased circulation of body fluids and achieves deeper cleansing. Hot and cold treatment is very refreshing and invigorating and creates an enhanced sense of well-being.

After heat treatment, the body becomes relaxed and you may feel lethargic. A cold bath or shower will invigorate the body, stimulate circulation, and give you a boost of energy.

The practice of combining heat and cold has been used for centuries in many cultures around the world. Sweat lodges were used among the Native Americans. In the dead of winter, they would heat the inside of a well-insulated lodge with a huge fire. Many of them, essentially naked, would crowd into the heated lodge. Here they would simmer in the sweltering heat. After producing a heavy sweat, they would rush outside and jump into a nearby river flowing with icy cold water. Quite an invigorating ordeal!

You can use any heat treatment you desire, then cool off in a number of ways—in the shower or bathtub, or walk outside in a swimsuit on a cold wintery day.

After a hot bath or steam bath, immerse yourself into a full tub of cold water from the tap. The first effect is a slight shock. The initial chill will dissipate followed by comfort. If you remain in too long, a second chill will follow. A few minutes is all that is necessary. Leave the bath while you are still comfortable and before the second chill sets in. You should remain in the cold water anywhere from 30 seconds to 4 minutes or so, depending on your tolerance level. As you gain experience with this, your tolerance will increase and you can remain longer. Bath temperature should be *below* 65 degrees F. Generally

cold water straight from the tap is at least this cool. Some people submerge themselves in water that is nearly freezing, so 65 degrees is warm in comparison.

You can also use the shower. If you do, start with hot water. Then turn off the hot and rinse yourself with cold water for a minute or two. Use the coldest water you can stand.

The effects of the hot and cold treatment can be enhanced by repeating this procedure a couple of times, ending with a cold rinse. Turn the hot water back on for a few minutes, then the cold, back to the hot, and again switch to cold. Always finish with the cold water.

PRECAUTIONS

Heat therapy is one of the simplest and most powerful natural detoxifying methods known. Inducing a fever can rid toxins so fast that you are thrown into a healing crisis, and for this reason you should generally approach these methods with caution. A healing crisis will not hurt you. It may be uncomfortable and may worry those who do not understand the healing process, but a healing crisis occurs only when the body is strong enough to expel toxins. It is a *healing* process which strengthens the body, not weaken it.

Large amounts of toxins are sometimes released into the blood by the treatment and may cause symptoms like difficulty in breathing, heart arrhythmia (irregularity of rhythm), nausea, and in the case of recreational drug users, flashbacks and hallucinations. For this reason the person attempting heat therapy should first take time to clean up his or her diet and generally improve health to avoid too severe of a cleansing reaction.

Because of the increase in cardiovascular activity caused by high heat, sweat therapy is not recommended for people with heart disease or other cardiovascular problems. Individuals with high blood pressure or a serious illness should first consult with their doctor. This treatment is not advised for pregnant women, small children, the elderly, or anyone with an open wound.

If you desire to engage in a heat treatment after vigorous aerobic exercise, let your body cool down first. Exercise also heats up the body and drains fluids. Doing one immediately after the other may be too demanding on the body.

Limit your time to about 30 minutes. Drink plenty of water before and after the sweat bath to replace fluids lost during the treatment. The sweat glands can secrete nearly a full pint in 15 minutes, so dehydration is a real possibility if you are not careful. Take mineral supplements and eat a little salt on your food every day, but don't overdo it; eat only natural or sea salt. Leg cramps can result due to a lack of minerals.

Enjoy the process. Do no push your body too far beyond its comfort level. Your goal is not to sweat out every toxin in your body in one day, but over a period of time gradually release toxins and improve health. Sweat therapy should be an ongoing process.

Research has shown that cancerous cells are destroyed at temperatures of 106 to 110 degrees F. But, if a person's internal temperature becomes too elevated it can destroy healthy cells. Prolonged temperatures over 106 degrees F can cause tissue damage. For brief periods, temperatures as high as 106 degrees F can be tolerated without harm. However, you should not attempt to raise your temperature this high without proper supervision.

If you are not suffering from any serious chronic disease, you can raise your temperature up to 104 degrees F without problem. Once you get away from the heat, your temperature begins to drop and will return to normal in an hour or so. A cold shower accelerates the cooling process so that normal temperature returns in a fraction of that time.

If you get dizzy or have headaches with the heat, use a cool damp towel on your forehead while you are in treatment. If you still are dizzy or your body becomes extremely fatigued, reduce the temperature or your time. People suffering from chronic conditions will generally have a lower tolerance to the heat. Some may have a slight cleansing reaction after the first treatment and their condition may temporarily worsen. After a while your body will be able to tolerate higher temperatures and more time. As health improves, a higher tolerance follows.

Don't use heat treatment if you have a deep cut or other injury. Heat increases inflammation and the production of tissue fluid which produces swelling. If you have an injury, wait at least a few days for healing to take place. Heat can then accelerate the healing process.

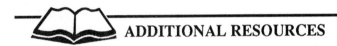 **ADDITIONAL RESOURCES**

Alternative Medicine. The Burton Goldberg Group. Fife, WA: Future Medicine publishing, 1994.

Home Remedies. Thrash, Agatha, M.D. Seale, AL: New Lifestyle Books, 1981.

Lectures in Naturopathic Hydrotherapy. Boyle, Wade, N.D. and Saine, Andre, N.D. East Palestine, OH: Buckeye Naturopathic Press, 1991.

Chapter 11

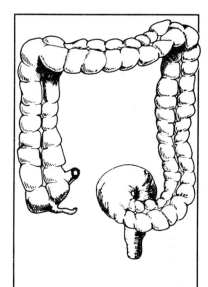

Each minute, 300 million of the body's cells die. If they were not replaced, all would be dead in about 230 days. Shortest-lived are the cells of the intestinal tract, lasting only a day or two.

COLON CLEANSING

The colon plays a vital role in the health of our entire body. The condition of this organ affects every other organ in the body and, consequently, our overall health. An unhealthy colon can have a direct relationship on the dysfunction or ill health of the liver, or the heart, or the brain, or any other organ. Having a healthy colon is vitally important for overall health and well-being. Keeping the colon healthy will prevent and even eliminate many "dis-ease" conditions in the body.

Most people in Western societies have unhealthy eliminatory organs. These organs are storage and breeding grounds for toxins and parasites. Detoxifying the bowels will greatly improve the way you look, feel, and act, and eliminate many unhealthy and annoying conditions.

TOXIC WASTE

The colon (also called the bowel) is the large intestine—the sewage pipe of our gastrointestinal tract. Its primary function is to collect and eliminate waste from the body. Another important function is its absorption of water and certain nutrients into the bloodstream.

Fecal waste enters the large intestine (colon) from the small intestine after most nutrient absorption has taken place. From here, muscles within the colon wall squeeze and push it along the intestinal canal. The colon starts on the lower right side of the abdomen, moves up toward the ribcage, crosses the body below the chest, and descends on the left side of the body where it bends up slightly and down again as it makes its way to the back of the pelvic area (see illustration on this page). Movement along this winding path is accomplished by what is called peristaltic motion—wave-like rhythmic contractions of the intestinal muscles.

It is easy to see that if the muscles do not work properly or the colon becomes distorted, movement of waste can bog down. And that is exactly what happens. A colon which becomes clogged becomes heavy with debris and can prolapse (that is distort by sagging), which further inhibits the flow of fecal material.

Through poor dietary habits, stress, insufficient exercise, illness, use of commercial laxatives, use of antibiotics, infrequent bowel movements, etc., the colon becomes sluggish and overburdened, and cannot function properly. Undigested food and body wastes accumulate, harden, and begin to adhere to the walls of the colon, further hindering elimination. When this occurs, an environment is established which encourages the growth of unhealthy bacteria, fungi, and parasites. Poisons from pathogenic organisms and decaying fecal matter slowly migrate through the mucous membrane of the colon and spread throughout the body.

The cells and tissues along the colon wall normally die, slough off, and are eliminated as a part of the feces. New cells regenerate and keep the colon new, fresh, clean, and alive. However, if the colon has excess waste accumulated and impacted on the canal walls, dead cells cannot be removed. They are stuck under the toxic feces and become toxic themselves as they decompose. Toxins from the fecal debris and dead cells seep through the colon wall and enter into surrounding tissues and the bloodstream. The dead, putrefying tissues and fecal waste decay inside the colon, giving off the odor of a decomposing carcass. This odor is often detected as body odor and bad breath. A healthy body does not have any unpleasant smell! The presence of body odor is one way you can tell if you or someone else is toxin laden.

Let me illustrate with an analogy. What would happen if you kept dumping waste from the kitchen into the garbage week after week without emptying it? After a couple of months what would it look and smell like? This is what happens to our colon when we are constipated. The garbage has nowhere to go, so it builds up in the bowel. Poisons eventually seep out and migrate into every cell in the body, setting the stage for "dis-ease." The immune system must work harder to remove these toxins, draining vital energy and lowering resistance to infections like colds and flus. Degenerative conditions begin to develop as the body's energy level is lowered and poisons accumulate. The fatigue, discomfort, and lack of overall health that results is blamed on aging. Degeneration of body and tissue is the result of autointoxication, not aging. There are many seniors who live vital, active lives without experiencing the pains and discomforts blamed on age. We blame age because autointoxication is a slow process and serious health problems that result from it are not always evident until later in life.

CONSTIPATION

Because fecal debris hardens and becomes encrusted onto the bowel walls, intestinal muscle integrity may be lost. Some areas of the bowel expand and grow large as they are engorged with fecal debris. Other segments may constrict or stretch thin, narrowing the canal and making passage more difficult. A weakened colon may balloon with accumulated waste and sag and stretch due to the excess weight, becoming distorted. The result is a badly

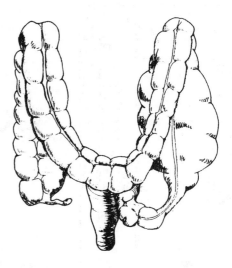

An unhealthy colon deformed by poor lifestyle and eating habits. In constrast, compare with the illustration of a healthy colon on page 142.

deformed colon where waste collects and putrefies; elimination of waste becomes ineffective and sporadic—a primary cause for constipation as well as colitis, colorectal cancer, and other colon diseases.

Most of us who live in affluent societies are chronically constipated—a consequence primarily of eating too much processed foods and not getting enough exercise. People may say they feel fine, they don't have stomach problems, so they believe they have a healthy colon. Yet, they suffer from constipation, as well as fatigue, skin blemishes, back pain, body odor, bad breath, poor digestion, gas, depression, etc. all of which can be caused by the absorption of toxins from a constipated colon.

People who are chronically constipated must strain to evacuate their bowels. The abdominal muscles must contract and a deep breath must be held as the diaphragm is forced downward in order to expel the small, hard fecal mass. The intra-abdominal pressures created by straining are also considered to be a cause of varicose veins, hiatal hernia, and hemorrhoids. Bowel evacuations should be very brief and effortless, not time-consuming, stressing ordeals. A healthy bowel will eliminate its contents in a matter of seconds. There will be no straining, no waiting, no discomfort.

How often should you have bowel movements? At what point would you be considered constipated? We can find the answer by observing people who have healthy digestive and eliminatory systems—people who are free from colon diseases. To find people of this type, scientists have studied primitive tribes. From these studies it was determined that a healthy digestive system will eliminate as often as food is eaten. Or in other words, you should have a bowel movement for every meal you eat.

To further substantiate elimination frequency, ask any mother—a baby will have a bowel movement after every meal. A baby's intestinal system is still young and healthy. It has not had time to develop digestive problems created by poor-quality foods, environmental toxins, or stress.

Most of us eat three meals a day, so ideally we should have three bowels movements a day. Generally, one to three bowel movements each day is considered the frequency necessary to maintain a healthy colon. For some people, even once a day is not enough. Aboriginal peoples can eliminate their entire bowel in one sitting. If you can do that, then once a day is enough. But if you must strain or if the evacuation produces little results, you are constipated.

Some people are surprised to learn that they should eliminate so often and so easily. They don't have a bowel movement every day, let alone three. They have become so used to being constipated that they don't realize they have a problem. For them it is "normal" to have one every second or third day, or even every five or six days. Some people don't do it any more often than every seven to ten days. That's only three to four bowel movements a month! Where does all the food go? It's certainly not absorbed to build body tissue, although some may be converted into fat.

Much of the food we eat is indigestible fiber. The body removes what it can from what is eaten and passes most everything else down the intestine and colon for elimination. If you eat three meals a day, day after day without a bowel evacuation, what happens to the undigested matter? This material doesn't just disappear. So what happens to it?—It stays in the colon! As fecal waste coats the inside of the colon, more is added, building up like the layers on an onion. The colon should have a canal about two inches in diameter, but when encrusted with fecal lining, this opening can be as narrow as the width of a pencil. Autopsies have revealed colons containing as much as 70 pounds of encrusted fecal material!

NUTRIENT ABSORPTION

One of the primary functions of the colon is the reabsorption of moisture from the feces. For proper elimination, the moisture content must not be too great, nor too little. Material which is too liquid moves so quickly through the intestines that nutrient absorption is poor.

Also, watery feces cannot clean or sweep the colon effectively. Too little moisture, on the other hand, plugs up the intestinal canal, and causes bloating, sagging, and distortion. The food we eat is moist. Additional juices are added in the stomach and intestine, making the undigested food mass quite runny. The colon reabsorbs much of this liquid to retain body fluid balance and to get the waste in a state which will allow easy movement and evacuation.

The product of a diet low in fiber (high in meat, dairy, and processed foods) is hard to eliminate. As fecal material builds up, movement through the colon becomes more difficult and slows down. This allows the colon to draw out more moisture than it normally would. As a result, the fecal material becomes encrusted along the lining, the walls of the colon turning hard and rubbery, making it almost impossible to remove. As a result, it creates a barrier which prevents nutrients from being absorbed through the intestinal wall. A person can eat like a horse and still be malnourished because the encrusted waste and mucus blocks nutrient absorption. The body, sensing a lack of essential nutrients, will signal food cravings to increase consumption in order to satisfy the body's need for balanced nutrition. Consequently, the person overeats, much of it going to fat, without significant nutrient absorption. So a person may be overweight, yet undernourished. Weight problems in some people may stem from an unhealthy colon and associated food cravings.

Clean out the colon and nutrient absorption improves, food cravings diminish and the compulsive need to eat diminishes, resulting in eating less food. The nutrients from the food that is eaten are absorbed more completely so you can function with more energy on less food. Energy is increased because less work is now required by the body to clean out toxins released from the colon.

COLON HEALTH
AND BODY HEALTH

Muscles that drive the peristaltic movement become weakened and ineffective if waste cannot be removed. The hardened, dense fecal lining prevents the muscles from completely contracting and thus movement in the colon is hampered even further. These muscles atrophy or lose integrity and more waste accumulates. This puts an unnecessary strain on the surrounding organs and the nervous system and also interferes with the absorption of nutrients from the colon.

As fecal material accumulates, excessive fermentation and putrefaction occurs, which leads to autointoxication. This material becomes a breeding ground for bacteria, fungi, and parasites. These organisms release poisons which are absorbed into the bloodstream and circulated throughout the entire body. The immune system constantly works to clean out these toxins. If enough of these toxins get into the bloodstream, the immune system will become overworked and, therefore, less effective, which can allow disease to gain a foothold. Toxins accumulate in the weakest areas of the body, since in these areas the organs and tissues may not be capable of removing them efficiently. These toxins accumulate and irritate surrounding tissues, often causing chronic inflammation, swelling, pain, and interfere with nerve impulses, which in turn may lead to degenerative conditions. These conditions may occur in any part of the body from the head to the toes. In this way, the health of the colon has a direct bearing on the health of the entire body. It is for this reason that the health of the colon is of major concern in achieving and maintaining good health for the entire body.

Besides contributing to all the problems associated with gaining weight (e.g., hypertension, heart disease, atherosclerosis, etc.), toxicity of the colon can manifest itself as headaches, excessive gas, skin blemishes, psoriasis, chronic fatigue, menstrual discomfort, prostate trouble, hemorrhoids, varicose veins, and heart problems, to name a few. A toxic colon can also affect the frequency and severity of colds and flus. A worn-out immune system will not be able to fight off infection as effectively as it otherwise could, so seasonal illnesses are more frequent.

Toxicity can also affect mental and emotional health. A person who is chronically constipated is often irritable, impatient, and moody, which can lead to marital and social problems. Cleaning the colon can have a pronounced effect on mental and physical well-being, making people much more pleasant to be around.

Fecal waste can be trapped in the colon for years. Yes, years. Once this material becomes encrusted onto the bowel walls, it is not easily removed and slowly poisons the body. This toxic accumulation of filth will remain in the colon for life if it is not removed by a detoxification program. If you are not eliminating completely and easily at least once a day, your colon is in trouble. Even if you have daily bowel movements, you could still have problems with your colon. If you experience any of the symptoms mentioned above, it is possible that they stem from putrefied waste trapped in your colon.

There are ways to detoxify and restore the colon and, in turn, our bodies to good health. Diet, exercise, and colonic flushes (e.g., herbal laxatives, enemas, and colonics) are the natural methods used to clean out the bowels and maintain good colon health. Natural laxatives are beneficial for minor problems, but chronic congestion may need more direct treatment. Enemas and colonics clean out the bowels by injecting water into the rectum. The water loosens the fecal matter which is then expelled. Enemas can be done at home. Colonics require a colonic therapist and special irrigation equipment.

Fermentation is a process that has been used for generations to make cheese, wine, yogurt, sauerkraut, pickles, miso, and other foods. One of the families of microorganisms involved in the fermentation of foods is Lactobacillus, which is a bacteria. Some Lactobacilli are harmful, such as the culprits that cause tooth decay; others, like acidophilus, are beneficial. Acidophilus is of great importance to us because it lives in the colon and helps with nutrient absorption and digestion as well as provide protection from harmful bacteria and other pathogenic microorganisms.

Studies performed in the 1950s were conducted to compare acidophilus with the drug neomycin sulfate to combat E. coli infection. Acidophilus proved to be 97 percent as effective as neomycin sulfate in combating E. coli infection. Acidophilus not only keeps harmful microorganisms in check, but prevents the development of many degenerative conditions of the digestive tract. Digestive disorders, including diarrhea, constipation, irritable colon and colitis, have been relieved by the administration of acidophilus.

British nutritionist K.W. Heaton reported in the *Journal of the Royal Society of Medicine* in 1986 about immigrants from Gujarat, India. When these Indians, primarily of the Hindu faith, move to London, they develop a variety of nutritional problems. One of the major foods in the diet of these people is kefir, a yogurt-like food fermented by acidophilus. Heaton noted that in India they eat imperfectly washed vegetables that are likely covered with acidophilus from the soil in their gardens. When these people moved to England, they eat well-washed British vegetables purchased from the local greengrocer. As time passes and the Indians become "more British," they begin eating an "endless variety of sugary foods and drinks," stop making kefir, and over a few years begin to "manifest a high prevalence of obesity, diabetes, and coronary heart disease." Although many dietary factors may be involved, the lack of acidophilus-containing foods and the consumption of foods which encourage the growth of harmful bacteria are major contributing factors in their ill health.

A healthy colon needs a healthy culture of "friendly" bacteria. This can only be done by eating a diet based on whole grains, fruits, and vegetables. Yogurt, kefir, and other soured milk products, which contain acidophilus, are also beneficial in moderate amounts. Acidophilus supplements, too, can help keep friendly bacteria in the

The Friendly Bacteria

Inside each of us live vast numbers of bacteria without which we could not remain in good health. There are several thousand billion in each person (more than all the cells in the body) divided into over four hundred species, most of them living in the digestive tract. If they were all placed together, the total weight of these "friendly" bacteria would come to nearly four pounds and, in fact, about a third of the fecal matter (less water) which you pass consists of dead or viable bacteria.

These bacteria are not parasites. And they do not exist as merely harmless inhabitants, but perform many important functions in the body. We live in true symbiosis with them. As long as we provide them with a reasonable diet and as long as they remain in good health, these bacteria provide valuable service in return.

However, not all of the friendly bacteria perform the same functions, some being far more useful and plentiful than others. Certain bacteria help to maintain good health while others have a definite value in helping us regain health once it has been upset.

Some beneficial functions of friendly bacteria include:

• They manufacture some important vitamins including niacin (B$_3$), pyridoxine (B$_6$), vitamin K, folic acid, and biotin.
• They manufacture the milk-digesting enzyme lactase which helps digest calcium-rich dairy products.
• They actively produce antibacterial substances which kill or deactivate hostile disease-causing bacteria. They do this by changing the local levels of acidity, by depriving pathogenic (disease-causing) bacteria of their nutrients, or by actually producing their own antibiotic substances which can kill invading bacteria, viruses, and yeasts. Naturally enough they are doing this to preserve "their" territory.
• Some bacteria (such as bifidobacteria and acidophilus) have been shown to have powerful anticarcinogenic features which are active against certain tumors.
• They improve the efficiency of the digestive tract—when they are weakened, bowel function is poor.
• They effectively help to reduce high cholesterol levels.

• They play an important part in the development of a baby's digestive function and immune system.
• They help protect against radiation damage and deactivate many toxic pollutants.
• They help to recycle estrogen which reduces the likelihood of menopausal symptoms and osteoporosis.
• Therapeutically they have been shown to be useful in treatment of acne, psoriasis, eczema, allergies, migraine, gout, rheumatic and arthritic conditions, cystitis, candidiasis, colitis, irritable bowel syndrome, and some forms of cancer.

Many factors influence just how healthy the bacteria are. While the type of friendly bacteria living in a region may seem much the same in health and disease, the tasks they perform change according to circumstances. For example, when bifidobacteria are in a good state of health, they will detoxify pollutants and carcinogens as well as manufacture various B vitamins. When in a poor state of health, however, they just cannot do these jobs as well or at all.

The type of diet you eat has a major influence on bacterial health. The bacteria are healthier on a diet rich in complex carbohydrates (vegetables, whole grains, legumes) and low in animal fats, fatty meat, sugars, and dairy products. Not surprisingly, the diet which is best for people is also ideal for healthy bacteria.

They are also influenced to a major extent by the degree of infection by yeasts and bacteria to which the bowel is subjected. Certain drugs, especially antibiotics, can severely upset this delicate balance (penicillin will kill friendly bacteria just as efficiently as it will kill disease-causing bacteria). Steroids (hormonal drugs such as cortisone, ACTH, prednisone, and birth control pills) also cause great damage to the bowel flora.

Damaged friendly bacteria can regain health and efficiency by detoxifying the intestinal canal, improving diet, reducing stress, and supplementing good-quality bacteria such as *Lactobacillus acidophilus* or *Lactobacillus bulgaricus*.

Source: *Alternative Medicine* compiled by the Burton Goldberg Group.

colon, but they are no substitution for fiber-rich, natural foods. Acidophilus supplements will have little effect on a person who continually eats poor-quality foods.

DIETARY FIBER

Meat and dairy products are some of the primary culprits in colon malfunction. They are mucus-forming. Eating too much of these foods causes the bowels to excrete a great deal of mucus. If movement through the bowels is slow, the mucus dehydrates and becomes thick and sticky, slowing down movement even further. The longer material remains in the colon, the more water is absorbed and the harder the fecal material becomes. Fiber-poor foods which are primarily the processed and refined foods (e.g., white flour, sugar, and foods made from these products), meat, and dairy which comprise the bulk of most people's diets, do not provide any aid in moving material through the intestines. In fact, if eaten in large quantities, some will go through the intestines undigested and contribute to the clogging of the colon. Fiber-rich foods (e.g., whole grains, fruits, vegetables, and legumes) work as a brush to sweep out the colon and keep everything moving along smoothly as it should. Eating primarily animal products and refined grains and other over-processed foods limits the amount of fiber in our diets. The lack of fiber has serious consequences on the function of the bowel.

Plants contain many different types of dietary fiber, predominantly as constituents of the cell walls. This fiber consists of compounds that, for the most part, are not digestible by the human body. Although fiber provides little nutritional value, it is important to digestion because it holds water, regulates bowel activity, and binds cholesterol, and carries it out of the body.

There are two types of dietary fiber: water-soluble and water-insoluble. Water-soluble fiber is found in abundance in fruit, oats, barley, and legumes. It has been shown to lower blood cholesterol and the rate of glucose absorption. Water-insoluble fiber found mostly in vegetables, wheat, and other grains, softens stools and accelerates intestinal transit time.

Observations by physicians working in Africa have led to the "fiber hypothesis," which states that consumption of unrefined, high-fiber, carbohydrate foods protects against many Western diseases, such as colon cancer and cardiovascular disease. Rural Africans who consume a diet high in fiber, show a low incidence of many chronic degenerative conditions. Some researchers, however, believe that these diseases result more frequently in Western countries due to the higher intake of meat, refined flour, and sugar rather than the absence of fibrous foods. Actually, both have a significant influence on our health.

Fecal bulk is largely a combination of undigested food, fiber, intestinal secretions, bacteria, and the remains of dead intestinal cells. Some of the foods we eat are not digestible because they are chemically altered by processing or cooking at high temperatures (e.g., barbecued or deep-fried foods) and the body cannot utilize them. Unlike dietary fiber, they do not aid in moving material through the colon, but plug it up.

Dietary fiber is that portion of plant food that cannot be digested by enzymes in the human digestive tract. Fiber is important because it absorbs cholesterol and water, providing a medium that is moist and mobile which can effectively sweep the inside of the bowel clean. A diet lacking in fiber will result in a toxic, constipated colon.

The colon absorbs water and some nutrients. If the walls of the colon are encrusted with fecal waste, water will be absorbed, dehydrating the fecal material making it hard and impenetrable. This creates a barrier which prevents nutrients from being absorbed. One of the major nutrients that enters the bloodstream through the colon is vitamin K. Vitamin K, an essential nutrient, is synthesized from dietary fiber by intestinal bacteria. A lack of vitamin K can cause serious health problems.

High-fiber foods also play a role in weight control. According to researchers, obesity is not seen in those parts of the world where people eat large amounts of fiber-rich foods. Foods high in fiber tend to be low in fat and simple sugars. Whole grain (high-fiber) breads provide less energy per pound than white (refined) breads. Fiber is removed in the milling process. Thus, a pound of whole wheat bread has more fiber and consequently less digestible carbohydrate (energy-producing nutrient) than a pound of white bread. The body receives more carbohydrate from white bread although less fiber, vitamins, minerals, and other nutrients. Overeating puts more energy-producing food (carbohydrate in particular) into the body than the body has need of; excess carbohydrate is then converted into fat and stored in the body. Most people eat far too much. They are eating refined carbohydrates that will be turned into body fat without supplying significant bulk, vitamins, or minerals. High-fiber foods, such as whole grains, because of their water-holding capacity produce a feeling of fullness. As a result, less food is eaten and less carbohydrate is turned into fat, yet more fiber and nutrients are consumed (since they were not removed in processing).

Many of the weight-loss products on the market are composed of bulk-inducing fibers such as methylcellulose. High-fiber foods reduce calorie consumption and consequently aid in losing weight.

Some types of fiber bind with cholesterol and carry it out of the body, thus reducing cholesterol. Knowing this, people have been buying pure fiber to sprinkle onto their foods. Not all fiber has similar effects. For example, wheat bran, which is an insoluble fiber, has no cholesterol-lowering effect, whereas oat bran and some of the fibers in apples (soluble fibers) do lower blood cholesterol. Unfortunately, the pure fiber they most often buy is wheat bran, the type with the least cholesterol-lowering effect. The fiber most effective at lowering blood cholesterol is found in abundance in fruit, oats, and legumes. On the other hand, wheat bran seems to be one of the most effective stool-softening types of fiber. Water-soluble fiber delays the time of transit of materials through the intestine, whereas insoluble fiber tend to accelerate transit time, thus alleviating or preventing constipation.

This does not mean that people should buy fiber in purified form. Whole foods, rather than processed, purified products, will offer the greatest benefits. Eating more fiber, like most other nutrients, is probably only better up to a point. Too much is no better for you than too little. Also, pure fiber is not as beneficial as the fiber in whole foods; the pure version is empty of nutrients, while the food version is loaded with them.

Health Benefits of Dietary Fiber

Weight control. A diet high in fibrous foods can promote weight loss if those foods displace concentrated fats and sweets. This is possible because fibrous foods offer less energy per serving than concentrated fats and sweets, thus providing fullness before too much energy-producing food is eaten.

Constipation and diarrhea relief. Some fibers attract water, thus softening the stools. Others help to solidify watery stools. By the one mechanism, they help relieve constipation, and by the other, they help relieve diarrhea.

Hemorrhoid prevention. Softer and larger stools ease elimination for the rectal muscles and reduce the pressure in the lower bowel, creating less likelihood that rectal veins will swell.

Appendicitis prevention. Fiber helps prevent compaction of the intestinal contents, which could obstruct the appendix and permit bacteria to invade and infect it.

Diverticulosis prevention. Fiber exercises the muscles of the digestive tract so that they retain their health and tone and resist bulging out into the pouches characteristic of diverticulosis.

Colon cancer prevention. Some fiber speeds up the passage of food residue through the digestive tract, thus shortening the transit time and helping to prevent exposure of the intestinal tissue to cancer-causing substances in food. Some fiber binds bile and carries it out of the body; this is also thought to reduce cancer risk. That fiber does have an independent protective effect of some kind is supported by evidence from Finland. The Finns eat a high-fat diet, but unlike other such diets, theirs is high in fiber as well. Their colon cancer rate is low, suggesting that fiber has a protective effect even in the presence of a high-fat diet.

Blood lipid and cardiovascular disease control. Some fiber binds with lipids (fats and oils) such as bile (which contains cholesterol) and is carried out of the body with the feces. Bile is made by the liver and stored in the gallbladder. It is excreted into the intestines to emulsify dietary fat, and then is reabsorbed. The removal of bile reduces the total amount of cholesterol remaining in the body. The lower cholesterol level consequently reduces the possible risk of heart and artery disease.

Blood glucose and insulin modulation. Monosaccharides (sugars) absorbed from some complex carbohydrates, in the presence of fiber, produce a moderate insulin response and an even rise in blood glucose concentrations. Insulin levels are high in obesity, cardiovascular disease, and diabetes (Type II), so this effect of fiber may be beneficial in all three diseases.

Diabetes control. Thanks to their effect on blood glucose concentrations, high-fiber foods help to manage diabetes. Persons with mild cases of diabetes, given high-fiber diets, have been able to reduce their inulin doses. Select complex carbohydrates from whole-grain breads and cereals, dried beans and peas, fruits, and vegetables. These foods provide fiber, and evidence suggests that diets high in fiber improve blood glucose control. Water-soluble fiber found in legumes, oats, barley, and some fruits slows the rate of glucose absorption for the GI tract into the blood.

Source: *Understanding Normal and Clinical Nutrition* by Eleanor Noss Whitney, Ph. D, et al.

People who increase their intake of high-fiber foods too rapidly may experience intestinal discomfort and gas. To avoid these side effects, increase dietary fiber intake gradually, and be sure fluid intake is adequate.

People in rural communities in Africa and India, who have healthy gastrointestinal tracts, consume approximately 60 grams of dietary fiber a day. Nutritionists recommend that we should eat at least 20 to 35 grams daily. This is about twice as much as the average intake in the United States, Canada, and most other Western countries. The diet can easily supply that amount, by replacing meat, dairy products, and refined, processed products with whole foods such as fruits, vegetables, legumes, and grains.

DO YOU NEED COLON CLEANSING?

How do you know if your colon is toxic and in need of a cleanse? If you eat a typical diet of meat, dairy, processed and refined foods, your colon is probably in poor health. Even those who eat primarily fruits and vegetables may be in need of colonic detoxification. Most people in modern Western societies were raised on typical grocery store and restaurant foods. Our intestines have been abused since childhood. Eating healthy high-fiber foods for a few months isn't going to clean it out. Even several years of healthy vegetarian eating may not correct many years of abuse.

Do you need to have your colon cleansed? Here are some signs which indicate colon detoxification is necessary.

Constipation. If you are not eliminating at least once a day. Evacuation should be effortless and brief. If you must force it or if it takes longer than a few seconds to completely evacuate your colon, you are more than likely constipated.

Diet. If you eat primarily meat, dairy, and processed foods. If your diet is low in fiber-rich foods like fruit, vegetables, whole grains, and nuts. If you have eaten low-fiber foods most of your life.

Overweight. Overeating puts a tremendous strain on the gastrointestinal tract. Food is not completely digested and passes into the colon where it can easily clog up the piping system. Rarely do people overeat fresh fruits and vegetables. Those who overeat consume poor-quality foods which tend to cause intestinal problems.

Stress. Stress affects every organ in the body, particularly the digestive organs. Stress slows down digestion and elimination. Chronic stress, anxiety, anger, fear, and agitation keep the digestive system operating at a reduced efficiency. Thus food is not completely digested, nutrients are not available for absorption, and food is passed along in the intestinal canal where it can lodge in the bowels.

Antibiotics. Antibiotics and some other drugs can slow down digestion and have the same effect as stress if used chronically. We all have bacteria in our intestines. Some bacteria are good and necessary for digestion and for the synthesis and absorption of vitamins. The good bacteria also keep the bad bacteria under control. Without the good bacteria, digestion and vitamin absorption would decrease and harmful bacteria could grow out of control. Antibiotics kill all bacteria, good and bad. If the bowels have become breeding grounds for pathogenic bacteria, the good bacteria will not be able to reestablish themselves.

Chronic health problems. Conditions such as fatigue, gas, acne, psoriasis, eczema, allergies, migraine, arthritis, vaginal or bladder infections, etc. Many of these problems are induced or aggravated by a toxic colon.

Body odor. Bad breath and body odor can be indicative of putrefied material in the colon and high degree of toxic accumulation throughout the body. A person who has a clean colon, is healthy, and bathes regularly will not have unpleasant body odors.

Lack of exercise. Exercise stimulates blood and lymph circulation (carrying nutrients throughout the body), aids the immune system (removes toxins and pathogenic microbes), and helps tone internal muscles (including the digestive organs). Indeed, all systems of the body are benefited by exercise. A lack of exercise slows down nutrient absorption, digestion, and elimination.

Most everyone can benefit from a detoxification of the intestinal canal. Even if you have a healthy colon, a *natural* cleansing treatment will do you no harm. People who have a greatly distorted intestinal canal will need to have regular cleansing. Some of the herbal detoxification methods and abdominal exercises will bring back a great deal of muscle integrity and restore function, but they are unlikely to create a toned twenty-year-old colon in a sixty-year-old body. A prolapsed (sagging) colon, for example, may be lifted back to some degree but it may never be completely restored to its ideal position. It all depends on how severely it was abused and distorted and how much effort the person puts into restoration and cleansing. So, for some people colon detoxification should become a regular process.

COLON EXERCISE

Muscular movement, internal massage, and fluid circulation aid in the digestive and eliminative processes. Physical exercise enhances intestinal movements, thus improving the transport of material through the canal. Exercise also helps maintain integrity of the intestinal muscles which keep the internal organs in tone and working properly.

Any exercise is beneficial to the body as long as it does not cause injury. Aerobics, jogging, weight lifting, etc. will all benefit the intestinal and abdominal muscles to some degree. Abdominal and deep breathing exercises are the best as they focus the activity in the abdominal area.

One of the best forms of exercise for the abdominal area and the intestines is slant board exercise. A slant board is a padded plank that is somewhat taller than the body. This board is set in a slanting position with one end on the floor and the other end elevated a foot or two. The board can be propped up on a chair, stool, or stair step. You would then lie down on the slant board with your head down toward the floor. You will feel almost as if you were on your head.

During the day we walk and sit with the force of gravity constantly pulling on us. Our internal organs, under this stress, are constantly being pulled downward, and may become distorted and even prolapsed. With the body inverted on a slant board, all of the internal organs, not just the intestines, are pulled back into place.

Inversion techniques have long been used in the Orient, especially India. Yoga exercises incorporate inversion positions to enhance the health of internal organs. Deep breathing is also an important aspect of yoga and an excellent abdominal exercise and intestinal toner.

You can gain a great deal of internal exercise by simply lying in an inverted position on the slant board—without doing anything else. You should maintain this position for 20 to 30 minutes. This is an excellent way to relax during a hectic day. Turn on some soothing music to help you relax. If you fall asleep and remain there an hour or more, that is all right. You won't harm yourself if you stay there longer. The only caution is, if you have heart problems or high blood pressure to check with your doctor before using a slant board.

You can enhance the benefits of inversion by practicing deep breathing while inverted. Breathe slowly from the diaphragm and consciously expand and contract the abdominal area with each breath (see Chapter 8, deep breathing exercises).

A more complete workout can be done by adding exercises. The following are a few examples.

Bicycle. Lift your legs into the air and peddle like you are riding a bicycle. You may want to time yourself. Do it for one minute, then rest for a minute; repeat the exercise three times with short rests in between. As your strength and endurance increase, you can increase the length of time you peddle, but keep the rest periods between them at about one minute.

Crunches. With you hands on top of your head or folded across your chest, bend forward as if to do a sit-up, but only lift your head and shoulders off the board. You come up only a few inches, stop, and drop slowly back down. Do as many repetitions as you can.

Twists. With hands over your head, turn your head to the right and twist your left shoulder over to the right as far as you can go. Stop and come back. Do the same thing on the other side. Twist your head and right shoulder to the left and then back. Try to keep your fanny flat on the board—do not lift it as you twist from side to side. This exercise can be done for a minute or so. You can do three sets of this exercise with short rests in between.

Slant boards can be purchased or made from scratch with a piece of wood and foam padding. Inversion tables and harnesses are also available from dealers. These devices clamp onto your feet and allow you to adjust the angle. You can simply step onto one, strap yourself in, and slowly flip yourself back. They are very convenient, but can be expensive. Check with your local health food store for more information on commercially made slant boards and inversion tables.

LAXATIVES

Constipation is commonly treated by taking a cathartic or a laxative. These medications loosen the bowels and promote evacuation. Cathartics are stronger than laxatives and work more rapidly; the two terms, however, are often used interchangeably.

Cathartics should only be used under medical supervision. The use of any drug to promote colonic evacuation is discouraged. Laxatives, if used habitually, contribute to, rather than relieve, constipation. They may cause excessive loss of fluid from the body, leading to dehydration. The loss of fluid resulting from dehydration affects every cell in the body. Lack of adequate water in the body slows down normal cellular processes (including the immune response) and in extreme cases can lead to death. Laxatives also speed motility (movement) of material through the intestine where most of our nutrients are absorbed. Forcing food through the intestines before digestion is complete may lead to malnutrition. In addition, commercial laxatives can have undesirable side effects, such as diarrhea, mucus in the stool, abdominal cramping, and even liver toxicity.

Most commercial laxatives act as chemical irritants and stimulate the muscular walls of the colon to contract abnormally to expel the irritating substances. It is very easy to become dependent upon these drugs and permanently destroy the normal ability of the colon to eliminate naturally. Castor oil has been commonly used as a strong laxative. This medicine causes irritation of the bowel, and is now used less frequently. Saline (salt-containing) laxatives produce their effect by causing the intestine to retain water that is normally absorbed into the blood. This causes fluid to accumulate in the bowel and aids in evacuation. Epsom salts and sodium phosphate are familiar examples.

Never take a strong laxative when there is abdominal pain. This pain may be a warning signal of appendicitis, and the laxative may cause rupture of the infected appendix.

No laxative should be taken regularly for the treatment of constipation. Constipation is best treated with a high-fiber diet and exercise.

Natural methods of evacuating the bowel can be used with beneficial results. A glass of hot water taken half an hour before breakfast has a very mild laxative action, as does a glass of fruit juice. Fruit, especially prunes, apricots, and figs have a mild laxative affect.

There are several herbal combinations that contain substances, such as cascara sagrada and psyllium seed, that are effective in cleaning the bowels, yet relatively harmless. Some commercially made herbal combinations can be purchased in health food stores.

I recommend an inexpensive combination you can put together yourself called the Ivy Bridges Formula. This formula makes a drink from natural sources which will help the body cleanse the bowels. It will cause you to empty your bowels frequently as it flushes encrusted and putrefied waste from your colon. The ingredients to the

Vitamin K

Vitamin K is made in your intestines—but not by you. It is synthesized by billions of bacteria which live harmlessly in your digestive tract. Bacterial syntheses in the intestines are our primary source of vitamin K. We also obtain some vitamin K through green leafy vegetables and members of the cabbage family.

A lack of vitamin K can lead to many deficiency conditions. Its primary importance is in the synthesis of blood-clotting proteins. Vitamin K is essential for the synthesis of at least four of the 13 proteins involved in making blood clot. If blood cannot clot, hemorrhage disease results. If an artery or vein is cut or broken under these circumstances, bleeding goes unstopped. (Many rodent poisons work because they counteract vitamin K which causes rodents to bleed to death.) Life-threatening vitamin K deficiency is seldom seen, but a combination of circumstances can bring it about.

Say, for example, a person is given antibiotics by his doctor to fight an infection. The antibiotics kill his intestinal bacteria which produce vitamin K. His diet lacks leafy greens and other vegetables that would also supply this vitamin. With his vitamin K stores depleted he suffers an injury from an accident. His blood fails to clot normally, and he bleeds to death.

The combination of antibiotics, vitamin K-poor diet, and injury leads to a potentially fatal situation. Taking sulfa drugs or antibiotics to combat bacterial infections (e.g., cystitis, strep throat, pneumonia, tetanus, syphilis, diphtheria, and other bacterial infections), destroys intestinal bacteria, which may lead to vitamin K deficiency. The routine prescription of antibiotics for any infection, including viral infections for which antibiotics are useless, kills helpful intestinal bacteria which supply essential vitamins.

Another very important function of vitamin K is the synthesis of blood protein that regulates blood calcium levels. Abnormal blood calcium levels can affect the health of the entire body. Calcium level in the blood is controlled by hormonal secretions from the parathyroid and thyroid glands which also affect bone density, and a deficiency in vitamin K can contribute to the development of osteoporosis. Without vitamin K, the bones produce an abnormal protein that cannot bind to the mineral crystal deposits that normally accumulate in bones. As a result bones may become weak.

Our cells are extremely sensitive to changing amounts of blood calcium. They cannot function normally with too much or too little calcium. With too much blood calcium, for example, brain cells and heart cells do not function normally; a person becomes mentally disturbed, and the heart may stop. With too little blood calcium, nerve cells become overactive, sometimes to such an extreme degree that they bombard muscles with so many impulses that the muscles go into spasms.

formula are readily available at most health food stores.
The formula is as follows:

½ cup apple juice
2 Tbs. liquid chlorophyll
2 Tbs. aloe vera juice
1 heaping tsp. psyllium powder
2 cascara sagrada capsules
1 glass of water

Mix the apple juice, chlorophyll, aloe vera juice, and psyllium powder together and drink it immediately, as the mixture thickens quickly. Follow with a full glass of water taken with two cascara sagrada capsules. This drink is best taken in the evening so it has time to work on during the night. In the morning when you awake, you will have your first bowel evacuation. You may experience a few more throughout the morning.

Drink the Ivy Bridges formula every day for about 30 days. If you have a serious constipation problem, you may extend this time up to 90 days. It is safe to use for this amount of time and promotes healing as well as cleansing.

The Ivy Bridges Formula is more than just an intestinal purgative. Unlike most commercial laxatives, it strengthens and promotes healing of the intestinal canal. The fiber-rich psyllium powder acts as a brush to sweep the colon clean. It provides bulk or fiber for the intestinal muscles to push and move fecal mass through the colon. It restores muscular integrity and promotes the return of regular eliminations.

Cascara sagrada is an herb that has long been used to relieve colon problems. It stimulates peristaltic muscular action of the intestinal canal. It is a natural laxative that can be used over an extended period of time without adverse effects. The formula recommends two capsules but if that causes abdominal discomfort or too strong of a laxative effect, you can cut down to using just one capsule.

Juice from the aloe vera plant is known for its ability to soothe and restore damaged skin tissue. For this reason, it is used in lotions and hand creams. In juice form it also has powerful healing and restorative properties on the intestines. It is a natural cathartic that has a strong stimulating effect on the muscles of the colon. It also kills and expels parasitic worms that may be inhabiting the intestines.

Chlorophyll is known to have revitalizing and refreshing effects on the intestinal organs. It is an antiseptic and promotes the growth of friendly bacteria in the intestinal tract. It provides intestinal nourishment and has a soothing or healing effect on the mucous linings.

Use of the Ivy Bridges Formula will help clean the colon, alleviate constipation, stimulate muscular contractions, and promote general intestinal health. It is far better than any commercial laxative and safe to use, even for extended periods of time.

Some people have thick encrusted mucus and fecal matter encasing their intestinal canal that prevents normal flow of intestinal debris. Purgatives and laxatives can do little to detoxify such heavy fecal accumulations. Even the Ivy Bridges Formula may not be able to penetrate and remove a thick accumulation of hardened debris. In such cases, an enema or colonic would be necessary to loosen and remove this highly toxic material.

ENEMA

An enema is an injection of liquid into the large intestine by way of the anal canal. The fluid soaks and loosens hardened fecal debris which sloughs off the intestinal wall and is flushed out of the body when the liquid is evacuated. Enemas have been used for therapeutic purposes for thousands of years. They have proven to be effective in removing hardened fecal material that otherwise would remain in the colon, poisoning the body and contributing to constipation.

Many people with intestinal problems have experienced almost immediate relief after having an enema. People who suffer from chronic headaches and migraines can often relieve their symptoms simply by having an enema. The headaches caused, at least in part, by toxic encumbrance in the colon. Once the noxious agents have been cleaned from the colon, the headache disappears. If the person has a great deal of fecal debris trapped in the colon, the headache may lessen, but not completely dissipate.

Enemas are more cleansing than laxatives. They do not have any of the side effects of laxatives and, unlike chemical laxatives, are completely harmless.

Enemas can, and usually are, administered without assistance and can be performed in the privacy of a bedroom or bathroom. Abdominal massage can enhance the emulsification of the intestinal debris, bringing about greater cleansing. In most cases more than one treatment is necessary to bring about complete cleansing. Generally, enemas must be repeated over a period of time. Some people do them once a day, others once a week, and others at no set interval, but as they feel the need.

The Ivy Bridges Formula will clean and tone a bowel that is not too encumbered with fecal waste. Enemas are needed if the Ivy Bridges Formula is not enough. Most people whose diet consists primarily of meat, dairy, fried foods, sweets, white bread, and other process and refined foods have serious bowel problems and trapped fecal waste. They may not even be aware of it. They have headaches, insomnia, skin blemishes, irritability, and other problems which can be directly related to a toxic colon. But they wouldn't know that these problems were caused by toxins seeping into their bloodstream from their colons because they may not experience any great pain in their colon. Most people, for example, wouldn't relate chronic psoriasis with the health of the intestines because they are unaware of the importance of colon health.

To clean out a toxic colon takes several enemas over a period of time in conjunction with the Ivy Bridges Formula. Both working together can bring about remarkable improvement in health. I can't tell you how often you should have an enema. Some people can become too dependent on them and do them every day, month after month, year after year. A more reasonable approach is to do two or three a week for several weeks, or months if necessary. At the same time, you should also be taking the Ivy Bridges drink and you should be eating lots of high-fiber foods such as fruits, vegetables, and grains—essentially the Natural Foods Diet. Eliminate or cut down on meat, dairy, fried foods, and other substances that promote intestinal blockage and mucus formation.

How to Do an Enema

Since enemas are a private matter, most people do not know how to do them. It is not something someone easily asks about. So I will explain in detail how to administer an enema yourself.

You can do the enema in the bathroom or bedroom, but you need easy access to a toilet. The materials necessary are few and inexpensive and can be obtained at a health food store. You will need:

- an enema bucket (or bag) to hold the enema solution (water)

- a tube with clamp that connects to the bucket (should be attached to bucket)

- natural lubricant such as vitamin E oil or K-Y jelly (not Vaseline)

- warm, distilled water (filtered water is okay)

Before administering the enema, try to empty your bowels first. This will remove the contents of the lower (sigmoid) colon and allow for better penetration of water. It will also allow you to hold the water longer which will aid in dissolving fecal matter.

Enemas are not difficult, nor do they cause pain (although you may experience some bloating similar to intestinal gas). You need to allow adequate time without being rushed. Give yourself 30 to 60 minutes to complete the process. Playing soothing music will help you relax and make the time spent more comforting.

Fill the enema bucket up with 32-48 ounces of warm water. Temperature should be like very warm bath water (about 102 degrees). The body's internal temperature is 101 degrees. This temperature is very warm to the touch, but is not hot. Clamp the tubing so it does not drain out. Place the bucket or hang the bag somewhere above your body. The water must run *downhill* into the rectum. You may hang the bag or bucket on a towel rack or hook. You could also try putting it on a high chair, music stand, or other piece of furniture.

You must lie down to administer the enema. This can be done in the bathtub, on the floor, or in bed. The bed is by far the most comfortable location. Since you will be holding the water internally, you need not fear making a mess on the bed. Put a bath towel down first, just in case some water drips.

After filling the container, undo the clamp and release a little water from the tube to let out any air bubbles. Reclamp. Lubricate the end of the tube with vitamin E oil, K-Y jelly, or another natural lubricant. Do not use Vaseline or any other petroleum-based or chemically manufactured substance.

Lie down on your left side. Take the lubricated tube and gently place it on the anal opening. The anus has two sphincter muscles that close to prevent the colon from leaking. One is at the anal opening and the other is just inside. Gently push the tube against the rectal opening. As the tube is pushed against the anus, the second sphincter muscle will constrict to prevent invasion by the tube. Stop and wait a few seconds. It usually helps if you gently spread the opening slightly to allow the tube to enter. The muscle will gradually relax; as it does, slowly push the tube with a twisting motion into the rectum. Push it in a couple of inches and stop.

Unclamp the tube to allow the water to flow. You will feel the warm water travel into your colon. The warmth of the water will cause the colon to expand slightly. With the tube still inserted, massage your abdomen, or flex and contract abdominal muscles. This will help the water flow further into the colon and relieve any bloating that might occur. When all the water has entered the colon, clamp the tube and slowly remove the nozzle.

Remain on your left side for another five minutes or so. Then turn face down into a knee-chest position with the weight of the body on the knees and one hand. Keep the head down so water will migrate to the top (transverse segment) of the colon. Use the free hand to massage the lower left side of the abdomen for several minutes. Massage is important because it helps break up encrusted fecal matter. Roll onto your back. Massage your abdomen starting on the lower left side (descending colon) and move up, then across just below your ribcage (transverse colon), and down your right side (ascending colon). This spreads the water as much as possible throughout the entire colon. Next, turn over to your right side for a few minutes, and massage the right side of your abdomen. Each portion of the colon is massaged, mixing contents as much as possible. Try to hold the water in as long as you can, up to 15 minutes is fine. If you need to expel it before then, do so. But the longer you can keep it in, the longer it has to work at dissolving and removing encrusted fecal matter.

During this process, you may experience some bloating or abdominal pressure. This is normal as your intestine contracts and cleanses. When you are ready to expel the fluid, get up and quickly go to the toilet. You will expel normal fecal matter as well as some unusual debris. Gray, green, or brown sticky mucus; small hard dark chunks; or long, tough ropy strands are frequently loosened and expelled during the enema. These toxic, putrefying substances are usually the obstacles interfering with normal bowel function.

After expelling the water, repeat the entire process a second time using cool (not ice cold) water instead of warm water. Heat is relaxing and warm water causes the intestinal muscles to relax and expand. This allows for deeper penetration of the water into the intestinal canal. Cool water has the opposite effect. It will cause the intestinal muscles to contract, encouraging them to move (improving tone and function) and break off and move out additional encrusted debris.

Enema Solutions

Water is the standard solution used for enemas. You should use pure distilled water to avoid injecting chlorine, fluorine, and other harmful chemicals into the body. Many people unknowingly use plain tap water. But tap water contains many toxic chemical and bacterial pollutants. It makes little sense to attempt to clean toxins out of the colon using a toxin laden solution.

You may add material, such as herbs, to the distilled water to enhance cleansing and healing. Herbal enemas can alkalize the typically overly acid bowel, help soothe irritation and inflammation, and promote healing of ulcerated tissues. There are several herbs that can be of benefit when added to the enema solution.

Garlic. This is a natural disinfectant. It helps kill

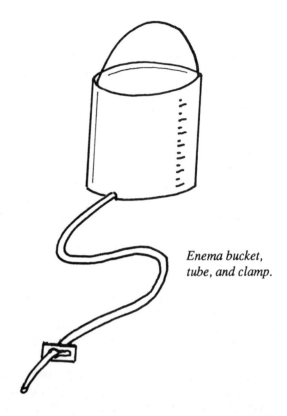

Enema bucket, tube, and clamp.

parasites and cleans out harmful bacteria, viruses, and fungi (which includes candida). Make an infusion by bringing a cup of water to a boil. Put five or six fresh chopped garlic cloves in a cup. Pour the water over the garlic and let it soak for about 15 minutes. Strain out the garlic (or use a tea ball). Discard the garlic pieces and add the tea to the enema solution.

Catnip. This herb, which is known for its hallucinogenic effect on cats, has many therapeutic uses in humans. It will detox and soothe the colon. Soak a teaspoon (you may also use a tea bag) of the herb in hot water for 15 minutes. Do not boil. Remove the herb and add the tea to the enema solution.

Pau d'arco. This South American herb has been used for centuries as a disinfectant. It is especially effective for yeast (fungal) infections. Make an infusion by soaking a teaspoon (you may also use a tea bag) of the herb in water brought to boiling temperature but removed from heat. Let it soak for 15 minutes. Remove herb and add the tea to the enema solution.

Aloe Vera. This valuable herb heals and soothes inflamed tissues and promotes growth of acidophilus—the friendly bacteria in the intestines which aids proper bowel function. Aloe vera juice is obtainable at most health food stores. Add one cup to the enema solution.

Acidophilus powder. When the colon is stopped up with encrusted debris, harmful bacteria and fungi can live and proliferate in the putrefying waste. Good bacteria, like acidophilus, cannot thrive in such conditions, and the harmful bacteria take over. Cleansing the colon will remove much of the material that encourages harmful microorganisms, but the good bacteria is still outnumbered. By adding acidophilus you encourage the reestablishment of the good bacteria. Mix four ounces of powder in four cups of water. It's also good for relief from gas and yeast infections.

Hydrogen peroxide. Hydrogen peroxide is an effective disinfectant. Mixed in the enema solution it provides a healthy dose of cleansing oxygen to the colon. Put eight drops of 35 percent food grade hydrogen peroxide per quart of distilled water for the enema solution.

The Coffee Enema

One of the best detoxifying agents used for the enema solution is coffee. Yes, ordinary coffee that people drink every day. In fact, using it as an enema solution is the only way coffee should be used in the body. Because of its cleansing action, coffee has become one of the most popular enema solutions recommended by holistic health care practitioners. It is not the coffee, per say, but the caffeine in the coffee that gives it its cleansing properties.

Using coffee in this way has been done for some time. Mention of it can be found in various folk medicine books. How it got started we don't really know. One account of its origin stems from the World War I era. Presumably, it was common during the war to administer opium as a rectal enema for use as a pain killer. This solution had a muddy brown color, very similar to coffee. As the story goes, during the height of a serious conflict, they ran out of opium. Soldiers wounded in the conflict looked to the opium enemas for relief from agonizing pain. In order to calm them as best they could, the medical staff administered coffee in place of opium to achieve a placebo effect. Apparently it worked and became general practice throughout the field hospitals at times when the opium supply was low. While coffee may not have actually had any pain-killing effect, its use apparently resulted in some benefit. Although this story may be apocryphal, using the coffee enema can lead to improved health.

Research on the use of coffee as an enema solution has demonstrated that caffeine is a very effective stimulant, fat emulsifier, and liver detoxifier. This is only true when injected rectally. Drinking coffee or other caffeinated drinks does not produce the same effects. It's as if nature made coffee for use in the rectum and not in the mouth, as most people use it.

When the coffee is injected into the colon, the caffeine is absorbed by the veins in the portal system and channeled directly into the liver. The caffeine stimulates

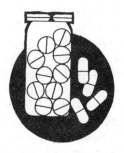

Crohn's Disease and Antibiotics

Although antibiotics have helped many people overcome infectious disease, it is also a harmful toxin to the body. Crohn's disease, which is an inflammatory condition of the intestinal tract that can cause diarrhea, abdominal cramps, or constipation, is believed to be caused by the buildup of intestinal toxins.

Crohn's disease was a rare condition prior to the 1950s. Since that time, there has been a rapid climb in developed countries and countries that have previously had virtually no reported cases. In fact, since 1950, Crohn's disease has spread like an epidemic. There is strong evidence that antibiotics are to blame. Penicillin and tetracycline have been available in oral form since 1953. The annual increase in prescriptions of antibiotics and the fact that there is a parallel increase in the annual incidence of Crohn's disease is harrowing. Comparative statistics have shown that wherever antibiotics are used early and in large quantities, the incidence of Crohn's disease is now quite high.

The widespread use and abuse of antibiotics is becoming increasingly alarming for many reasons, including the development of "supergerms" that are resistant to currently available antibiotics. However, prescriptions for antibiotics are not the only source of concern. Antibiotics have also been added to animal nutrition since the 1950s. Administration of sublethal amounts of antibiotics has been shown to induce a capacity for toxin production in intestinal organisms. This action may be playing a greater role in Crohn's disease than prescription antibiotics.

Over the years researchers have sought to identify Crohn's disease as an infectious process. There is some evidence to support the hypothesis that the pathogen is a component of the normal intestinal flora, for example a coliform bacterium, which suddenly produces immunostimulatory toxins or becomes invasive as a direct result of sublethal doses of antibiotics.

—*American Journal of Natural Medicine*, Vol. 2, No. 10

the liver and gallbladder to excrete toxins, open bile ducts, and encourage peristaltic action of the intestines. It breaks down the accumulated fat in the liver cells, encourages excretion of bile and removal of gallstones, and cleans the intestinal walls. All of these actions promote cleansing of the liver, gallbladder, and intestines. The liver is the main detoxifying organ of the body. When it is overworked and burdened with a toxic pileup, poisons circulate in the bloodstream and throughout the body. The coffee enema will cleanse the liver of much of these toxins so that it can function more efficiently. The coffee enema is used primarily to clean the liver and gallbladder rather than the colon.

Use one-fourth cup of regular (not decaffeinated) coffee in four cups of water. Heat to boiling. Filter out and discard the grounds. Use the liquid for the enema. Follow the coffee enema with another enema using only pure water. The second enema will remove remnants of the coffee solution as well as additional intestinal debris.

COLONIC

A colonic is similar to an enema except it cleans more thoroughly and must be administered by a trained colonic therapist. One problem with enemas is that it is difficult to adequately clean the entire colon. Enemas can clean the lower bowel (sigmoid and descending colon), but for some people the solution does not penetrate well into the upper two thirds of the colon (the transverse and ascending segments). Although you may put a substantial amount of water into the colon and massage it the best you can, the solution may not penetrate and dissolve matter from the entire organ. Colonics, on the other hand, inject the solution into the rectum by a hose. The fluid flows into the colon and travels all the way to the cecum (where colon and small intestine join). The water continually flows into the colon around and back out. This results in a more complete cleansing process.

A colonic machine pumps the water into the body and drains the waste water out. The colonic therapist aids in the process by massaging the client's abdominal area to ensure thorough penetration and to break up fecal debris.

For people who are chronically constipated and have serious toxic accumulations in their bowels, colonics are the preferred method of intestinal detoxification. For a badly distorted colon, an enema cannot penetrate effectively. Accumulated fecal debris blocks off complete circulation of the enema solution. In such cases enemas are not effective in cleaning the upper portions of the bowel. As the colon becomes cleaner and the canal widens and becomes less distorted, enemas become more useful. Herbal laxatives, such as the Ivy Bridges Formula, can be of benefit to anyone, whether they have major or relatively minor constipation problems. The Ivy Bridges Formula can (and should) also be used on a regular basis for a period of time along with colonics and enemas. Colonics and enemas will clean out the colon, but they will not restore muscle integrity. Exercise and herbal stimulants (such as cascara sagrada) will help to bring back muscular tone and function to atrophied intestinal muscles.

Since the colonic flushes out and cleans the entire colon, some people may wonder if the intestinal flora will be disturbed by this treatment. The intestinal flora are billions of microscopic organisms that include bacteria and fungi which inhabit the bowel and play a very important role in health and disease. Bacteria synthesize valuable nutrients, regulate acidity, and inhibit growth of harmful organisms. The proper balance of the friendly microorganisms is essential to a healthy colon. Even though a colonic removes a great deal of material, including good as well as bad bacteria, enough friendly organisms remain to easily repopulate the colon. In fact, colonics will enhance the growth of helpful bacteria since they thrive in an environment that is clean and healthy.

 **ADDITIONAL RESOURCES**

Gastrointestinal Health. Perkin, Steven, M.D. New York: Harper Perennial, 1992.

Healing Within: The Complete Guide to Colon Health. Weinberger, Stanley. Larkspur, CA: Healing Within Products, 1988.

Irritable Bowel Syndrome and Diverticulosis. Trickett, Shirley. London, England: Thorson's/Harper Collins, 1992.

Tissue Cleansing through Bowel Management. Jensen, Bernard, Ph.D. Escondido, CA: Bernard Jensen, 1981.

Chapter 12

KIDNEY CLEANSING

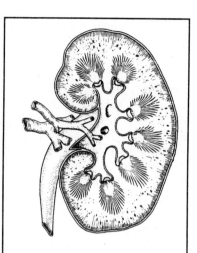

From a medical standpoint Roger was sick. He was 52 pounds overweight, retained water which caused swelling in his legs and feet, and had a severe psoriasis problem which produced red patches of scaly skin over parts of his body. The problem that concerned his doctors the most was kidney disease and the presence of kidney stones. The doctors told him his condition was too advanced for ordinary forms of treatment and that he would die. His only hope was to surgically remove his kidneys, put him on a dialysis machine for the rest of his life or attempt a kidney transplant.

The diagnosis did not give him much hope. At only 27 years of age, he considered himself too young for this type of disease. How could he have such health problems? These are degenerative conditions that happen to 72-year-olds, not 27-year-olds. He did not relish the idea of surgery and its consequences. Ignoring his doctor's advice to attempt a surgical solution, he turned to natural methods.

Roger visited a naturopathic physician who explained to him that his condition was treatable without surgery. Roger had grown up on a dairy farm and had lived most of his life on milk, ice cream, creamed cereal, beef, and processed flour and sugar. He continued to eat these foods as an adult. The naturopath modified his diet. Dairy and meat was restricted, and fruits, vegetables, and whole grains emphasized. Roger started a detoxification program. The program involved a kidney and bladder detoxification process consisting of herbal supplements and vitamins.

The process of detoxing the kidneys only took a few weeks, but Roger continued with the diet. He went back to his doctor for a checkup and reevaluation. His doctor was amazed. Roger's kidneys were functioning normally and there was no sign of kidney stones. The doctor did not believe the results and attributed them to errors. The tests were run again, but with the same results. The doctor could not understand.

Improved kidney health was just one of the benefits Roger gained while on the detoxification program. He also lost annoying excess weight; the swelling problem in his legs and feet subsided, and his psoriasis cleared up. He felt like a new man—a healthy 27-year-old man.

Most of Roger's health problems stemmed from his kidneys. The kidneys are one of the body's channels of elimination as well as one of the body's organs of regulation. If the kidneys cannot remove waste, toxins remain in the body and the body is forced to attempt to eliminate them through other channels. The skin

The physician is nature's assistant.
— Galen, 2nd Century AD

Chlorinated drinking water is directly responsible for more than 4,200 cases of bladder cancer and 6,500 cases of rectal cancer every year.
—Am. Jour. of Public Health

is also an organ of elimination, excreting uric acid and waste products in sweat and oil. If the kidneys are not functioning at full strength, toxins will be eliminated through the skin. This may cause rashes and psoriasis when irritating poisons are excreted through the skin.

The kidneys also regulate chemical balance and water content of the body. If the kidneys are not doing that job, chemical balance and water content are obviously affected, which can lead to numerous symptoms and health problems. When Roger cleaned up his diet, preventing new toxins from entering his body, and detoxified his urinary system, his body chemistry became normal, channels of waste elimination were able to function properly, and, consequently, his health improved.

THE URINARY SYSTEM

The urinary system produces and excretes urine from the body. It consists of the kidneys, bladder, and urinary ducts. The bladder is a storage tank for the urine. Urinary ducts are the tubings between the kidneys, bladder, and body orifice. The kidneys are the most important organs in this system. They regulate many functions vital in maintaining homeostasis (physiological balance between all body organs).

The primary function of the kidneys is to remove waste and other toxins from the blood, but they also maintain electrolyte, water, and acid-base balances in the body. These processes are vitally important to maintaining homeostasis. If the urinary system does not operate as it should, the normal composition of the blood cannot be maintained, and serious health consequences result.

You can locate the position of your kidneys on yourself; stand erect and put your fingers on the bony ridges of your hips with your thumbs meeting on your backbone. In this position, your kidneys lie just above your thumbs. Usually the right kidney is a little lower than the left. The kidneys lie just above your waistline under a layer of muscle. Often, when people complain about lower back pain, it is not their back or spine that is hurting, but their kidneys. Dehydration, due to illness or not drinking enough liquids, will cause your kidneys to become painful and you may complain of a "backache."

Just as our bodies produce waste from the food we eat, each of our cells produces waste as a result of metabolism. Cellular waste, certain drugs and other toxins are picked up by the blood and carried to the kidneys where they are filtered out and eventually excreted. Metabolic waste must be removed from the blood, or it quickly accumulates to toxic levels. This condition is called uremia or uremic poisoning.

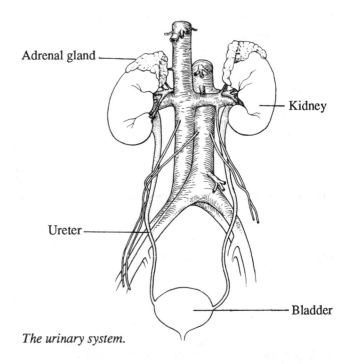

The urinary system.

The kidneys provide an important function in maintaining fluid and electrolyte balance as well. Electrolytes are substances such as salts that dissolve or break apart into ions when mixed in water. Health depends on maintaining a proper balance of water and the electrolytes within it.

Our bodies are composed mostly of water. The water content varies with each individual but is determined by age, gender, and weight. In a newborn infant 75-80 percent of the body weight is water. In an adult male, water comprises 55-60 percent, and in an adult female, 50-55 percent. Water is used by every cell in the body and is necessary for proper metabolism. Water provides the medium in which chemical reactions take place. If we have too much water, the kidneys remove more by excreting more urine. If we are deficient in water, the kidneys remove less in order to conserve fluid. In this way the kidneys work to maintain fluid balance.

The electrolytes in the body fluids are kept in a delicate balance. The kidneys regulate the levels of many chemical substances in the blood such as chloride, sodium, potassium, and bicarbonate. They also regulate the proper balance between body water content and salt by selectively retaining or excreting both substances as requirements demand.

The acid-base balance of the blood is maintained by the kidneys. Normal pH for blood is between 7.45-7.35. If the blood becomes either too acidic or too basic, body

The Kidneys:
- Maintain fluid, electrolyte, and acid-base balance
- Eliminate metabolic waste products.
- Help regulate blood pressure.
- Produce a hormone that stimulates red blood cell production.
- Activate vitamin D and so help regulate calcium and bone metabolim.

functions deteriorate and death may result. The kidneys control the absorption and replacement of certain ions in order to maintain this delicate balance. The types of foods we eat largely determine the body's acidity. A person who eats a lot of high-protein foods, such as meat and dairy, will add more acids to the body fluids and blood, thus increasing acidity. Over the long term this can lead to acidosis which can affect the function of every cell in the body and lead to numerous degenerative health conditions.

Kidneys also function in blood pressure regulation. When blood pressure is low, cells in kidneys secret a hormone that initiates constriction of blood vessels and thus raises blood pressure. High blood pressure may in fact be a sign of underlying kidney disease. The kidneys produce hormones which stimulate bone marrow to make red blood cells. It is easy to see why the kidneys are considered to be the most important homeostatic organs in the body.

KIDNEY HEALTH

The kidneys are among the body's most important organs. If it were not for their constant filtration of the blood, we would be poisoned by our own waste products. In order to clean toxins out of the blood effectively, the kidneys must be functioning properly. If they are filled with bacteria, calculi deposits, and accumulated toxins, they cannot filter the blood or regulate chemical and pH balance effectively. For this reason, cleansing and detoxifying the kidneys is an important step you should take in a holistic detoxification program.

If your kidneys are in poor health, you should not undertake any herbal cleansing or serious detoxification program until they are functioning properly. The use of cleansing herbs and other detoxification methods can draw out of the tissues massive quantities of toxins. These toxins are dumped into the bloodstream for elimination from the body. If the kidneys are filled with toxins themselves and not healthy, they will not be able to remove the additional toxins pumped into them and may become overworked and weakened. The blood will remain at an overly toxic level, creating a prolonged period of discomfort. If the toxins cannot be removed, they will redeposit themselves in tissues throughout the body. Thus, the cleansing accomplishes little and may further damage the kidneys.

The Natural Foods Diet will help to both clean the body and restore kidney health. Exercise and heat therapy will also strengthen the kidneys. Anyone who does the kidney cleanse program described in this chapter should first be on the Natural Foods Diet for at least a few weeks. If you know or suspect that you have kidney problems, one of the first detoxification programs you should go on is the kidney cleanse, and it should be repeated often. This cleanse will strengthen the kidneys so they will be able to adequately handle the elimination created by other detoxification programs.

The health of the kidneys depends on several factors. Stress and cardiovascular disease can influence kidney health as can inherent weakness. Diet and exercise exerts the strongest influence on urinary health. High-protein diets, for example, can lead to gout (formation of uric acid crystals in joints and kidneys) and acidosis (which affects all body systems including the urinary system).

Infections are the most common urinary disorders. Most urinary tract infections are caused by bacteria. Microorganisms can infect the bladder, urinary ducts, or kidneys. These infections can be very painful. Infections of the kidney are responsible for a number of diseases. The commonest are those caused by the tubercle bacillus, the colon bacillus, and various types of staphylococcus and streptococcus. Infection may come from the bloodstream, the lymph channels, or by direct ascension to the kidneys from an infected bladder. Ultimately such infections may cause abscess in or on the kidneys or result in pus formation (pyelitis). Such diseases are frequently serious and are accompanied by prostration, fever, and prolonged ill health. Since most infections are caused by colon bacteria, maintaining a healthy colon is important to the health of the urinary system.

Renal calculi or kidney stones can cause even greater pain and discomfort than infections. Kidney stones and gravel (smaller deposits) are crystallized mineral deposits that develop in the kidneys. Calculi develop when calcium

The kidneys can lose 80 percent of their functional ability before symptoms appear. This is why kidney disease is often far advanced before its presence is detected.

and other minerals, such as uric acid, crystallize in the collection ducts of the kidneys. They remain attached to the ducts unless broken off.

If the stones are small, they will simply flow through the ducts and be voided with the urine. Larger stones may obstruct the passageway in the ducts. When this happens, it causes an intense pain as rhythmic muscle contractions of the urinary ducts attempt to dislodge them. Kidney stones often have sharp edges that scratch and cut the urinary ducts as they pass down the canal, causing bleeding. Kidney stones can be extremely painful. It has been described as excruciatingly painful as childbirth.

Kidney stones can cause obstruction anywhere along the urinary canal. Obstruction usually results in backing up of the urine, that can extend all the way to the kidney. The severity of the obstruction depends on the location of the obstruction and the degree to which urine flow is impaired. This condition produces an environment which encourages bacterial growth, leading to urinary infections.

Kidney stones can be caused by several factors. An infection of the urinary tract can cause cellular debris to act as seeds on which crystals can form. Bacteria make the urine more alkaline, resulting in the deposit of phosphates, which form calcium phosphate stones. Stones can also be formed if your body is low in water due to low fluid intake or profuse sweating. Lack of fluid can make the urine more concentrated, causing urinary salts to solidify and stones to form. Many people have a mild form of chronic dehydrations which can lead to stone development. Drinking adequate amounts of water will help relieve this problem. Excessive uric acid and increased calcium in the urine can also cause stones to form. Long-term confinement to bed or even a chronic lack of exercise may encourage calcium to leach from the bones and into the blood and thus increase calcium levels in the urine. Nitrogen from protein-rich foods (meat and dairy) is a principle ingredient of uric acid. People whose diets are high in protein increase their risk of developing stones. Research shows that soft drinks containing phosphoric acid encourage the formation of kidney stones. Sugar and refined flour stimulate the pancreas to release insulin, which, in turn, stimulates increased calcium excretion through the urine. People who suffer from osteoporosis are losing calcium from their bones which is being discarded in the urine. The increased levels of calcium in the urine make the formation of kidney stones more likely.

One of the problems with kidney stones is that those who have them may have no symptoms, depending on where the stone is located and its size. Small stones and gravel may pass out of the body without any symptoms or discomfort. Larger stones, however, can cause a great deal of trouble. In such cases you may experience sudden severe and excruciating back pain which may come and go. At first you may think it is simply muscular cramping or a spinal problem and seek medical or chiropractic treatment. The pain will often radiate from the back to the abdomen and genital area. This pain may be associated with nausea, vomiting, abdominal bloating, blood in the urine, painful urination, and chills and fever. Because kidney stones are a result of lifestyle choices, stones tend to reoccur. About 60 percent of those who have had stones will develop them again within seven years.

Improving the diet by eliminating stone-forming foods and drinks and getting adequate exercise will help keep stones from forming. Diet alone, however, will not get rid of stones once they have formed. Once stones have developed, the only way to get rid of them through natural means is by kidney detoxification.

KIDNEY DETOXIFICATION

Since the kidneys are the most important organ in our bodies in maintaining homeostasis, the health of all the organs in our bodies relies on the proper functioning and health of the kidneys. When the kidneys malfunction, the entire body suffers, not just the kidneys. For this reason, it is of prime importance to keep the urinary system in good health. Since autointoxication and infection cause most kidney problems, the solution to gaining good kidney health is detoxification. Remove all irritating chemicals, crystal deposits, and metabolic waste, and replace damaged cells with new healthy tissues.

Conditions Associated with Kidney Stones
Malabsorption of nutrients

Cystinuria

Glucocorticoid excess

Gout

Hyperparathyroidism

Hyperthyroidism

Immobilization

Malignancies (some types)

Osteoporosis

Paget's disease

Recurrent urinary tract infections

Renal tubular acidosis

Vitamin D excess

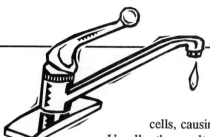

Water

Next to oxygen, water is the most vital element to human life. On average, the body consists of about 60 percent water, about 50 quarts in an averaged-sized man. About two and a half quarts are lost each day through exhalation, perspiration, and excretion. If this loss goes unreplenished and the body loses seven to ten quarts of water, death is inevitable. Eleven days is the maximum a person can live without drinking any water.

Water is also a powerful solvent necessary to wash and carry metabolic waste out of the body. Too much water, however, can upset the body's mineral balance. Excessive water intake can dilute the mineral concentrations in the fluid outside body cells; this fluid enters the cells, causing them to swell.

Usually, the result is an uncomfortable bloating. When brain cells become this engorged, however, the result may be an excruciating headache, convulsions, or even coma.

Drinking too much water has not been a problem in the past because water always contained salts and trace minerals. When you drink filtered or distilled water it is important to include in your diet an adequate amount of salt, especially sea salt because it contains important trace minerals.

You don't need to suffer the pain and discomfort of urinary infections, or the agonizing torture of passing kidney stones; nor do you need to subject yourself to the damaging effects of drugs or surgery. Nature has provided us an abundant number of cleansing herbs that are gentle, yet will detoxify and restore health to the urinary system, including removing stones (the results of autointoxication).

Herbs can remove toxins, dissolve stones, kill infection, soothe tissues, and encourage healthy cellular growth. One of the best herbs for overall health, yet one that is not generally considered for its medicinal properties nor even recognized as an herb, is the common everyday apple. Yes, the fruit of the apple tree is considered one of the best all-around healing herbs nature has provided mankind. Dr. Edward E. Shook, one of America's foremost authorities on herbs, states in his classic herbal textbook *Advanced Treatise in Herbology*, "We say, after an exhaustive study of its chemistry, that in our opinion there is no other remedial agent or herb in the whole range of known therapeutic agents that can compare with the apple tree."

Some may question calling the apple an herb. By definition an herb is any plant or part of a plant that is used for food or medicine. This is the definition the Bible gives to herbs in the Book of Genesis. The apple has long been known for its therapeutic effects on health. We are all familiar with the old saying, "An apple a day keeps the doctor away." This wise old proverb has been repeated for generations. And although most of us don't normally consider the apple a healing herb, it is both a healing herb and a valuable food.

The apple is rich in vitamins, minerals, and complex carbohydrates and contains protein, fiber, and organic salts and acids. Therapeutically it is a purifier, vitalizer, cleanser, antiseptic, disinfectant, germicide, respiratory stimulant, cardiac stimulant, brain and nerve stimulant, and tonic. Dr. Shook says, "It has been shown that in countries where unsweetened cider is used as a common beverage, stones (calculi) are unknown. A series of inquiries made by doctors in Normandy, where cider is the principal drink, brought to light the fact that not a single case of stones had been met with in more than forty years."

Fresh apples, whether they be raw, cooked, or juiced, are all beneficial. Much of the nutritive value is contained in the skin, so it is advisable to eat the whole fruit, but eat only organically grown apples to avoid pesticide residue and paraffin wax coating that is found on ordinary produce.

Another herb which is of great benefit to the health of the urinary system is the hydrangea plant. This plant is commonly used as an oriental shrub around homes. The part of the plant that is used medicinally is the root. Hydrangea root is one of the, if not the most, powerful herbs known for dissolving calculous deposits in the kidneys as well as other parts of the body (e.g., gallbladder, joints, etc.). For this reason it is beneficial for use by those who suffer with kidney stones, gallstones, arthritis, arteriosclerosis, and similar conditions. Its greatest value is in dissolving kidney stones.

The following formula is one recommended by Dr. Shook and has been proven effective as a stone solvent.

1 quart pure apple juice (organic)

2 ounces hydrangea root (chopped)

Soak hydrangea root in the juice for 12 hours. Put the juice and root on the stove and bring to a boil. Slowly simmer for 30 minutes. Let cool, strain out hydrangea root, and bottle. Keep juice in the refrigerator. Drink a cupful three to four times a day. There are no side effects or danger of overdose as this formula is completely harmless.

Hydrangea root can be purchased whole at good health food stores. It can also be obtained as a tincture (liquid extract). In tincture form it is most convenient. To prepare a dose, simply fill a cup with apple juice and add 20-30 drops of hydrangea tincture. Drink it warm or cold. This way you avoid the trouble of heating the juice/hydrangea mixture and straining out the root afterwards.

There are many other herbs that will detoxify the urinary system and dissolve kidney stones and relieve infection. Combining several of these herbs together can increase the effectiveness of each one and bring about quicker detoxification and healing. The following combination will detoxify and strengthen the urinary system. Kidney stones will completely dissolve and be passed in the urine unnoticed and without pain. This formula includes herbs which are soothing to the kidney and encourage growth of healthy tissues.

Apple juice

Hydrangea root (tincture)

Gravel root, also known as queen of the
    meadow (capsule)

Parsley (capsule)

Marshmallow root (capsule)

Uva ursi, also known as bearberry (capsule)

Vegetable glycerin (liquid)

Ginger root or cayenne pepper (capsule)

Vitamin B$_6$, 100 mg (tablet)

Magnesium oxide, 300 mg (capsule)

The apple juice and hydrangea alone will dissolve kidney stones and improve the health of the urinary system. Combining the other ingredients will enhance stone removal and kidney detoxification and health. Use as many of the ingredients as you can find, the more the

better, but you will still gain results if you have only apple juice and hydrangea root.

Apple juice, hydrangea root, and gravel root are stone dissolvers. Parsley is a strong diuretic (increases urine flow), suitable for treating urinary infections and stones. Marshmallow root is soothing and healing to tissues and useful for inflammation and ulceration of the urinary tract. Uva ursi is a diuretic and urinary disinfectant. Vegetable glycerin softens and protects tissues and enhances healing. Ginger root and cayenne pepper are stimulants which enhance the effectiveness of the other ingredients. You can use either ginger or cayenne in this formula. These two spices when packaged and sold as seasonings are usually less potent than the capsulated form sold as dietary supplements. Vitamin B$_6$ and magnesium oxide help to prevent stones from forming.

These ingredients can be obtained in various forms—tablet, capsule, tincture, powder, tea, etc. The most convenient form is as a pill (tablet or capsule). Hydrangea root usually is more readily available as a tincture. Vegetable glycerin comes as a thick, syrupy liquid.

Combine one cup of organic apple juice with 20-30 drops of hydrangea extract and one teaspoon of vegetable glycerin. Stir well. Use this liquid to help you swallow the pills. Take one pill of each herb three times a day before meals along with the apple mixture. Take one vitamin B$_6$ and one magnesium oxide pill once a day (just before breakfast is a good time). Drink plenty of water throughout the day as the cleanse will cause you to urinate more frequently.

Take this combination for at least three weeks. In that time stones will be dissolved and voided. If you have had a history of kidney infections, stones, or other problems, you should remain on the kidney cleanse for five weeks.

This kidney cleansing formula should be repeated once or twice a year, or more often if you have had kidney problems, to keep the urinary tract detoxified and functioning properly.

During the cleanse, refrain from meat, dairy, coffee, black tea, soft drinks (particularly colas), chocolate (drink or candy), rhubarb, and raw spinach, as these substances can encourage the formation of stones.

 **ADDITIONAL RESOURCES**

Alternative Medicine. The Burton Goldberg Group. Fife, WA: Futute Medicine Publishing, 1994.

Chapter 13

LIVER CLEANSING

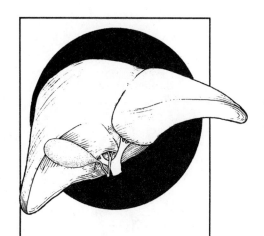

At first, Noreen thought it was just an upset stomach. Later when nausea turned to vomiting and fever, she decided it was time to see the doctor. She was diagnosed with cholelithiasis—inflammation of the gallbladder accompanied by gallstones. In most cases, gallstones are not life threatening and inflammation can be treated by rest and diet. Noreen's skin was yellow with jaundice, indicating that one or more stones were blocking the bile ducts causing bile to back up to the liver. Ordinarily, the doctor would have suggested surgery, but Noreen's case was different. Her general health was not the best. She was 62 years old and obese. The doctor feared that her heart would not hold up under the stress of an operation.

Noreen was hospitalized and given an assortment of drugs to treat her symptoms and, hopefully, either dissolve the stones or give her enough strength to withstand surgery. She stayed in the hospital for a couple of weeks, each day growing weaker and weaker. Finally, after some days in a state of delirium, they decided she was not going to pull through and discontinued the treatments. She was left to die in peace.

But she didn't die as expected. Once they stopped their procedures to save her life, she began to improve. Delirium left and her senses returned. She was able to sit up and talk. She was getting better with each day.

On seeing her drastic return to health, the doctors, in their wisdom, attempted to save her and again resumed treatment. She promptly relapsed into delirium and died a few days later. As is often the case, the supposed cure can be worse than the sickness. It appears that way with Noreen.

The sad thing about this story is that Noreen did not have to die. She did not need surgery to recover her health. If started early enough, she could have rid herself of the troublesome gallstones completely by natural means—without drugs, surgery, pain, hospitalization and, most of all, without dying.

THE LIVER

The liver is located on the right side of the abdominal cavity just beneath the ribcage. This large organ fills the entire right section of the abdominal cavity and even extends part way into the left side. Because it secrets a substance called bile, the liver is classified as a gland, and in fact, it is the largest gland in the body. In adults it weights as much as four pounds.

The liver performs hundreds of functions, more than any other gland, necessary for us not only to maintain good health, but to sustain life itself. The

Health is a matter of choice, not a mystery of chance.
—Robert A. Mendelssohn, M.D.

The greatest single curse in medicine is the curse of unnecessary operations, and there would be fewer of them, if the doctor got the same salary whether he operated or not.
—Richard Cabot, M.D., Harvard Medical School, 1938

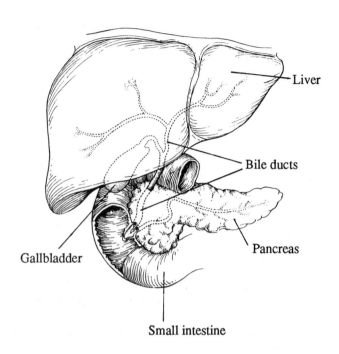

Liver

Bile ducts

Pancreas

Gallbladder

Small intestine

liver is the body's primary detoxification organ and manufacturing plant. It cleans alcohol, drugs, bacterial products, poisons, various waste products, and worn-out red blood cells fro the body. The liver is also the main factory and storehouse of the body. It produces amino acids, proteins, and fats, and stores fat and glucose (the energy source for cellular metabolism).

The liver is unique among the organs in the body in that it is the only one that receives a double blood supply. One of the sources of blood to the liver comes directly from the heart and lungs. This blood source supplies the liver with a rich source of oxygen. The liver receives about one fourth of the arterial blood pumped out of the heart at every beat. The other source of blood comes from the veins in the intestinal area; this blood contains the digested nutrients absorbed through the intestinal wall. This allows the blood coming from the gastrointestinal tract (containing absorbable products of digestion) to pass through the liver before entering the general circulation. This gives the liver first access to nutrients, as well as toxins. Blood containing poisons absorbed from the intestinal tract, is first sent through the liver before entering the general circulation, providing a means of protecting the rest of the body from a myriad of harmful and even deadly substances.

The liver plays a major role in the metabolism of carbohydrates, fats, and proteins—the three nutrients that supply the body with energy. It converts simple carbohydrates to glucose (the basic energy source for all

bodily functions), removes excess glucose from the blood, and makes and stores glycogen (which provides a ready source of energy between meals).

In addition to carbohydrate metabolism, the liver is also of considerable importance in the metabolism of protein. The formation of urea from dietary protein is an important liver function. The liver manufactures many types of amino acids that are in short supply. It removes from circulation amino acids that are present in excess of need and dismantles them or converts them to other amino acids. It removes ammonia (a toxic byproduct of dietary protein) from the blood and converts it to urea (less toxic than ammonia) to be sent to the kidneys for excretion. It makes other nitrogen-containing compounds the body needs such as bases used in DNA and RNA, plasma proteins, antibodies, clotting factors, and anticlotting factors.

The liver also controls the metabolism of dietary fat. It manufactures bile, which is stored in the gallbladder, and is necessary for the digestion of dietary fat. It builds and breaks down fats as needed by the body and packages extra fat for export to other body organs.

The liver is a valuable storehouse for the material from which blood pigment (hemoglobin) is made. Liver cells also store several other substances, including vitamins (notably A, D, E, and K), minerals, and fat. These substances are released to the body as required. The liver also functions in the formation of lymph—a vital body fluid which provides the medium in which white blood cells circulate throughout the body, fighting infection and removing toxins. Thus a healthy liver is essential to the immune system. The liver helps to maintain the hormone balance in the body by destroying or inactivating hormones that are not needed. At the same time, hundreds of lesser functions are performed by the liver. It is plainly evident that the health and proper function of the liver is vital to the health and life of the entire body.

BILE

Bile is most commonly associated with the gallbladder. The gallbladder, while not a part of the liver, is an important accessory organ to the liver. The gallbladder is a hollow, pear-shaped organ, three to four inches long. It rests under the liver on the upper part of the abdomen. This organ serves as a storage tank for bile.

One of the primary functions of the liver is to make bile. The liver is composed of a complex network of millions of canals called biliary tubing. Liver cells manufacture and excrete bile into the tiny biliary tubes which join with larger and larger tubes as bile volume increases. The bile drains from the biliary tubes into a single large tube called the common bile duct. This duct drains (through the cystic duct) into the gallbladder which servers as a reservoir for the bile.

The liver secretes bile more or less continuously, the amount varying from a pint to more than a quart in 24 hours. In a fasting state little bile is formed. Bile is a liquid containing, among other substances, bile pigments, bile salts, and cholesterol. Bile is essential for the digestion of fats and oils. Bile does not contain digestive enzymes. Its purpose is to emulsify fat so that enzymes excreted by the pancreas can break them down.

When a meal is eaten, the presence of fat and oil in the duodenum (first segment of the small intestine) triggers the liver and gallbladder to release bile into the intestine. Water and oil do not mix. You can clearly see this in oil-based salad dressings where a layer of oil will float on top of the water or vinegar. When you eat fat and oil, the same thing happens in the intestines—the fat and oil separate from the water-soluble digestive juices. This separation would create a barrier, preventing digestive enzymes from coming into contact with all the fat molecules, and thus the fat would not be completely digested. Fats and oils supply essential fatty acids and vitamins that are necessary for health. Bile emulsifies or breaks the fat apart so that the fat molecules can mix freely with the digestive juice.

Between meals, a lot of the bile moves up the cystic duct from the liver into the gallbladder where it is concentrated and stored. The gallbladder is often a site for the collecting and calcifying of gallstones. The gallbladder is considered a nonessential organ and is often surgically removed if gallstones are detected and inflammation is present.

GALLSTONES

The most common abnormal condition associated with the gallbladder is the accumulation of gallstones. Gallstones are solid, but not necessarily hard, masses composed primarily of cholesterol. Crystallized bile pigments and calcium salts can harden the stones. They often accumulate in large numbers. Gallstones were once thought to form in the gallbladder, hence the name "gallstone." This is still the general belief among those trained in traditional medicine. But many holistic physicians and alternative health practitioners believe they are actually formed in the liver and migrate to the gallbladder with the bile where they collect. In the gallbladder they continue to grow and may even calcify or harden.

Many people have gallstones without realizing it. The typical diet in Western countries promotes gallstone formation. The biliary tubing within the liver becomes clogged with stones which prevents bile (and toxins and cholesterol) from draining from the liver. This backup causes numerous symptoms.

X-rays may not show the presence of gallstones because most of them are not calcified, which is necessary in order to be detected by x-rays. Gallstones may be found in both the gallbladder and the biliary tubing of the liver. There are several types of gallstones. Most of them are composed primarily of cholesterol. Color varies from black, white, tan, or red, to green. Uncalcified stones are like little balls of clay. At the center of the stones may be found a particle of bacteria or some other contaminant which provides the seed upon which the stone begins its growth.

Stones may or may not be accompanied by symptoms. If they are small enough, they may pass through the biliary tubing and bile duct without notice and eventually be expelled from the body. But stones that get trapped in the gallbladder or bile tubing and ducts can cause inflammation and infection. Autopsies show that many people have gallstones without having had any symptoms. In fact, most people may have gallstones and not know it because there are no direct symptoms. Symptoms manifest themselves in other areas of the body which seem unrelated to the liver and gallbladder, for example, as digestive problems, hormonal imbalances, headaches, skin problems, etc. However, gallstones may cause chronic inflammation of the gallbladder, accompanied by intense pain in the upper abdomen, fever, nausea, vomiting, and extreme exhaustion.

Acute, intense pain may be experienced if a large gallstone passes through the common bile duct. This is especially likely to occur after a meal high in fats, which stimulates the flow of bile from the gallbladder. Sometimes a gallstone becomes lodged in the bile duct, blocking the flow of bile into the intestine. If this happens, the person develops jaundice and serious inflammation of the gallbladder and the duct. Without bile going to the intestines, the feces appear gray-white because pigments from bile give feces its characteristic brown color. Excessive amounts of bile backed up in the gallbladder and liver would be absorbed into the blood. Jaundice, a yellowish skin discoloration, would result. Pain often accompanies this condition.

Obstruction of the biliary tubes within the liver may also occur and, in fact, may be a more common condition than most realize. Small stones, some nearly as tiny as the head of a pin, inside the liver block the flow of bile through the liver's biliary tubing, which drains into the common bile duct. While many of the small biliary tubes may be clogged and cut off, others continue to release bile. This causes a decrease in the total amount of bile excreted and, in turn, hampers digestion and nutrient absorption, thus contributing to malnutrition. Bile locked up in the clogged tubes is reabsorbed and may lead to various degrees of jaundice. Mild jaundice may not be readily noticeable, except the skin will not be a healthy, pinkish color. A liver filled with numerous small stones can be as bad as a single large stone blocking the entire bile duct which feeds into the intestine. If a person has large stones, many smaller ones are certain to be present. These stones continue to multiply and grow in size if conditions that cause them are not changed.

LIVER HEALTH

Every day we consume poisons (preservatives, chemical food additives, pesticides, molds, etc.). Additional toxins are absorbed through the skin, inhaled in the air, and even produced within us. Many of these deadly poisons are filtered through the liver where they are destroyed or neutralized. Without the constant work of the liver to detoxify these substances, we would quickly die. The liver, however, can only handle so much. If more poisons are channeled through it than it can adequately process, the toxins pass through and circulate with the blood throughout the body. Filled with toxins itself, the liver slowly deteriorates and the multitude of important life-sustaining processes it performs are not effectively performed. Toxins, for example, which are not removed, circulate and accumulate in the body where they may cause problems and degeneration of other tissues. When the liver is burdened with toxic accumulation, it becomes diseased.

The most common liver problem is the accumulation of stones. This may lead to more serious conditions including hepatitis. A considerable number of liver conditions are grouped under this term. Hepatitis is characterized by inflammation, degeneration, and death of liver cells. Hepatitis may be accompanied by jaundice, liver enlargement, anorexia, and abdominal discomfort. Sometimes vomiting and diarrhea are present. The temperature may be slightly elevated (seldom above 101 F). The urine becomes dark and the stools gray-white after a time, indicating a total absence of bile in the digestive tract. The liver loses it ability to function so bile is not produced, nor are many of the hundreds of other functions of the liver performed.

A number of different conditions can cause hepatitis. Alcohol, drugs, or other toxins may initiate hepatitis. It may also result from a bacterial or viral infection or parasite infestation. Hepatitis A, for example, is caused by an infection from the hepatitis A virus. Contaminated food is often a source of infection. Hepatitis A occurs commonly in young people because of poor dietary habits and ranges in severity from mild to life-threatening. Another viral infection, hepatitis B, is usually more severe. It is also called serum hepatitis because it is often transmitted by contaminated blood serum. There is often no apparent clinical difference between this disease, which is of infectious origin, and the hepatitis caused by poisons (for example, chloroform, phosphorus, certain drugs, mushrooms). Hepatitis can seriously interfere with liver functions. Medical science has no cure for it and there is little that can be done. Most cures must come from within the body itself with rest and careful attention to diet.

Hepatitis, chronic alcohol abuse, malnutrition, or infection may lead to a more serious degenerative liver condition known as cirrhosis in which liver cells harden and die, accompanied by serious loss of liver function. Advanced stages of cirrhosis are usually nonreversible and fatal. Cirrhosis is common among alcoholics. The liver's ability to regenerate damaged tissue is well know, but it has its limits. For example, when the toxic effects of alcohol accumulate faster than the liver can regenerate itself, damaged tissue is replaced with fibrous or fatty tissue instead of normal tissue. No matter what the cause of liver cirrhosis, the symptoms are the same: nausea, anorexia, gray-white stools, weakness, and pain. If the cause of cirrhosis is removed, in time the liver may be able to repair itself.

Certain medications may cause abnormalities of the liver. In fact, many drugs have adverse affects on the function of the liver. The liver identifies the chemicals in most drugs as foreign substances, which they are, and will try to remove them. Removing the chemical constituents of these drugs poisons the liver just as much as contaminated food. Too much medication can place a great deal of burden on the liver hampering it from adequately performing its many functions and further deteriorating it.

Chemicals in foods (preservatives, colorings, artificial flavorings, etc.) are likewise contaminants to the body which must be removed by the liver. The liver can and does become overloaded with poisons from food, drugs, microorganisms, and other contaminants. The buildup of these poisons decreases the ability of the liver to function. Often our livers are just barely able to keep up with the contaminants we feed into the body every day. When additional contaminants or microorganisms appear, the liver cannot handle them and it begins to break down. This is how cancer is often transferred to the liver from other areas of the body. The liver is sometimes the primary site of cancer and is often invaded by metastasis when cancer occurs in other parts of the body.

The good news is that the liver has a remarkable power of regeneration and restoration. It can reverse the conditions of disease and deterioration better than any other organ in the body. Thus, a seriously damaged liver can be restored to health. Experiments have shown that after the removal of as much as 70 percent of the liver from some animals, the organ can regenerate itself within a few weeks. The human liver has the same ability. A liver that is seriously damaged by poisons, microorganisms, parasites, and stones can recover if these disease-causing agents are removed. Detoxification of the liver removes toxins and allows the liver to regenerate and function as it should.

LIVER DETOXIFICATION

Detoxification of the liver releases huge amounts of toxins. Most are flushed down the intestines and out of the body. Some are dumped or absorbed into the bloodstream. This puts a heavy burden on the kidneys which will filter out much of this debris. The liver cleanse program described here will purge your liver of gallstones and other toxic matter, promote healing and repair, and stimulate proper liver function. Cleansing the liver bile ducts is one of the most powerful things you can do to improve your overall health. Because the kidneys are put under stress during the liver cleanse, you need to have healthy kidneys to handle the job. For this reason, before doing the liver cleanse, you must first do the kidney cleanse described in the previous chapter.

Gallstones in the liver and gallbladder absorb toxins and can be breeding grounds for parasites and bacteria. As long as stones are present, they continue to enlarge and can block biliary passageways in the liver, shutting off the flow of bile to the gallbladder and to the intestines. As stones increase in number and grow in size, they block the biliary tubing which causes the liver to make less bile. This not only hampers digestion, because without bile the body cannot effectively digest fats and oils, but it also increases the cholesterol level of the body. The liver becomes stagnant and begins to deteriorate. Liver cells die without new ones regenerating. Gallstones provide a breeding ground for microorganisms which leads to frequent infections, further inhibiting the function of the liver.

By detoxifying the liver and removing harmful toxins, the liver will be able to do its job better, and the whole body will gain better health. Your digestion will improve; acne and psoriasis may clear up; even many allergies could disappear. You may also see shoulder, upper arm and upper back pain, due to bursitis, vanish. Your energy level will increase as energy will not be continually drained to fight off infections and remove toxins.

Herbalists have used a variety of methods to clean and detoxify the liver. There are many excellent herbs

useful for restoring liver health and removing gallstones. The method discussed here is one herbalists have used successfully for years. It is by far the quickest. Most herbal liver detoxifiers work slowly, gradually dissolving stones over a long period of time. The method given here will remove the stones quickly, without dissolving them, along with other toxins and without pain or discomfort.

Unlike the kidney cleanse, which dissolves the stones, the liver cleanse flushes the stones from the body and you will be able to see them. They will be expelled into the toilet with your bowel evacuations. They are clearly identifiable because they will float, since they are made primarily of cholesterol, and will usually be a pea green color, from bile pigment. The liver cleansing process described here is very simple; you will need the following:

Olive oil
Fresh grapefruit
Epsom salt
L-ornithine capsules
Milk thistle capsules

The Epsom salt is a laxative and causes diarrhea-like symptoms the morning after it is taken. It also dilates the biliary ducts which allow stones to loosen and flow freely out into the intestine. Epsom salt is sold in most drug stores.

The olive oil stimulates the liver and gallbladder to expel bile, thus forcing the stones out of the ducts. The grapefruit juice makes the oil easier to drink and also acts as a liver cleanser.

The L-ornithine capsules are used to help you sleep. L-ornithine is an amino acid which aids in digestion and metabolism. If you do not take it, you may have a difficult time getting to sleep, which will make for a long night. You can get a bottle of capsules from your local health food store.

Milk thistle is an herb which is known for its ability to clean and rejuvenate the liver. The active ingredient in milk thistle is silymarin. Some herb companies sell silymarin extract in pill form. Another herb that scientific studies have shown to be a super-potent liver cleanser is Picrorhiza kurroa. This is an herb, native to the Himalayas, has a long traditional use in Ayurvedaic medicine of India.

The liver cleansing process will cause you to empty your bowels frequently for part of a day. You will need easy access to a bathroom. So choose a day that will be convenient for this purpose. You will fast for two meals; start by skipping dinner one night and continue past breakfast the next day. By lunch time you can resume eating normally again.

If you choose Saturday as the day to be near to the bathroom, you will start the cleansing process on Friday the day before. After lunch Friday eat and drink nothing else, except water. Do not take any vitamins, dietary supplements, or medications that you can do without. No beverages of any sort. On Friday for breakfast and lunch eat only non-fat foods. Eat nothing that contains any fat or oil—no butter, oil-based salad dressing, cheese, meat, etc. Eat absolutely nothing past 2:00 p.m. If you do, you may feel ill later. You want to avoid fat on this day because fat stimulates the excretion of bile. Avoiding fat will allow bile to build up so that it will create a more complete evacuation when you start to cleanse the liver and gallbladder Friday night.

At 6:00 p.m. Friday, mix 1 tablespoon of Epsom salt with $^3/_4$ cup of water. Drink this mixture. You will eventually make four doses of the Epsom salt and water. Two will be taken Friday night and two Saturday morning. Epsom salt has an unpleasant taste. Using a straw to drink it will make it easier to get down. You may also add a little vitamin C powder to mask the taste somewhat. Drink the entire thing quickly. You may wash residue of the solution down your throat with a few swallows of pure water afterwards.

At 8:00 p.m. Friday, drink another mixture of 1 tablespoon of Epsom salt with $^3/_4$ cup of water. For best results, you should adhere strictly to this time schedule.

Just before 10:00 p.m. and before going to bed, you will prepare a mixture of olive oil and grapefruit juice. Measure out $^1/_2$ cup of olive oil into a glass. Squeeze the juice out of one grapefruit, making $^2/_3$ to one cup full. Remove and discard pulp. Add the juice to the olive oil. Mix the two together vigorously and drink it. Take four L-ornithine capsules at the same time. Do not leave out the L-ornithine capsules or you may have a long sleepless night. Drink all of the solution within a couple of minutes. It does not taste bad. Some people enjoy the taste of the oil-grapefruit mixture. Go *immediately* to bed.

You need to lie down as soon as you drink this mixture. If you don't, you may not effectively expel the gallstones. Lie flat on your back for at least 20 minutes and go to sleep. As you rest, you may feel the liver and gallbladder working and the stones traveling through the bile ducts. If you follow these directions, you should not feel any pain or discomfort.

In the morning after you awake and sometime after about 6:00 a.m., take a third drink of 1 tablespoon of Epsom salt with $^3/_4$ cup of water.

Wait two hours (no earlier than 8:00 a.m.) and take one final dose of Epsom salt and water.

Wait another two hours. You can now resume eating. In brief, the process consists of six steps:

(1) Stop eating after 2:00 p.m.

(2) At 6:00 p.m. drink $^3/_4$ cup of water with 1 tablespoon Epsom salt.

(3) At 8:00 p.m. drink $^3/_4$ cup of water with 1 tablespoon Epsom salt.

(4) At 10:00 p.m. drink mixture of $^1/_2$ cup olive oil and juice of one grapefruit along with four L-ornithine capsules. Go immediately to bed.

(5) After 6:00 a.m. the next morning drink $^3/_4$ cup water with 1 tablespoon Epsom salt.

(6) Two hours later drink $^3/_4$ cup of water with 1 tablespoon Epsom salt. Wait another two hours before resuming eating.

If you follow these instructions exactly as they are given, you will experience no discomfort or ill effect. However, you should expect frequent loose stools in the morning. Notice the debris which floats in the toilet bowl with each evacuation. These are stones from your liver and gallbladder! They will vary from pin head to marble size and maybe even a bit larger. Most will be greenish in color from the bile pigments. You can imagine how the larger stones, some measuring 3/4 inch or more can plug the flow of bile in the biliary tubing and ducts.

Your first bowel movement of the day will probably contain the most stones. Count them. You will remove a total of anywhere from 100 to 1000 or more stones. Along with the stones the bile will pull out toxins that will be either flushed out through the bowels or carried to the kidneys and eliminated. The liver and gallbladder will be flushed clean of a great deal of toxic debris.

Some people are amazed at the number of stones that are passed during the liver cleanse. Some people will pass a thousand or more. All of various sizes. "In three different people, reports one therapist "I have seen stones as large as golf balls come out. My own mother passed one this size. My mother had this terrible gallbladder attack. It almost killed her. She was scheduled for emergency surgery. I said, 'No you're not!' I flew down to Florida right away and gave my mother this same program.

"She passed a stone as large as a golf ball. She heard it fall in the toilet. I scooped it out with rubber gloves. I dissected it. It was covered with dark green. I cut into it with a sharp knife. The inside was like white plaster. I peeled that off. Inside it was hard and white, the size of a nickel. My mother avoided surgery. To this day she has been fine."

The liver cleanse is perfectly safe and will cause no adverse effects, unless you neglected to do the kidney cleanse beforehand. Some people who do not do the kidney cleanse first may feel ill after the liver cleanse because their kidneys are not able to adequately remove the toxins that have been dumped into the bloodstream. People in their seventies and eighties can do the liver cleanse without problem. Children can as well, but depending on their age would take smaller dosages. For preteens the dosage should be cut in half for all ingredients.

If you have lots of stones, a single cleanse will not remove them all. Stones and debris deeper within the liver will remain. After your initial cleanse, they will gradually move forward as bile is excreted with meals and can be removed with a second liver cleanse. The liver cleanse can be repeated again in a week or two. By this time, most of the remaining stones should have loosened up and be in a position where they can be expelled easily by another liver cleanse. The flush can be repeated a third time if necessary.

It is recommended that after the liver cleanse, you clean any remaining stones and toxins from the colon with an enema or colonic. This is particularly important if you have had problems with constipation. If the colon does not completely eliminate the toxins expelled by the liver and gallbladder, they will remain in contact with intestinal tissues. Toxins from this debris can be absorbed into the bloodstream and end up back in the liver or accumulate in other tissues. People can and do benefit even without

cleaning the colon, but the more thorough the cleanse, the better the results.

After you have completed the first liver cleanse, start taking the milk thistle capsules, as directed on the label. You may begin with the smallest dosage listed at first, but within a week increase to the maximum. For example, if the bottle says to take one to three capsules three times a day, start by taking one capsule three times a day (three per day) and gradually add one a day until you are taking three capsules three times a day (a total of nine a day). When you do the second liver cleanse, do not take the milk thistle or any other supplements for the two days you do the program. Resume taking the maximum dosage when you finish the second liver cleanse. Continue until the bottle is empty.

There are several excellent herbs that help to detoxify and stimulate healing of the liver. Milk thistle and Picrorhiza kurroa are perhaps the best of them all. They are completely safe to use and will encourage the removal of additional toxins and the regeneration of healthy new cells.

QUICK LIVER FLUSH

The above liver cleanse will purge the liver and gallbladder of a great many toxins. However, it involves fasting and purging of the intestinal tract which requires some time and energy. It is recommended that you do the complete liver cleanse at least once and repeat as often as needed.

Since the liver is the body's main defense against dietary toxins, it is a good idea to keep it as clean and healthy as possible. After the doing the liver cleanse program, you can benefit by periodic, and less involved,

Epsom Salt

Epsom salt is a naturally occurring mineral composed of magnesium, sulfur, hydrogen, and oxygen. It is commonly sold in drugstores as a muscle relaxant and laxative. Added to warm bath water it has a relaxing effect on sore or tired muscles and aids in healing damages tissues. Taken internally it relaxes digestive muscles, producing a laxative effect.

Epsom salt derives its name from the village of Epsom, England where it was found in spring water. Henry Wicker came across the small spring in 1618 while looking for a source of water for his cattle. Wicker enlarged the opening, but the cattle refused to drink the bitter-tasting water. People in the area discovered that the magnesium-rich spring had health-restoring properties and began using it medicinally, both externally and internally. The water's reputation as an internal remedy quickly spread.

The mineral spring at Epsom became so popular for its medicinal properties that during the late 17th and early 18th centuries, the village of Epsom was a fashionable health and water resort visited by as many as 2,000 people a day. Epsom salt, the mineral in the Epsom spring water is found in many places around the world, most notably in limestone caves where it resembles snowballs clinging in loose masses to the roof and walls.

simple liver flushes. The liver flush is much like the liver cleanse just described, but can be easily done at any time without fasting and without taking a strong laxative.

The ingredients are as follows:

½ fresh lemon

2 grapefruits

2 tablespoons olive oil

2 cascara sagrada capsules (or other herbal laxative)

Cascara sagrada, a relatively mild herbal laxative, is recommended because it is non-habit forming and completely safe. It is readily available in capsule form or as a tincture at health food stores. Any herbal laxative can be used in the liver flush. Herb companies sell laxative teas which contain senna, another natural laxative. You could use this if you prefer. The herbal laxative will loosen the bowels and help speed intestinal contents through the system. Toxins expelled into the small intestine by way of the gallbladder and biliary ducts will be quickly removed. If toxins are simply dumped into the intestines and allowed to sit in a sluggish colon, many of the poisons will be reabsorbed into the bloodstream. So taking an herbal laxative is important. Do *not* take pharmaceutical laxatives like Ex-lax.

The laxatives take time to work, so take them after your evening meal but several hours before bedtime. Just before going to bed blend together the juice of 1/2 lemon, 2 grapefruits (apple juice can be used in place of grapefruit, if you prefer), and 2 tablespoons of olive oil. Remove pulp. Mix well and drink. Go to bed immediately.

This drink is always taken at night because the liver is most active between the hours of 11:00 P.M. and 1:00 P.M. Greater detoxification will occur during these hours.

The liver flush as described here is not meant to be a replacement for the more thorough liver cleanse described earlier. It serves as a supplementary method of cleansing the liver and can and should be done periodically as you feel the need. Some people feel they benefit by doing the complete liver cleanse once a year and the liver flush every couple of months.

HEALTH BENEFITS

The liver cleansing process described here has been criticized by doctors because it contradicts traditional medical beliefs. The biggest point of contention is regarding the stones that are removed by this process. Gallstones are thought to be formed only in the gallbladder and not the liver. They are believed to be few in number, not hundreds

Milk Thistle

Two hundred scientific research experiments, clinical studies, and biopsy data show that milk thistle contains the most potent liver-protecting compound known — silymarin.

In human studies, silymarin heals and protects the liver from chronic stress, free radical-caused hepatitis, acute and chronic hepatitis, and from cirrhosis induced by either toxins, drugs, or alcohol. Silymarin normalizes chronic inflammatory liver disease, fatty infiltration of the liver (chemical- and alcohol-induced fatty liver), and inflammation of the bile duct.

Another significant benefit of silymarin is its ability to increase production of new liver cells to replace damaged old ones. Thus, it protects, regenerates, and regulates the liver.

Silymarin is rapidly absorbed as a supplement with no toxicity, even for pregnant women.

The first response to treatment of liver disease usually occurs within a few weeks (as determined by standard blood tests). Because liver functions directly affect the rest of the body and the emotions, there is often a distinct improvement in a patient's general physical condition. To judge its effect, treatment with silymarin should last at least one to three months.

—Steven R. Schechter, N.D. *Let's Live*, December 91.

or thousands. They are thought to be only in select individuals, not most people. They are not linked to any symptoms or illness other than those directly relating to the gallbladder. Current medical practice to treat this problem is to surgically remove the entire gallbladder. If there are stones in the liver, they remain and so do the digestive problems, skin problems, bursitis, and other conditions.

We hear the word "stone" and we automatically think of something hard and dense. Most gallstones surgically removed from gallbladders are hard. They are calcified because the stones have developed to an advanced stage, which seriously affects the health of the body. Softer stones are less troublesome and undetectable on x-rays, therefore, they are not removed.

Critics claim that the stones removed by the liver cleanse are not really gallstones because they don't look like the typical calcified stones removed from gallbladders. They suggest that the stones removed by the liver cleanse are particles of food or sponified oil. The fact they are colored by bile pigments suggests a bile origin. Whether the green stones you expel from the liver cleanse fit the medical definition for gallstones or not doesn't matter. The Epsom salt and olive oil has pulled toxins out of the liver and gallbladder. These "stones" were removed as part of the cleansing process along with other toxins. Removing them from the body has resulted in marked improvement in health. Skin problems, digestive problems, aches and pains, fatigue, chronic muscle pains, chills and poor circulation, and other problems disappear after the liver cleanse. If removal of the stones and other toxins results in improved health, what does it matter what they're called? I prefer to simply refer to them as "stones" rather than identify them as gallstones. Others call them liver stones. Whatever you call them, the body does better without them.

The liver flush is the quickest, most powerful way to cleanse the liver and gallbladder. The health benefits are numerous. Those who criticize it have never tried it. Those who have tried it know it works.

"I have saved literally hundreds of gallbladders that were scheduled for surgery," says therapist Marge Kapsos in an interview reported in *The Last Chance Health Report*. "Just the other week I had a 22-year-old girl come in. She was desperate because her doctor, a female surgeon, had scheduled her for gallbladder removal surgery. As a last resort, she went on a liver flush. She lost hundreds of stones. She was immediately relieved of her symptoms and has not suffered an attack since.

"When she went back to the doctor for an ultrasound, there were no stones present. The girl told her doctor that she had gone on a liver flush. The doctor went crazy, demanding to know what kind of quackery was that, and who on earth had advised her to do such a thing. After she calmed down, the doctor told her, 'There was no need to do something like that. We do have medication that can dissolve the stones.'

"But of course she had never mentioned that option before! Hardly anybody in this situation is advised of that. Doctors want to do the surgery for the money, and that's all there is to it."

The liver flush, unlike drugs, does not have any harmful side effects. And surgery would seem to be unnecessary in many cases.

The liver cleanse will bring about improved health to the entire body, not just the liver and gallbladder. "When I first heard about the liver flush," says naturopath Nathalie Tucker, "I did it on myself and was most impressed with the results—I passed 269 stones . . . I have five patients that are long-time sufferers from Epstein-Barr syndrome; in other words, chronic fatigue syndrome. I am one of the five, so I was particularly interested in whether the liver flush would relieve some of the disease's more debilitating symptoms.

"One of these women had been suffering for seven years. In and out of hospitals, mostly bedridden, in fact, she almost died twice. An osteopath told her that one lobe of her liver had completely quit functioning.

"I did a liver flush on her and got 395 stones, one of them quite large. All three lobes of her liver are working fine now, and she is out and about, working, able to handle her life."

Many people have gotten amazing results from the liver cleanse, even alleviating chronic conditions like Parkinson's disease. Nathalie Tucker says, "One man who did it was in his mid-sixties and had been suffering terribly from Parkinson's disease for eleven years. He had deteriorated to the point where he was trembly all over and could not function well enough to work—even for part of a day.

"Within two weeks of flushing his liver he was back to working a full day. He can now run, bend, squat, stoop. He is able to do whatever needs to be done in his job, which is running a backhoe on a banana plantation."

Jan Ellison reports, "I have suffered from chronic fatigue syndrome for more than seven years. It has been agony. At the time I got really interested in the liver flush, my liver was swollen and painful on top of all my other symptoms. It hurt so much that a lot of the time I was walking around with one hand pressed against my liver.

"I got the most incredible results from just one flush—lots of green stones—one the size of a cherry tomato. And the relief from the pain in my liver was immediate. I feel normal again for the first time in years.

"Incidentally, my appearance got a real lift from doing the flush as well. My eyes got very clear and didn't have a yellow tinge anymore, and my skin got pinker. I also got an immediate sense of well being and relief from the exhaustion of fighting my illness. Doing the flush was a great experience."

Liver detoxification is one of the most beneficial procedures you can do for your health. It is simple and inexpensive and causes no pain.

 ADDITIONAL RESOURCES

Natural Liver Therapy: Herbs and Other Natural Remedies for a Healthy Liver. Hobbs, Christopher. Capitola, CA: Bontanica Press, 1993.

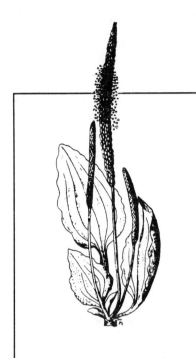

And God said, Behold, I have given you every herb bearing seed, which is upon the face of the earth, and every tree, in which is the fruit of a tree yielding seed; to you it shall be for meat.

—Genesis 1:29

Chapter 14

HERBAL DETOXIFICATION

Doctors had given up hope of curing Yong Ki Hong, a 46-year-old Korean father of four, and said he had only three months to live. Yong Ki lived in Pung Tak, a Korean city about sixty miles from Seoul. He drank socially, at least every other day, and he smoked a pack of cigarettes a day.

His job as a truck driver required him to undergo periodic physical exams. In 1988, during a routine exam, doctors discovered a problem with his liver. Further testing showed that he was a chronic hepatitis B carrier. The doctor requested that Yong Ki get a blood test and CAT scan every few months. He was given some medication for his liver and dismissed. Yong Ki continued to drink socially as before.

For six years Yong Ki went regularly to the hospital, to be tested. Then, in 1994 the CAT scan revealed 11 small tumors in his liver. Most were pea-sized, the two largest, however, were about the size of golf balls. Doctors immediately took a biopsy and found them to be cancerous. Chemotherapy was the prescribed course of action.

After his first treatment, Yong Ki was to come back in three months. However, he developed a fever, was unable to sleep, felt miserable and developed a rash all over his chest. His brothers were concerned, and they made an appointment for him in the Samsung Medical Center, the largest and most modern hospital in Korea. At the same time they called members of the family in the United States and asked for any information about alternative treatments for liver cancer.

Yong Ki went to Samsung and was given a CAT scan and blood test. The doctors there confirmed earlier tests. However, instead of chemotherapy, the doctors wanted to treat him with injections of alcohol, which was more commonly used at the Samsung Medical Center than chemotherapy. In alcohol treatment, the alcohol is injected directly into the tumors. They gave him one treatment, but the doctor had said even alcohol wouldn't do much for Yong Ki because his tumors were too many and too large.

At this time, Yong Ki's niece, who lived in the United States, learned of his condition. She called a Seattle Hospital with liver cancer specialists who told her that since the doctors in Korea had said the cancer was inoperable, they could do nothing either, though they would be willing to see the patient if he came with all the medical records. Yong Ki was not able to come, so his niece began researching natural therapies. She gathered information about herbs which included methods of detoxification and cancer treatment, and immediately flew to Korea.

Yong Ki was in the hospital undergoing alcohol treatment when his niece arrived. She saw him undergo the effects of one injection; it was awful. The doctors told her there was no hope for him and that he wouldn't live more than three months. They told her he would probably become jaundiced and lose consciousness as his last days approached. Seeing that there was little more that they could do for him, they discharged him from the hospital and sent him home, without medications. They told him to come back in three weeks for a checkup.

His niece asked the doctors if there was anything else they could do, and they told her no. She asked if she could give him the herbs and vitamins she brought from the United States They told her, "You can give these to him when Yong Ki gets home."

Yong Ki started taking them immediately, according to the instructions and schedule his niece wrote out for him. He does not speak or read English, so she removed all of the labels and replaced them with numbers 1, 2, 3, etc. She translated the instructions about taking the remedies for him. He followed the instructions religiously.

Yong Ki's niece left Korea the next day to return to her job. After twenty-one days, Yong Ki went back to the hospital, and the doctors did another CAT scan and blood test. They found some improvement, but the liver function test was still abnormal. The CAT scan, however, showed that the nine pea-sized tumors were gone!

The three largest tumors had become whitish and loosely defined on the edges, instead of round and well defined as before. The doctor said, "This is amazing. What are you doing?" Yong Ki told them about the herbal formulas and vitamins he was taking, but he didn't know what they were, because the bottles were only labeled with numbers.

One month later Yong Ki became very ill, with flu-like symptoms, a high fever, and aches all over his body. He was still taking the herbs. His brother became concerned, and went to the local hospital to talk to a doctor. The doctor, amazed at the results of the CAT scan at Samsung hospital and overall improvement, said that Yong Ki was probably just getting rid of the cancer, and his current symptoms were probably the body's way of removing toxins from his body (e.g., a healing crisis).

Despite the doctor's assurances, Yong Ki worried that he might have gotten worse. His next CAT scan, however, showed improvement. The doctors at the Samsung hospital became so interested in Yong Ki's case that they ordered another CAT scan fifty-one days later. They even offered to do it for a greatly reduced price. This scan showed that the three largest tumors had now disappeared, leaving only a shadow effect where they had once been.

Another CAT scan eighty-one days later showed no sign of cancer.

The last CAT scan performed some months later revealed no shadow or trace of the tumors. Yong Ki is ecstatic about the whole experience. He tells all his friends about alternative ways to heal illness and how he regained his health with herbs after traditional medical treatments failed.

HERBS AS MEDICINE

Herbs have a long medical tradition. They were the standard remedies before the advent of drugs and radiation. Herbs can be used for most illnesses and, at proper dosages, have proven to be effective without causing harmful side effects like drugs. The problem with using herbs is that people use them like drugs. They feel that if you take a few capsules or cup of herbal tea a day, all your troubles will be gone, so still live their normal, unhealthy lifestyle. Herbs will help, but if you eat junk food (loaded with toxins), don't exercise, breathe polluted air, drink polluted water (containing chlorine, fluorine, etc.), smoke, drink alcohol and otherwise expose your body to poisons, you cannot overcome illness. Herbs can help to rejuvenate damaged tissues, speed detoxification, and promote healing, but if you continue to pump poisons into the body, they will have little effect. You may meet people who say as they drink their sixth cup of coffee and gulp down a sugary donut, "Oh, I tried herbal remedies, but they didn't seem to help me." The reason they didn't help is because this type of person is overloading his or her body with toxins. If a person truly wants to gain better health, he must make a lifestyle change and stop as many poisons from entering his body as possible. When you can do this, you are on the road to recovery.

Many herbs work as detoxifiers and cleansers. These herbs will accelerate internal cleansing and speed recovery. Next to fasting, herbs are the oldest method used for detoxification. Throughout the world where people live close to nature, they have learned to use the herbs growing around them. Many different herbs that grow in different areas of the world have been used for similar purposes. Some are more effective than others. In our modern society we have the advantage of using herbs from all over the world, not just the ones growing near us. This way, we have access to the strongest, most effective herbal detoxifiers the earth has to offer.

Herbs contain vitamins and minerals which in themselves may be very beneficial to the body. Many people are vitamin and mineral deficient even though they consume "enriched" white bread and eat three big meals a day. Poor-quality foods do not always supply a complete range of nutrients. And farm soils are sadly depleted of trace minerals which are necessary for good health. Most herbs are not grown on commercial soils; in fact, many are harvested in the wild. Therefore, they provide trace minerals the body doesn't get from foods. Each herb has its own combination of chemical constituents that act on the body to promote healing and cleansing. The combination of vitamins, minerals, and unique chemical compounds makes herbs effective detoxifiers.

No adverse side effects occur as with over-the-counter and prescription drugs, as long as you follow recommended dosages listed on labels. Most herbs are non-toxic even at very large dosages, and are non-habit forming. A few can cause unpleasant reactions if taken in excess, but you would have to consume a far greater amount than the recommended dosages. Even moderate overdoses are harmless. Only mega doses far beyond recommendations will bring discomfort or unpleasant reactions. Most are safe at even mega doses, although large quantities of any supplement are discouraged. Their biggest drawback is taste. While some herbs like cinnamon, cloves, peppermint, chamomile, etc. have a pleasant or mild flavor, others have a strong, bitter or pungent taste. Teas and extracts from the latter are easier to take if combined with a little honey or juice. Herbs in tablet or capsule form are no problem as their taste is not noticeable in this form.

There are hundreds of medicinal herbs. Herb companies make supplements using a mixture of them. Some herbs which complement each other are said to be synergistic, and the combination of them works better than either one alone. The classic example of this is echinacea and golden seal—blood purifiers and immune boosters.

This chapter describes some of the most useful and potent herbs for detoxification and healing. You can go to a health food store and find preparations using these herbs in tea or capsule form. Many herb companies make their own combinations and they are generally all good (depending on the freshness and quality of the herbs used).

Some herbs, such as ginseng, can be used every day as a tonic. Others, like echinacea, have a powerful effect on the body and should only be used periodically when there is a specific need. Most of the detoxifying herbs are of the latter group. Time of use can extend from a few days to a few months. If herbs are to be used for several months at a time, they should be taken no more than six days a week. One day each week the herbs should not be taken. This gives the body time to adjust without the stimulus of the herb, which enhances natural processes of healing.

A few herbs should not be used by people with certain conditions. For example, barberry should not be used during pregnancy as the alkaloid berberine stimulates the uterus. Such precautions are listed on the labels.

Large doses of many herbs may cause headache, nausea, vomiting, diarrhea, abdominal cramping, etc. Never overdo it. A little bit is good, more isn't always better. Stick to recommended dosages listed on bottles, unless told otherwise by a health care provider experienced with herbs.

Just because a, herb is natural doesn't mean it can be abused and taken indiscriminately. Any substance taken in excess will cause harm—anything, even water. People have lost consciousness and nearly died from drinking too much water!

HOW TO USE HERBS

Herbs can be used as teas or they may be ground and put into capsules. They can also be made into a concentrated liquid called a tincture. Some herbs have strong, unpleasant flavors. Drinking tea made from these less palatable herbs can be a bit unpleasant. In these cases you may want to use them in capsule or tincture form.

Teas can be purchased prepackaged in tea bags or in bulk out of a jar. You can use either. Some companies make premixed herbal combinations (in both tea and capsule form). These can be very good as they combine herbs that complement and enhance each others' cleansing properties.

To prepare the tea, heat water to boiling and pour it into a cup. Add the tea to the cup and let it soak. Do not boil the tea in the water! Boiling breaks down some of the beneficial chemical constituents of the tea which can decrease the herb's effectiveness. Let it soak in hot water for 10 to 15 minutes.

Some people may not like the taste of herbal teas and admittedly, some of them are hard to swallow without a bit of doctoring. You can make such teas more palatable by adding a little honey. Some prefer, however, to combine the benefits of fruit juice with the tea. You can do this by mixing a half cup of juice with a half cup of tea. The juice will mask the disagreeable taste of most strong-flavored herbs.

Tinctures come in small bottles with an eyedropper lid. Tinctures tend to be very strong flavored because they are concentrated herbal extracts. Put the recommended number of drops (see directions on label) of the tincture into a cup of juice. If the flavor is too strong with the recommended number of drops, cut it in half. Add the other half to another glass later on in the day. This way you still get the full daily dosage.

For many people, capsules are the easiest way to take herbs. Some people just don't care for tea and prefer the ease of just swallowing a few capsules. At times where hot water or juice is not readily available, capsules are most convenient.

TOTAL HERBAL CLEANSE

Detoxifying means to remove harmful substances. These substances can be animal (protozoa, parasites), mineral (lead, arsenic, mercury), vegetable (fungi, bacteria), chemical (environmental pollutants, artificial food additives), or degenerative and nonfunctional cells (cancer). There are herbs that you can use to clean all these from the system.

Hundreds of different herbs are useful in detoxifying the body. Any number of these can be used. Herb companies make combinations of these herbs that you can buy in capsule form. Many of these are good and beneficial. Some herbs are stronger or more effective than others. Combining different compatible herbs together can enhance the cleansing power of the herbs. Below is a list of some herbs that have proven to be among the most effective detoxifiers. These herbs taken together will provide full body cleansing and promote cellular rejuvenation. The combination of the following herbs has a powerful cleansing action on the body. They may initiate a healing crisis and pull toxins out of the tissues. If you have a lot of toxic debris stored in your body, you may experience a severe cleansing reaction. All channels of the body will be working to eliminate debris and you can expect discharges from the sinuses, lungs, kidneys, bowels, skin, eyes, and ears. It is recommended that before doing a cleanse of this magnitude, you prepare yourself first. Preparation involves cleansing the body of toxins and strengthening the major organs of elimination. A kidney, for example, that is not functioning at full strength cannot handle the increased load of toxins dumped on it from the detoxifying process. The toxins will then remain in the body without being removed, and symptoms of illness will result. A weak kidney overloaded with an influx of toxins may degenerate even further as a result. So, before doing the total herbal cleanse described below, you should do the following:

- Be on the Natural Foods Diet
- Complete colon cleanse
- Complete the kidney cleanse
- Complete the liver cleanse

After being on the Natural Foods Diet for a few months and cleansing the colon, kidneys, and liver, your body should be strong enough to handle the total herbal cleanse. After doing these other cleanses, your body may be strong enough that you will not experience any discomfort or cleansing symptoms. This does not mean that the herbs are not doing any good, it means that your organs are strong enough to handle the removal of toxins that are being pulled out of your tissues without overloading other organs. So you may or may not experience a full healing crisis after doing the total herbal cleanse. But it is likely that you will notice an increased discharge from sinuses, kidneys, and bowels. This may be slight or significant. Fever and headaches and other symptoms may also temporarily manifest themselves. This is the consequence of cleansing and not adverse or allergic reactions to the herbs. The herbs will not hurt you.

Herbs in the total herbal cleanse each focus on different parts or systems of the body, although there is some overlap as many herbs work on several areas of the body to enhance overall health. The herbs work on the organs of elimination, since those are often clogged and diseased with toxic accumulations and are where most toxins are channeled by the body. The blood is the lifestream of the body. It carries oxygen and nutrients to every cell. The blood often contains toxic material including parasites, bacteria, fungi, heavy metals, etc. that are circulated throughout the body. Candidiasis, a fungus, is spread through the bloodsteam and affects the entire body, not just mucous membranes. The same is true for many other microbes and parasites. Flatworms, for example, are commonly found in the bloodstream. Formaldehyde, lead, mercury, aluminum, and other poisons are also found to some degree in most people. If the body is to be healthy, the blood must be cleansed. Herbs which act as antimicrobiotics that kill microbes are a necessary part of the cleansing process as these organisms are toxins and their presence leads to frequent and chronic illness such as yeast infections, bladder infections, colds, etc. The herbs in the total herbal cleanse are as follows:

Milk thistle. Liver detoxifier and cell rejuvenator.

Barberry. Works on the liver, gallbladder, stomach, and digestive organs. Also has antibacterial and antifungal properties.

Juniper berries. Detoxifies the kidneys and bladder. Also acts as an antiseptic on the urinary system.

Cascara sagrada. Strengthens intestinal muscles and improves bowel elimination. Also increases secretions of the stomach, liver, gallbladder, and pancreas. It is one of the very best and safest laxatives available.

Mullein. An excellent herb for the release and

expulsion of toxins in the bronchial tubes and lungs. Soothes mucous membranes. Also good for the urinary system.

Hawthorn berries. Strengthens the heart and improves blood circulation. Dilates blood vessels increasing circulation and improving ability of circulatory system in delivering nutrients and removing toxins.

Echinacea and golden seal. Both of these herbs enhance the immune system. Excellent blood and lymph detoxifiers. Commonly sold in combination with each other because together they provide a much stronger effect. Also effective antimicrobiotic.

Garlic. Antibiotic, antifungal, and blood cleanser.

Cayenne. Circulatory stimulant. Enhances the effects of all the other herbs.

All of these herbs are available in capsule form including the garlic and cayenne, which would otherwise be too strong to swallow. The other herbs on this list may also be obtained in bulk and used to make into tea. Take the herbs as directed on the bottles' labels.

Along with the herbs listed above, you should also add a complete set of antioxidants. There are many companies which produce antioxidant formulas. Many of them are good. Look for one that has a variety of antioxidant vitamins. The one you choose should contain as many of the following as possible: Vitamin C, vitamin E, beta-carotene, bioflavonoids, rutin, CoQ10, zinc, selenium, Pycnogenol (or grape seed extract), bilberry extract, gingko biloba extract, green tea, and quercetin. It is best to use a combination of these because they work together and enhance each others' antioxidant properties. Find a single supplement that has most of these and take that (according to instructions on the container) along with the herbs.

This is a very powerful combination of herbs and vitamins that will detoxify and cleanse the body thoroughly. Drink lots of water as bowel and urine flow will increase, both of which will release a lot of fluid from the body. Keep in mind that herbs are not like drugs. Drugs work almost immediately on relieving symptoms without affecting the root cause of the problem. Herbs work on the cause and require a longer time to see results, but symptoms of ill health will disappear as the cause is removed. For this reason, this combination of herbs should be taken for at least a month and may extend for several months. Take all these supplements six days a week, and then give your system a break on the seventh day. This will give better results. Don't take all the herbs all at once, but spread them out throughout the day, preferably just before meals.

Depending on your health, this herbal cleansing formula may push you into a healing crisis, so be conscious of this fact. It may take only a few days to reach a healing crisis or may take a few months. It all depends on the condition of your health. It is recommended that you go through some of the other cleansing programs first, like the kidney cleans and liver cleanse, and be eating a Natural Food Diet before going on this herbal cleanse. In order to eliminate toxins properly, the kidney and liver must be healthy enough to handle the job.

The herbal cleanse should not be used during pregnancy. Some of the ingredients will stimulate uterine contractions. The cleansing process may be too severe for those who are pregnant or have a serious disease, such as kidney disease.

PARASITE PURGE

After suffering for some time with abdominal pain, Brenda was scheduled for an appendectomy. She was diagnosed with appendicitis. Appendectomy is a routine surgery with little to fear. During surgery to remove the appendix, doctors found the organ healthy. Before sewing her back up a nematode (parasitic worm) crawled out of her abdomen.

In New England, several orthodox Jews all developed symptoms of Parkinson's disease within months of each other. Examination revealed the cause to be parasites in their brains. The fact that parasites had infected their brains was not unusual; what was unusual is that the parasites were commonly associated with eating undercooked pork. Orthodox Jews do not eat pork. Investigation revealed that the parasites were transmitted to the Jews from their housekeeper and cook, who was not Jewish and had parasite eggs under her fingernails from touching pork. These eggs were later transferred during food preparation by the cook.

Cathy suffered from chronic fatigue, memory loss and itchy ears and nose, and thought she had ulcers. These symptoms troubled her for about four years. Doctors examined her and even checked for parasites, but tests were negative. They had no solution for her except the standard medications to treat her symptoms. A holistic minded physician recommended she go on a parasite cleanse even though the lab test showed no evidence of parasites. She began taking the herbs he recommended, soon developed a severe breathing problem, and was admitted to the hospital. The doctors assumed she was having an allergic reaction to the herbs. After two days, she passed a 15-inch tapeworm. She continued with the herbs and over the next five days passed four more tapeworms as well as some tiny round red worms. It took 90 days to get rid of all the parasites in her body.

Parasites cause more human devastation and kill more people worldwide than does cancer. Probably half of the human population is infected by parasites, such as roundworms, hookworms, and whipworms. Even in Western countries that have good sanitation practices, parasites are much more common than we might expect. Some health experts claim that 80 percent of us are affected. Tests do not always detect their presence. Labs test for only 40 or 50 kinds of parasites out of the thousands that can live in the body. Also, most tests are performed on stool samples, but many parasites do not live in the digestive tract. Parasites can infect any part of the body without leaving a trace in the intestines. Tests are unreliable.

Parasite infection can cause a host of problems ranging from intestinal discomfort to back pain, vision problems, and emotional disturbances. Many of the health problems people suffer from are actually a direct consequence of parasites.

Bacteria, viruses, fungi, worms, and microscopic insects are living, breathing, and crawling all around us, on us and even inside of us. Tiny mites live on our skin, eating our dead flesh.

We have other parasites living inside of us, in our intestines, in our blood, and could be inhabiting almost any organ in the body. Parasites are found in the liver, heart, pancreas, even the brain. No organ is safe from these creatures. Many of these organisms are relatively harmless. Those that aren't are kept under control by our immune system.

Parasites come from many sources. We breathe in eggs, put contaminants in our mouth, or rub an eye, and the eggs find a warm moist place to incubate and hatch. Any mucous membrane can provide an opening into the body. Even handling bedding from an infected person can spread parasites. Some intestinal worms come out of the rectum at night when the host is asleep to lay their eggs, so sheets and underwear are contaminated. We can live for years with parasites without knowing it. We may have stomach pain and call it indigestion or ulcer, pain in joints and call it arthritis, constipation and call it colitis, uncontrollable nervous movements and call it Parkinson's disease, or any other number of conditions, but heaven forbid—it can't be parasites! It is assumed that parasites affect people in underdeveloped countries, not those in clean, healthy environments.

Parasites are everywhere. If you have a pet, your pet probably has them, and if you allow your pets into your house, you very likely have been exposed to them. You may not know it as you don't recognize symptoms of parasite infestation. Look at a dog, for example, what do they eat? Where do they go? Dogs will kill a squirrel and bury it for a week or two, then dig it up and eat it. Is this a possible source for worms? They sniff old animal droppings, inhaling eggs. They drink water from ditches and puddles contaminated with who knows what. They eat just about anything that may be lying around, rotting and harboring parasites or their eggs. Cats and other pets are the same. Worms will leave their host to lay eggs at night. We come in contact with them by petting the animal or touching its bed, or anything the dog has come in contact with. You may pick them up when visiting a friend who has pets, or even when just going outside. The floor and even your shoes can infect you. You rub your eye, or eat something without washing your hands, and the eggs are transferred to you. In order to be completely free of them, we would need to live in a sterilized environment, which none of us do. The only other way to fight them is with a healthy immune system and antiparasitic herbs.

Parasites are toxins. They are foreign to the body and cause health problems. A complete detoxification program will include a method to remove parasites. Parasites themselves are harmful as they suck your life energy and excrete harmful waste into your body. Parasites in you heart, for example, like the dog heartworm (Dirofilaria), produce ammonia as a waste product. Ammonia, their equivalent of urine, is very toxic, especially to the brain.

Nature has provided us with many natural deworming or deparasitic herbs. But most all parasites that affect the human organism can be treated with just three herbs. Unlike drug parasiticides, herbs do not have harmful side effects. Also, drugs treat only a few types of parasites, so you would need to take many different types in order to completely rid yourself of these menacing creatures.

Of all the herbal parasiticides you need only use three. These three will kill all the parasites usually found in humans (as well as pets). They are:

- Black Walnut Hulls
- Wormwood
- Cloves

The walnut hulls and wormwood kill adult and developmental stages of parasites; the cloves kill the eggs. Used together, they kill adults and eggs. Obviously, if you kill just adults, their eggs will hatch, causing reinfection. If you kill just eggs, the adults will simply lay more.

Black walnut hulls are the green fibrous casings surrounding the black walnut shell. It is one of nature's best parasiticides. Hulls must be harvested green before they begin to decay and turn black. Once they have turned black, the essential chemical constituents that make the hull useful as a parasiticide have decayed. The best way to take this herb is as a tincture mixed in juice.

There are many plants called wormwood. The one with the scientific name *Artemesia* is the one with the most parasite-fighting ability. As the name implies, this plant has a reputation for killing and expelling worms. The FDA has regulated this plant because they consider it could become toxic if taken in large dosages over extended periods of time, yet it has been used for centuries with no ill effect. Wormwood is very bitter and is best taken in capsule form. You must buy the herb in bulk. Sometimes you may find it in combination with other herbs in capsule form. Using bulk herbs you can put them in capsules yourself. Use size 00 or, if not available, size 0 gelatin capsules, obtainable at any health food store. If you can stand the taste, you can also just make a tea and drink it that way.

Cloves are the ordinary spice used in pastries and such. The ones sold in spice racks at the grocery store have usually been ground and have been sitting around for months. Essential chemicals necessary for killing eggs have long evaporated. Use fresh, ground cloves in 00 or 0 gel capsules. It has a much stronger aroma and taste. Or just buy capsules already made; both are available in health food stores.

There are no side effects with these herbs at the dosages recommended. You do not need to stop other medications or herbal therapies.

Take all three herbs together three times a day. Add 30 drops of black walnut hull tincture to one cup of organic apple juice. Drink this with one capsule each of wormwood and clove. Take this combination three times a day before meals or on an empty stomach. Most parasites will die within a week, but continue this formula for at least three weeks, and you may continue it for up to three months. Take it every day. You must be consistent, especially for the first week. On the second week take two capsules three times a day. The third week take three capsules three times a day. Following weeks, remain at three capsules, three times a day. Both wormwood and black walnut hulls have a strong pungent taste, that's why they expel parasites.

Children are more susceptible to parasites than adults as they are always sticking things into their mouths and are less concerned about proper sanitation. Teenagers can take adult dosages. Reduce quantity for preteens to 10 drops of black walnut hull tincture, one capsule each of wormwood and clove a day. For very small children, you can reduce this.

You are always being exposed to parasites. You get them from other people, your family, your pets, food, and drink. Reinfestation will occur. So do the parasite cleanse once or twice a year.

FUNGAL INFECTIONS

John had been on the Natural Foods Diet for a full year. He had undertaken the kidney and liver cleanse programs described in this book and was doing extended (over seven-day) fasts. During the year he lost 25 pounds in excess weight. He was now at the ideal weight for his height and bone structure. He noticed great improvement in his overall health but still was troubled with persistent skin rashes.

Along with the fasting, John began to do enemas. He noticed unusual objects in the stools after the enemas. The most significant was when he expelled large (up to $1/2$ inch) pieces of hairy root-like balls of fungus. The balls were segments of a larger growth that had been thriving in his colon for some time, probably many years. The entire growth was estimated to have been at least as large as a man's hand. This growth was clogging his intestines, releasing toxins into his body, and making him susceptible to recurring fungal infections in other parts of the body, thus the reason for the skin problems. Herbal treatment with additional enemas removed the growth from his bowels and cleared up his persistent skin rash.

One of the worse plagues of Western culture is fungus. Most of us are probably infested with it to some degree. Yeast is a fungus that affects the mouth as thrush, the urinary and vaginal canals as candidiasis, and the skin as ringworm, jock itch, and athlete's foot. Meningitis, which is an inflammation of the membranes of the brain or spinal cord, can also be caused by a fungal infection. The fungus that causes meningitis, *Cryptococcus neoformans*, commonly affects people undergoing chemotherapy and radiation treatment for cancer. Fungus also infests the bladder, intestines, lymphatic system, and blood. It can affect virtually any organ system in the body. San Joaquin fever, which is caused by a fungal infection, can disrupt the entire body.

Fungi are a group of simple organisms similar to plants, but without chlorophyll. Without chlorophyll, pathogenic fungi cannot produce their own food, so they must parasitize other organisms. Yeasts are small single-celled fungi, and molds are larger, multicellular organisms. Most pathogenic fungi parasitize tissue on or near the skin or mucous membranes as in ringworm or vaginal yeast infections. But many can affect organs and tissues throughout the body.

We *all* have fungus growing in or on our bodies. Yes, every one of us, not just those in poor health or who live in unsanitary conditions. Fungi and their spores are everywhere. We come in contact with them on our skin, breathe them in the air, and eat them in our food every day. There is no way we can avoid them.

The reason we all don't have hideous fungal infections is because our immune systems keep them in check. All of us have in our bodies the fungus Candida albicans which causes yeast infections (candidiasis). But our immune systems prevent it from growing, spreading, and getting out of control. When the immune system is weakened by illness, medications, poor eating habits, and lack of exercise, the fungi proliferate. Many times we will be unaware of the presence of a fungal infection. We attribute symptoms—urinary problems, constipation, lack of energy, frequent illness, etc.—to the natural deterioration of the body as it grows older. If we are healthy, we should not have problems like this as we age.

Most people in Western society have fungal infections to one degree or another because of their lifestyle. The body is put under strain, constantly battling these parasitic invaders. Every time we get sick or use medications, the infection gains greater strength. Fungal spores circulate in the blood and lymphatic system and can affect any part of the body. A significant step towards achieving good health is to remove the fungus from our bodies. Eating good healthy food is a major step in this direction. As we eat right, the body's immune system will be strengthened. But this is a long process. We can accelerate the removal of fungi from our bodies with the use of herbs.

One of the most common herbs for treating candida and other fungal infections is garlic. In clinical studies garlic, particularly raw garlic, has proven to be effective in reducing and relieving fungal infections. Eating raw garlic and taking garlic supplements (capsules and extract) can aid in ridding the body of troublesome fungi. As a fungal detoxifier, fresh garlic juice is one of the best. The obvious problem with consuming fresh garlic is the strong taste and the lingering smell. After eating fresh garlic, or supplements made with fresh garlic, the breath reveals the fact, and even the body can emit a faint scent. This can be inconvenient if you work with people every day and your appearance and hygiene are important. Some garlic supplements have been deodorized so that you don't have that lingering odor with you throughout the day. You may also try taking garlic in the evening so that by the next day the odoriferous effects have worn off.

Another herb that has become popular as an antifungal remedy is pau d'arco. This herb can be purchased in capsule form or as a tea.

By far the most effective natural antifungal remedy is caprylic acid. Caprylic acid has proven to be just as effective in controlling yeast infections as the most popular antifungal medications prescribed by physicians. But unlike most medications, caprylic acid is a product of nature and has no undesirable side effects. You will often see natural antifungal or candida fighting supplements in the health food store that combine garlic and pau d'arco, with caprylic acid. Used as directed on the container these are effective in cleansing candida from the body.

Caprylic acid is a fatty acid derived from coconut. Coconut also contains other similar fatty acids that make it a powerful antifungal herb. Simply eating fresh coconut every day has helped people rid themselves of systemic candida infections. The medicinal properties of coconut come from a unique group of fatty acids found almost exclusively in tropical plants. This is discussed more fully below.

BACTERIAL AND VIRAL INFECTIONS

In the 1960s food scientists discovered one of nature's most potent natural antibiotics. Researchers looking for a functional food which could be used as an additive to retard spoilage found an herb that surpassed all expectations. That herb was the seed of the coconut palm. The fatty acids in the oil of the coconut seed proved to be the magic ingredient. Coconut oil was found to act as an antioxidant that could prevent oxidation and food spoilage but even more remarkable was that the fatty acids in the oil could also kill disease-causing bacteria, viruses, and fungi.

The antimicrobial properties of coconut oil are activated during digestion. Our bodies transform the oil into powerful germ-fighting fatty acids called medium-chain fatty acids. Caprylic acid which in now used to combat yeast infections is one of these fatty acids.

These unique fatty acids are also produced in the mammary glands of nursing mothers and form a vital part of her breast milk. Their purpose in milk is to provide nourishment as well as protect the infant from infectious organisms. The immune system of newborns is still immature and vulnerable to a host of disease-causing microorganisms. Medium-chain fatty acids in the milk protect the baby from infection for the first few months of life.

These medium-chain fatty acids are created by nature for the purpose of fighting infections. They are more powerful than herbs traditionally used to combat infections such as garlic, echinacea, goldenseal, and elderberry.

Babies are not the only ones who can benefit from the antimicrobial properties of medium-chain fatty acids. No matter what your age, you can cleanse disease-causing microorganisms from your body by consuming a source of medium-chain fatty acids. Other than breast milk the only other commonly used food source for these fatty acids is from the tropical oils, particularly coconut oil.

Coconuts and coconut oil have been used for thousands of years in tropical regions of the world as both food and medicine. Coconut oil is probably the most popular traditional medicine in the world. Ayurvedic medicine of India holds coconut oil in high esteem for its healing properties. Only recently has the medicinal value of coconut oil been verified by modern science.

In recent years scientific research has demonstrated that medium-chain fatty acids from coconut oil are effective in killing viruses that cause influenza, measles, herpes, mononucleosis, hepatitis C, and AIDS; bacteria which cause stomach ulcers, throat infections, pneumonia, sinusitis, ear infections, food poisoning, urinary tract infections, gonorrhea, meningitis, and toxic shock syndrome; and fungus which cause ringworm, candida, and thrush.

The amount of coconut oil recommended to ward off infection is 3.5 tablespoons or more taken every day until symptoms are gone. Some people take this much daily whether they are sick or not just to prevent illness from occurring. The best way to take coconut oil is with food. Simply prepare your meals using coconut oil. You may need to add more oil than you ordinarily use. You may split the dosage between two or more meals during the day.

Many people hesitate to use coconut oil for fear of eating saturated fat. The saturated fat in coconut oil is totally different from the saturated fat in meat. Fats in meats and even most plants are composed of long-chain fatty acids. The fats in coconut oil are predominately the beneficial medium-chain variety. Recent medical research has shown that medium-chain fatty acids may actually help fight heart disease. So eating coconut oil will *lower* your risk of heart disease and improve your health.

For a more complete discussion on the health aspects of coconut oil and how to use it, I highly recommend you read the book *The Coconut Oil Miracle.*

 **ADDITIONAL RESOURCES**

The Coconut Oil Miracle. Fife, Bruce, N.D. New York, NY: Avery, 2004.

Guess What Came to Dinner: Parasites and Your Health. Gittleman, Ann Louise. Garden City Park, NY: Avary Publishing Group, 1993.

The Healing Herbs. Castleman, Michael. Emmaus, PA: Rodale Press, 1991.

The New Holistic Herbal. Hoffmann, David. Rockport, MA: Element Books. 1992.

Weiner's Herbal. Weiner, Michael, Ph.D. Mill Valley, CA: Quantum Books, 1990.

Chapter 15

CLEANSING THE MIND

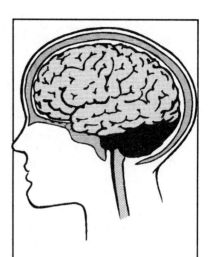

Although mental and emotional cleansing is the last detoxification process listed in this book, it is certainly not the least important. In fact, psychological cleansing and stress management are probably the most important steps toward achieving and maintaining good health.

The mind has tremendous power over our physical health. How we perceive ourselves and our outlook on life affects our health. In this chapter you will learn how to cleanse poisons from the brain and purge toxic emotions and stress from the mind.

In an article on centenarians for *Parade* magazine, Caryl Stern noted from her interviews that people who live to be a hundred years old and more have one striking similarity—they are all happy, bright, and exuberant. They think positively about themselves and about life. In other words, they have a positive mental attitude about themselves and about life. Our psychological health and outlook on life has a lot to do with our physical health—more so than most people realize.

It is more important to know what sort of person has a disease than to know what sort of disease a person has.
—Hippocrates

NUTRITION AND MENTAL HEALTH

Many people are surprised to discover that our diets play an important part in our mental health. If the health of our entire body can be adversely affected by poor-quality foods, isn't it logical to assume that the brain and nervous system can also be affected? The brain, in fact, is very susceptible to foods, drugs, and toxins.

According to Melvin Werbach, M.D., a faculty member at the UCLA School of Medicine and author of *Nutritional Influences on Mental Illness*, "It is clear that nutrition can powerfully influence cognition, emotion, and behavior. It is also clear that the effects of classical nutritional deficiency diseases upon mental function constitute only a small part of a rapidly expanding list of interfaces between nutrition and the mind." A deficiency of any single nutrient can alter brain function and lead to depression, anxiety, and other mental disorders.

Food additives can have numerous adverse effects. Caffeine is one that has been extensively studied and is well known to affect the nervous system, including our minds. It is a stimulant. A person's response to caffeine will vary; however, people prone to depression or anxiety tend to be especially sensitive to caffeine. The term "caffeinism" is used to describe a clinical syndrome similar to generalized anxiety and panic disorders that include such symptoms as depression, nervousness, palpitations, irritability, and recurrent headaches.

Several studies have looked at caffeine intake and depression. For example, one study found that among healthy college students, moderate and high coffee drinkers scored higher on a depression scale than did low users. Interestingly, the moderate and high coffee drinkers also tended to have significantly lower academic performance. Several other studies have shown that depressed patients tend to consume fairly high amounts of caffeine (i.e., greater than three or four cups of coffee a day). The intake of caffeine has been positively correlated with the degree of mental illness in psychiatric patients. In other words, the more caffeine consumed, the greater the mental illness in these patients.

When refined sugar is combined with caffeine the symptoms intensify. In one particular study subjects described themselves as feeling depressed and didn't know why, often felt tired even though they slept a lot, were very moody, and generally seemed to feel bad most of the time. When caffeine and sugar were taken from their diet, subjects reported substantial improvement and, in subsequent testing when given supplements in a double-blind study, those that took caffeine and sugar supplements reported a significantly higher rate of depression during the test period. Other studies have shown similar results.

The average American consumes 150-225 mg of caffeine daily, or roughly the amount of caffeine in one to two cups of coffee. Although most people can handle this amount, some people are more sensitive to the effects of caffeine than others. Even small amounts of caffeine, as found in decaffeinated coffee, are enough to affect some people adversely and produce caffeinism. People with depression or any psychological disorder should avoid caffeine completely.

Caffeine is just one of many substances that can affect the mind. Drugs, alcohol, nicotine, food dyes, preservatives, and other chemical additives can all affect how we think and act.

The mind can be affected by the health of other organs in the body. The colon is the body's sewage pipe, removing metabolic waste and toxic debris from our bodies. When fecal matter gets clogged or pathogenic organisms proliferate in the bowel, toxins are absorbed into the bloodstream, affecting every part of the body—including the brain. Toxins in the brain can affect thought, reason, judgment, memory, patience, temper, rationality, mental and physical energy, concentration, sex drive, equilibrium, senses, and coordination. Eating low-fiber, high-protein, fatty, and chemical laden foods is the primary cause of colon autointoxication.

Behavioral Effects of Some Vitamin Deficiencies

Deficient Vitamin	Behavioral Effects
Thiamin	Korsakoff's psychosis, mental depression, apathy, anxiety, irritability
Riboflavin	Depression, irritability
Niacin	Apathy, anxiety, depression, hyperirritability, mania, memory deficits, delirium, organic dementia, emotional liability
Biotin	Depression, extreme lassitude, somnolence
Pantothenic acid	Restlessness, irritability, depression, fatigue
B_6	Depression, irritability, sensitivity to sound
Folic acid	Forgetfulness, insomnia, apathy, irritability, depression, psychosis, delirium, dementia
B_{12}	Psychotic states, depression, irritability, confusion, memory loss, hallucinations, delusions, paranoia
C	Lassitude, hypochondriasis, depression, hysteria

Carbohydrates in our food are converted by the liver into glucose. The level of glucose in our blood is closely regulated by the pancreas. Either too much or too little glucose in the blood can have serious health consequences. Diabetes, for example, is a condition resulting from too much glucose in the blood. Glucose is the fuel by which the brain, as well as the other organs of the body, derives its energy. The brain functions at a social level when it has plenty of fuel; when the blood sugar drops below the critical level, as in hypoglycemia, the brain ceases to function at a social level, leading to irritability and hyperactivity to explosive behavior and even violence. A pancreas hampered by toxins and other negative factors can cause adverse psychological changes.

The liver—the body's main processing plant—can also affect the mind. Here elements from digested food are stored, synthesized, distributed, and poisons detoxified. A poor-quality diet puts a tremendous burden on the liver. Too much stress can lead to degenerative liver disease and infection.

For centuries, traditional Chinese doctors have linked the liver with hot tempers. Researchers at the University of California Los Angeles Medical Center have found that when a liver is diseased by hepatitis, cirrhosis, or some other condition, it releases toxins into the bloodstream. These toxins travel to the brain and trigger bouts of irritability, anger, and even rage. These toxins may also be responsible for feelings of disorientation, anxiety, and apathy. This may explain, in part, the outbursts commonly associated with alcoholism. Among alcoholics with liver disease, it is the diseased liver, say researchers, rather than the alcohol abuse, which seems to determine the more volatile behaviors.

A poor-quality diet contributes directly to many mental and emotional problems. It also affects the way we handle stress. Stress is one of the major causes of dis-ease.

STRESS
A Cause of Dis-ease

Stress is often said to be the most destructive element in people's lives, but that's only partly true. The real element is the way we react to stress. Some people have a high stress tolerance and can withstand situations that would drive others crazy. Others have a very low tolerance to stress and, as a result, their reactions are more severe.

Your thoughts and emotions have a big impact on your health. Stress-related symptoms continue to account for 70 percent of all physician office visits, according to a leading research and educational institute in northern California. According to the Institute of HeartMath (IHM),

$200 billion each year is spent by businesses throughout the United States on stress and stress-related illnesses. In addition, estimates show that at least 40 percent of employee turnover is due to stress, according to *California Business* (April 1993).

More importantly, the link between stress and disease has been firmly established. In a landmark 20-year study conducted at the University of London, researchers found that negative reactions to stress were the single most dangerous risk factor for cancer and heart disease—worse than smoking or eating high cholesterol foods.

Stress weakens the immune system, slows down vital body functions, drains nutrients, and overworks organs, making us more susceptible to the effects of toxins and malnutrition. Stress can also contribute directly to the toxic load on the body by increasing harmful acid accumulation (i.e., acidosis) from metabolic processes. Stress can make a significant impact on health, causing numerous dis-ease conditions regardless of our diet or environment. We may eat clean, healthy foods and live in an unpolluted environment, but if we are over-stressed, vital nutrients are quickly used up, immune response decreases, digestion slows down—releasing toxins into the blood—and harmful metabolic acid accumulates, all precursors to disease.

Aches, pains, and dysfunction of organs can be directly caused by psychological factors resulting from stress. Stress can cause high blood pressure; headaches; facial, neck, leg, and back pain; stomach aches, constipation, colitis, ulcers, and other digestive problems; behavior problems; learning difficulties; sleep disturbances (including nightmares and bed-wetting); skin diseases; and infections. Stressful events often precede bacterial and viral infections. Research studies suggest that even conditions like asthma, allergies, and diabetes are adversely affected by stress.

Fight-or-Flight Response

If you came face to face with a tiger, almost instantly your glands would kick into feverish activity and your sympathetic nervous system would take over. Glucose, the body's cellular energy source, would be vigorously pumped into your bloodsteam, super-charging many of your bodily functions. Your heart would beat faster, your blood pressure would rise, more blood would be pumped to your skeletal muscles, and respiration would increase. Non-essential functions, such as digestion, would slow down. The body would be ready to either fight the tiger or flee for life. Thus the term "fight-or-flight."

We don't have to be face-to-face with danger to trigger the fight-or-flight response. This action is a natural consequence to any type of stress. Stress is brought on by fear, anger, hate, greed and even passive emotions such as grief, anxiety, worry, or feelings of failure.

Stress is caused by many negative factors, but can also be caused by positive events such as a new job, marriage, or winning the jackpot. Some stress is beneficial. After all, our bodies were designed to handle stress at appropriate times. Stress sharpens our minds and bodies to improve performance. An athlete, for example, can perform much better during competition when he is nervous. Likewise, a businessman has more spunk and enthusiasm when making an important deal or giving a demonstration. These actions are enhanced when the body is under stress, but the proper response is for the body to relax once the stress stimulators are removed—the athletic event is over or the demonstration is finished. It is when the body is continually stimulated, particularly by negative factors, that stress becomes detrimental.

The stress response can be activated by numerous daily situations—rushing to work, fighting traffic, facing unpleasant bosses and annoying co-workers, dealing with work related problems, meeting deadlines, satisfying customer demands, struggling with family problems, solving financial difficulties, and coping with illness. The list is endless. All of these create tension and stress and can evoke the fight-or-flight response. For some people, these situations are a constant occurrence throughout the day, every day. They are under stress more than they are not. Our bodies are capable of responding to stress for short periods of time without causing any undue problems. But if the stress is prolonged, and especially if physical action is not a permitted response to the stress, then it can drain the body of its reserves and leave it weakened, worn, and susceptible to illness.

During the fight-or-flight response a healthy body is capable of handling great physical demands for short periods of time. Functions not immediately necessary to deal with the cause of the stress are temporarily slowed down. When stress is prolonged, the overstimulation of some organs and the understimulation of others can lead to serious health problems.

Stress stimulates the adrenal glands to secrete hormones at a feverish pace. These hormones, in turn, stimulate the stress response in other tissues. Some of these hormones suppress the immune system. This is all right in dealing with occasional emergencies; however, when the tension and anxiety of modern life keep the stress response on continually, the hormones suppress our resistance to disease, even withering away the lymph nodes. The adrenal glands also secrete a testosterone-like sex hormone that can cause the development of male secondary sexual characteristics such as beard growth, development of body hair, and increased muscle mass on both men and women. Stress thus produces masculine effects, including an increase in aggressiveness, which can intensify or prolong stress and intensify its effects.

Overstimulation can deplete the adrenal glands of vital elements, causing them to malfunction. This can lead to the over- or under-secretion of several different hormones. Excessive stress can wear out the adrenal glands, thus causing a chain reaction leading to a whole host of diseases and adverse side effects.

During times of stress, the heart rate increases. Most blood vessels that feed internal organs constrict, causing an increase in blood pressure which, in turn, puts a great deal of stress on the rapidly beating heart and the circulatory system. Prolonged stress aggravates cardiovascular illness and undoubtedly is a factor in the extraordinarily high death rate due to heart disease. Restricted blood flow to the internal organs also causes a decrease in the delivery of nutrients and the removal of toxins in these vital tissues. This situation promotes stagnation of internal fluids which leads to degenerative conditions and the promotion of diseases such as cancer.

Stress also causes digestive muscles to slow down and the glands to secrete sparingly. During emergencies digestion is unnecessary; we function on nutrient reserves. If stress is prolonged, digestion remains suppressed. Food is not digested fully so nutrients are not available for absorption. Even though a person may eat normally, if he or she is continually under stress, nutrient deficiencies can result. During times of stress the body requires greater amounts of nutrients, especially the B vitamins. Since nutrient absorption is decreased at this time the problem of nutrient deficiency is compounded. Nutrients are necessary to fuel metabolism, growth, repair, hormone production, and numerous other functions vital to health. Lack of essential nutrients signals food cravings in an attempt to get these vital nutrients. Eating may increase, but digestion and absorption remain suppressed. With most people, increased eating means consuming more poor-quality foods filled with sugar and fat which only add more stress to the body.

When food is not digested completely, more material is moved through intestines, leading to constipation and stagnation of feces in the colon. Putrefying fecal debris releases toxins and carcinogens into the body and provides an environment which encourages the proliferation of pathogenic bacteria and parasites.

Anger Kills

While you are driving, a car recklessly pulls in front you. Do you honk your horn and say a few choice words? Maybe even flash on your high beams or consider tailgating to get back at him for his rudeness? It's not a pretty picture. Too many of us overreact to the countless aggravations of everyday life by boiling over.

Researchers are telling us that although anger creates stress, the most unhealthy consequences result if you act out that anger. It's okay to think that the person who just turned in front of you in traffic is a jerk, and go on your merry way. What's not okay is to scream at him and pound the steering wheel. Researches say that blowing your stack or even seething silently can put your heart at risk. Expressing anger intensifies the stress reaction, setting the heart racing and blood pressure soaring. Tests show that when no outward displays of anger occur, the body displays little reaction.

A few years ago we were encouraged to vent our anger by letting it out. This way, it was reasoned, anger would be dissipated. According to the theory, doing nothing would only create more internal stress. This has been shown to be dangerously inaccurate. Some people who do not openly vent their anger hold it inside and keep it burning. For such people, openly expressing anger may be less harmful than constant brooding. But those people who let stress-causing situations pass without expressing anger openly or silently brooding about it, tend not to build up stress.

Anger and other stress factors can literally kill you. Studies have shown that people whose blood pressure shoots up during stressful mental challenges are more likely to get hardening of the arteries, which can lead to heart attacks and strokes. Experts have long known that people with consistently high blood pressure risk getting atherosclerosis, the cholesterol-clogging of blood vessels commonly called hardening of the arteries. As blood surges through your arteries and stress hormones pour from your adrenal glands, once-smooth artery walls begin

Would You Like to Live to Be A Hundred?   100

When asked if they would like to live to be a hundred, many people say they would not because then they would suffer too long with degenerative diseases that afflict the aged.

But the truth of the matter is, most of those who live to be a hundred do not experience long periods of debilitating degenerative disease. They are in relatively good health. That is why they live so long. After the age of 85, the odds that you will die in the next year or two actually level off. And half of today's centenarians are in good health, both physically and mentally. Those people who are prone to degenerative disease die long before they reach life expectancy, which is in mid 70s. Many even die in their forties and earlier.

Genetics plays a part in the life potential, but its influence is greatly overrated. The real deciding factors are diet, lifestyle, and degree of exposure to environmental toxins. You can have strong genes and die young for lack of a healthy diet, competent medical care, or the ability to cope with stress. "That's the good news," Leonard W. Poon says. Dr. Poon, director of the University of Georgia's Gerontology Center and head of the nation's biggest centenarian study. "We all have a chance of becoming centenarians."

The assumption that the older you get, the sicker you get, is incorrect. Age does not cause disease.

Many people claim advances in medicine like antibiotics have helped get today's elderly past killers like pneumonia. But, for the most part, centenarians have *not* been saved by new medical technologies like heart-bypass surgery, because they have managed to avoid major illnesses like heart disease.

"They're able to handle dietary problems and environmental insults that would devastate the rest of us," says Dr. Perls of Harvard University. "Over their whole life-span, these people have seldom spent much time with a doctor," says Dr. Perls. "When they finally get sick, they die quickly, and it costs relatively little." The good news is that there are a growing number of centenarians. If they can make it in a polluted world, we can too, if we take care of ourselves. It won't happen by chance and it won't happen if we neglect our health and expose ourselves to harmful influences.

When you look at the lives of centenarians here and around the world, what common dominators are there? The three most common denominators are avoidance of harmful toxins, adequate physical activity, and maintaining a positive mental attitude.

Plainly, good health and the key to looking and feeling years younger require more than following a set of rigid rules. It also involves achieving an exuberant, hopeful, fun-loving state of mind, free from harmful stress. Scientists are increasingly proving that celebrated pianist Arthur Rubinstein was right when he said, "I have found if you love life, life will love you back." Rubinstein lived to be 95.

to scar and pit. Then fatty cells clump on that pocked surface, like mineral deposits in an old water pipe. Arteries narrow, blood flow decreases, and your body is starved of oxygen. The final result is chest pain, strokes, or heart attacks.

This conclusion rests on some compelling findings. In one study, for example, 255 doctors who had taken a standard personality test while attending the University of North Carolina's medical school were tracked down 25 years later. Those whose hostility scores had been in the top half were four to five times as likely to have developed heart disease in the intervening decades as were those whose hostility scores had been in the lower half.

A similar study that looked at 118 lawyers found equally striking results. Of those lawyers who had scored in the top quarter for hostility, nearly one in five was dead by age 50. Of those in the lowest quarter, only one in 25 had died.

Dr. David Krantz, a psychologist at Uniformed Services University of the Health Sciences, in Bethesda, Md., says, "People would say, 'You're telling me I can't be competitive? I shouldn't meet deadlines? How am I going to explain that to my boss?' Now the message is more manageable: Ambition is not the problem. Aggressiveness is not the problem. Hostility is the problem. What your boss wants is for you to get the work done. He doesn't necessarily want you to act like a SOB."

While stress factors, including anger, are often portrayed as uniformly bad, effects of stress vary dramatically from person to person. Some handle frustrations with little change in blood pressure, yet it soars in others. Researchers have found that those who react most powerfully to mental stress develop the most deposits in their arteries. Even when they looked at all the other known contributors to this disease, such as smoking and diabetes, the reaction to stress was the most potent contributor to atherosclerosis.

Centuries before, physicians recognized that cancer and other diseases tend to follow tragedy or crisis in a person's life. Studies have confirmed that stress caused by negative emotions such as anger, grief, worry, anxiety, fear, and depression lowers the efficiency of the disease-fighting cells of the body's immune system. Divorce is one of the most devastating stressors. Divorced people have higher rates of cancer, heart disease, pneumonia, high blood pressure, and accidental death than married persons. Married men also have one-third the lung cancer of single men.

A study at the Albert Einstein College of Medicine in New York found that children with cancer had twice as many recent crises as other children matched to be similar except for their disease. Another study showed that 31 of 33 children with leukemia had experienced a traumatic stress (a traumatic loss or move) within the two years before their diagnosis.

Not everyone who suffers a tragic loss or crisis in life develops an illness. An important deciding factor seems to be how one copes with the stress. Those who can effectively deal with a stress-causing situation and don't let it bother them, generally stay well. Those who get angry and let it eat at them, wear down their immune systems, making them susceptible to disease. Depressed people are twice as likely to get cancer as those who are not. Stress may not necessarily be the primary cause of disease, but stress opens the door.

The simple truth is, happy people generally don't get sick. Attitude is the single most important factor in reducing stress and staying well. Those who are at peace with themselves and the people they are around have far fewer serious illnesses than those who are not.

We have learned that stress directly or indirectly contributes to cardiovascular disease, gastrointestinal problems, hormonal dysfunction, and numerous other degenerative diseases, as well as suppresses the immune system, which opens the door to infection from harmful microorganisms and lowers the body's ability to ward off diseases of all types.

PSYCHOLOGICAL CLEANSING AND STRESS MANAGEMENT

Most of us probably aren't aware of how much tension we hold. We go from being wound up and tense to collapsing into our couch or easy chair by the end of the day. This is the result of overstimulation and exhaustion. Our vital energy and nutrient stores are depleted. Some people are so wound up, especially if they consume sugary foods and caffeine, that it takes a long time for them to relax and they suffer from insomnia. In the morning they are exhausted because they didn't get enough restful sleep, but force themselves to get up for work. The cycle continues over and over each day. The weekends become a welcome chance to get away from the rat race and catch up on badly needed rest. Such people seem to live just for the weekends.

People who handle the stress of daily life well don't live for the weekends. Monday morning is not a dreaded event. They meet each new day with a smile. They are glad to be alive. If you are one of those who hate Mondays, constantly looks forward to the weekends, comes home exhausted from work, or who may have insomnia even though physically tired, you are badly overstressed and in danger of developing the conditions described in this chapter. If you find yourself cursing thoughtless drivers or getting uptight by the actions of others, you also may have far too much stress.

Good health requires the detoxification of stress and other negative psychological factors. Seven keys to psychological cleansing and stress reduction are: (1) nutrition, (2) exercise, (3) play and laughter, (4) relaxation, (5) visualization, (6) positive mental attitude, and (7) love and forgiveness.

Nutrition

Eating nutritious, clean food is the first step you should take to combat stress as well as any mental or emotional problem. A good diet is often all that is necessary to break harmful addictions, change your perception on life, bring dramatic improvements in stamina, and sleep more restfully.

Besides eating clean, wholesome foods and avoiding toxin laden ones, some natural dietary supplements can be useful in supporting the body to help it cope with the stress. Vitamins are rapidly drained from the body during stress, particularly the B-complex vitamins. B-complex vitamins are necessary for healthy nervous system function. They are crucial in the production of energy, adrenal gland hormones, and serotonin (which serves as a buffer against stress). Damaging free radicals are also produced by stress. Antioxidants such as vitamin E, vitamin C, beta-carotene, and bioflavonoids fight free radicals. Minerals are also important, especially calcium, magnesium, and potassium. These minerals have a relaxing effect on the body; they relieve muscle tension and calm the emotions. Taking a vitamin supplement rich in B vitamins, antioxidants, and minerals could be of great benefit.

A number of herbs have been found useful in dealing with the effects of stress. Two herbs that support and strengthen the adrenals, the glands affected most by stress, are licorice root and parsley. The herb ginkgo biloba has antioxidant properties that directly affect brain function. It helps to reduce harmful free radicals as well as increase the delivery of oxygen to the brain, which improves mental function. Siberian ginseng is another herb that can help counteract the effects of stress. Ginseng can raise our tolerance to stress by normalizing various organ functions. For example, it can increase or decrease the secretion of hormones, raise or lower our blood sugar level, and raise or lower our blood pressure. Ginseng also stimulates the immune system, increases physical stamina, and improves mental alertness.

For depression, the herb that has shown the best results in clinical studies and in practical application is St.

John's wort. It is perhaps the most effective natural antidepressant currently available. In studies St. John's wort extract was shown to produce improvements in many psychological symptoms including depression, anxiety, apathy, sleep disturbances, insomnia, anorexia, and feelings of worthlessness. To be effective the St. John's wort extract must be standardized to contain 0.3 percent hypericin and be taken at the dosage of 300 mg, three times daily.

Many herbs have a sedative effect and are useful in easing stress and helping to achieve a peaceful night's sleep. Taken in reasonable doses they have no adverse side effects and can be used along with most of the detox methods discussed in this book. The following herbs are known to be effective in calming nerves, relieving stress, and promoting sleep: hops, valerian root, kava kava, scullcap, catnip, chamomile, lemonbalm, and passion flower. Any of the above mentioned herbs can be taken as a tea or in capsule form. Combinations can enhance the effects of all ingredients. You can combine valerian, for example, with lemonbalm or passionflower. These herbs are packaged alone or in combination by a variety of tea and herb companies.

The herb and vitamin supplements should be used only as crutches until dietary, lifestyle, and psychological adjustments take hold. Once the body has overcome nutrient deficiencies and repaired itself, it should be able to function normally even when exposed to a moderate amount of stress.

Exercise

Vigorous exercise is a natural release for the body's fight-or-flight response during periods of stress. You can work off the epinephrine overload that accompanies stress, and afterwards, your body returns to its pre-stress state. In addition, as your heart and lungs become more efficient through aerobic exercise, you also build up your stamina and endurance. This makes it easier to cope with stress for longer periods of time without becoming burned out.

Regular exercise may be the most powerful natural antidepressant available. It also increases energy, improves digestion and absorption of nutrients, and releases tension. Various studies have clearly indicated that exercise has profound effects. These studies have shown that increased participation in exercise, sports, and other vigorous physical activities is strongly associated with decreased symptoms of restlessness, tension, depression, fatigue, and insomnia. In addition, people who exercise regularly have higher self-esteem, feel better, and are much happier compared to people who do not exercise.

Aerobic exercise affects the chemical processes in

the brain by increasing blood flow, releasing hormones, stimulating the nervous system, and raising the levels of morphine-like substances called endorphins. Endorphins, which are more potent than morphine, are released during exercise and can trigger a neurophysiological "high." When endorphin levels are low, depression occurs. Conversely, when endorphin levels are elevated, so is mood.

A wealth of research confirms the effectiveness of exercise in dealing with moderate depression and anxiety. For example, in one classic study, Dr. John Greist, psychiatrist and professor at the University of Wisconsin, divided depressed patients into three groups. The first group took up running. The second group used time-limited psychotherapy (i.e., the date the treatment ended was predetermined). The third group used time-unlimited psychotherapy. Levels of depression were evaluated before, during, and at the conclusion of the study. At the end of the study, Dr. Greist found that patients who had time-limited psychotherapy were slightly depressed. Patients in time-unlimited psychotherapy were moderately depressed. However, the patients who ran reported almost no depression.

Drs. Ismail and Trachtman, two physiologists at Purdue University, developed an exercise program for middle-aged men. They wrote, "After a while, we articulated what at first we only felt: we were fairly sure that our paunchy, sedentary, middle-aged businessmen were undergoing personality changes, subtly but definitely . . . The men often seemed more open and extroverted. Although many of them had known each other well before the program started, by the time they reached the end of the program they seemed to be interacting more freely and to be more relaxed. Their whole demeanor seemed to us to be more even, stable, and self-confident."

The state of your muscles also affects mood. You may hold your shoulder or neck muscles stiff with worry. You may clench your lower jaw with resentment. Fear may tie your stomach up in knots. Stretching promotes circulation and relieves muscle stiffness. When the muscle fibers are elongated, there's an increase of blood to the muscle and a decrease of tension. When you develop better muscle tone and blood supply through regular exercise, your muscles are less susceptible to the fatigue and soreness that can result from chronic stress.

Lifting the spirits and calming the nerves isn't all exercise does for the emotional health. It also enhances clarity of thought, powers of concentration, and memory. Students who exercise regularly also do better academically. Likewise, job satisfaction and performance is enhanced. Some companies recognize this and encourage employees to exercise by providing aerobic classes and even exercise equipment or facilities.

Any type of exercise will be beneficial at any time of the day. Some people like to exercise after work to help them unwind and relax. Others like to do it during their lunch hour to freshen their minds and recharge their bodies. Still others work out in the morning to prepare them for the day. A few combine these, doing light to moderate physical activities during the day followed by a more vigorous workout later on.

The most beneficial exercise is one that gets your heart pumping, lungs blowing, and sweat glands flowing. In other words, you need to get vigorous! Light to moderate exercise is okay and can help reduce stress throughout the day if done often, but if you want to enjoy the real benefits of exercise you need to work up a sweat and get out of breath. A leisurely stroll around the block won't do this. But fast, vigorous walking can.

Any aerobic exercise that increases heart rate and respiration can be of benefit. This isn't always possible during the day when stressful situations are at their peak. Mild activities that you can do at work can be beneficial to help diffuse tension throughout the day. Examples would be to walk up a few flights of stairs. Make it a routine to use stairs instead of the elevator. Take walks at lunch time. Take any opportunity you can to get up and move.

You can also do chair exercises to help relieve stress while sitting at a desk. To do this, sit comfortably in a chair with your back gently against the back of the chair and both feet flat on the floor, legs uncrossed. Take several deep breaths, bringing air deep into the lungs by first expanding the stomach and then the chest and lungs. Hold momentarily and slowly expel the air from the top down from the lungs to the stomach ending by tightening the abdominal muscles (see pages 114-115). Relax the muscles and begin again by expanding the abdomen. This alone can do wonders in relieving stress.

Start at the top of your head and work down your face, tightening and relaxing the muscles. Wrinkle your forehead. Open and close your eyes tightly. Wiggle your nose. Clench your teeth and unclench them, open your mouth, make faces, and move every muscle in your face.

Continue down the body. Twist your head from side to side and then up and down; shrug your shoulders several times. Tighten the muscles in your arms. Open and close

> Fear less, hope more; eat less, chew more; whine less, breathe more; talk less, say more; hate less, love more; and all good things are yours.
>
> —Swedish Proverb

your fists. Shake them out. Tighten muscles in thighs, knees, and calves; flex your feet and toes. Finally, get up and walk around if you can.

Play and Laughter

We normally associate playing with childishness, but play should not be restricted to children only. Adults need time to play just as much as children. As the saying goes, "All work and no play makes Jack a dull boy." We might add, "a sick boy" as well. This saying is true regardless of Jack's age. Play can have a strong therapeutic effect on our minds and bodies. It is one of the pleasures of life, and a great stress reducer.

Play can be described as an activity that you usually do with other people that brings pleasure and often laughter. What you do is not so important as how you feel while you're doing it. It should be relaxing, even though it may be physically demanding, like hiking, swimming, volleyball, tennis, skiing, or other recreational activity. It can be social, like card or board games with friends or family. Window shopping, playing a musical instrument, singing, visiting friends, dancing, gardening, and surfing on the internet, are other examples. Any type of activity that pulls you away from the daily grind and which you enjoy can be classified as play. Any activity counts as long as the reward lies in the doing of it.

Take time to enjoy life. Learn new skills and develop new interests. Do something you enjoy every single day. If you can't think of anything, then you need to open your eyes to what life has to offer. Look around you and find things you would like to do. Often, just learning a new skill will develop appreciation and enjoyment for new activities. Try new things and give them a chance; in so doing you will also meet people and make new friends.

Play often involves laughter. Laughter in itself has therapeutic benefits and can be a powerful medicine. The healing power of humor was recognized in ancient times. The wisdom of King Solomon recorded in the Bible states, "A merry heart doeth good like a medicine" (Proverbs 17:22).

Scientific evidence demonstrates the health benefits of laughter. It relaxes the muscles, increases oxygen in blood, stimulates circulation, and reduces tension. All muscles of the chest, abdomen, and face get a workout. Physiologists have found that muscle relaxation and anxiety cannot exist together, and the relaxation response after a good laugh has been measured as lasting as long as 45 minutes.

According to some studies, laughter also increases the production of chemicals in the brain which activate the immune system and increase the production of endorphins.

Humor also diverts attention away from stressful thoughts, allowing us to relax.

Take time to watch or listen to humorous television programs, movies, radio programs, and tapes. Read light-hearted books and magazines. Associate with people who have a sense of humor. Cultivate your own sense of humor.

Relaxation

In our modern, hectic world we often do not take time to relax. In the warm, tropical climate of the Caribbean relaxing is considered an art. In fact, they have a special word for it—liming. Liming is the art of doing nothing, guilt free. Like the Caribbeans, we should be able to sit back and relax without feeling that we need to be doing something else. Give yourself a break—take a nap, read a book, meditate, go for a walk, smell the roses, enjoy nature, stare out the window, daydream. You'll return to your daily chores feeling more refreshed and less stressed.

An excellent way to facilitate relaxation is with a massage. Therapeutic touch relaxes the muscles, soothes stiff joints, improves circulation, remove toxins, eases tension, and refreshes the mind. Massages can be relaxing or invigorating, depending on the type you get. An invigorating deep tissue massage can be stimulating and increase energy, while a Swedish massage will melt you like butter. Massage therapists are trained to give either one. Although a trained massage therapist can give you the best treatment, you can gain a great deal of benefit with a massage from your spouse or a friend.

The healing properties of music have been known since biblical times. Harp players would perform as a means to relax. Young David played the harp for King Saul to help him recover from his frequent bouts with depression.

As the saying goes, "Music soothes the savage beast." Music has great power with its effects on emotions and mood. A lively tune will get your body moving and your foot tapping. A mellow piece will calm you down. Loud rock music will wind you up into a frenzy.

Music can be a great help in relieving stress. Listening to the right type of music on your way home from work can help soothe your nerves and ease stress by the time you arrive home. Listening to background music at work can also help.

Not all music has calming, healing qualities. Soft, easy listening music is best. Jazz and pop music and such will invigorate and get blood flowing and epinephrine pumping throughout the system, energizing you. Hard rock, rap, and other high-beat music aggravates the nerves and mind, intensifying stress. If you've been on edge all day at work, your adrenals are shot, and you feel exhausted; the last thing you want to do is listen to invigorating music, including pop and soft rock. It will force adrenal glands to squeeze out more stress hormones and add to the eventual burnout of the body. Instead, listen to easy listening music, particularly classical, and baroque music especially.

Baroque music is a form of classical music written by composers covering a period of time from 1600 to 1750. The most famous baroque composers were Johann Sebastian Bach and George Frederick Handel. Baroque music has a high degree of order and symmetry; for this reason it is very soothing to the mind. Studies have shown that it enhances learning and healing. Even plants grow faster and become healthier when exposed to classical, and especially baroque, music. These beneficial results are not evident with other types of music, especially rock, which has been shown to decrease the ability of the mind to learn, agitates nerves, and stifles healing. Plants exposed to rock music grow deformed and twisted. People who work in a stressful environment and play such music are actually weakening and wearing their bodies down and leaving themselves open to disease. Believe it or not, rock music affects rational thought, often leading to bizarre behavior. On the other hand, baroque and other classical music is in harmony with nature and helps relieve stress and normalize body functions. For a more in-depth look at the effects of music on the mind, see the references at the end of this chapter.

Many kinds of music have relaxing, beneficial effects besides classical. Soft instrumentals, easy listening music, and spiritual music can also work well. The main element is that the music must be quieting rather than stimulating.

Visualization

Visual imagery harnesses the mind's healing power and focusing it on a specific problem. It involves belief or faith that the body can heal itself, and cultivates that belief. Visualization, hypnosis, meditation, and biofeedback are all really part of the same process—deep concentration. The mind focuses on one thing so intently that it is oblivious to the environment or surroundings.

Visualization and similar techniques have been successful in treating patients with cancer, arthritis, impotence, and a host of other diseases. In fact, a person with any type of disease or illness can benefit from visualization techniques. One of the important reasons for doing visualization is to build faith in whatever treatment program you pursue. If you keep telling yourself that you are getting healthier every day and visualize it in your mind, you will convince yourself of it and your body will respond by becoming healthier.

The power of hypnotherapy has long been established. It has been used to eliminate fears, change bad habits, aid in recovery from surgery, speed healing of injuries, and overcome degenerative and infectious illnesses. The mind wields great power over the health of our bodies. We can use this power to speed detoxification and enhance healing. Even serious degenerative conditions such as cancer can respond.

You don't need a visualization coach or hypnotherapist to aid you, although these people can be helpful. You can do it on your own, using self-hypnosis techniques in conjunction with other treatment regimens, such as diet and exercise.

Self-hypnosis can be induced in many ways. The methods described in the bestseller *How to Hypnotize Yourself and Others* by Rachel Copelan offers simple effective techniques you can use on yourself to enter a hypnotic state. Once in this state you can use methods of visualization to support and enhance cleansing and healing.

Dr. Robert Becker, an orthopedic surgeon and researcher, has demonstrated that the body flows with electrical energy. His work led directly to the use of electricity to accelerate the healing of broken bones. Dr. Becker found that hypnotized patients can consciously produce voltage changes in specific areas of the body. It is believed that electric currents control the chemical and cellular processes of healing, which provides a scientific explanation for hypnotic cures and even the placebo effect.

Scientists don't understand the full power of the mind and its power of involuntary functions like heart rate and digestion. But it is known that the mind can consciously affect involuntary functions such a blood pressure, heart rate, dilation of blood vessels, etc. It's known that people under hypnosis can control bleeding after surgery without affecting the flow of blood to other parts of the body. We can channel healing electrical energies into any part of our body.

Visualizing changes in your body can help the body bring those changes about. It has been found that during hypnosis, healing is much more effective when visual imagery is incorporated into the process. Simply trying to get an organ to function better, like telling the stomach to secrete digestive enzymes, isn't nearly as effective. Rather than tell the stomach to perform these operations, with visualization you "see" in your mind the digestive enzymes being formed and secreted. The body would then respond to the visualization by producing the enzymes. This reaction is similar to when you think of eating your favorite foods and your mouth begins to water. Saliva, which contains digestive enzymes necessary for proper digestion, is secreted by the simple process of visualization.

How does one go about visualization? There are many methods. The main idea is to visualize and experience, as much as possible, something happening in your body. Begin by selecting a place where you can be undisturbed. Get into a comfortable position either sitting or lying down. If sitting, place both feet flat on the floor in front of you with your arms resting comfortably in your lap or on arms of a chair. If lying down, stretch out on a bed or some other appropriate surface, even the floor will do. Take off glasses and jewelry and get totally comfortable.

Close your eyes. For some, *soft* background music helps them relax, but this isn't necessary. To get your mind and body to relax, begin with some slow deep breathing exercises. Inhale by first expanding the abdomen; this pulls the diaphragm down which expands the lungs. Slowly fill your lungs to capacity, hold briefly, then slowly let the air out as you contract the abdominal muscles. Tightening the abdomen will aid in the expulsion of the air. Repeat this cycle several times without straining. Deep breathing will release tension, allowing you to relax and focus the mind on your body and away from daily concerns. After a few minutes of deep breathing, let the breathing become natural.

To further relieve tension and develop deeper concentration, focus your thoughts on the top of your head and begin relaxing each part of your body from the top down an inch at a time. Picture in your mind each body segment as you move down your face, relaxing each muscle, to the neck and shoulders, the arms, and hands. Then go down the spine, vertebra by vertebra, to the hips, thighs, knees, calves, ankles, and toes. Concentrate on relaxing each one in turn. By now your body should be completely relaxed and your mind tuned into visualization. This is similar to the induction process of self-hypnosis.

At this stage, you will concentrate all your thoughts and energy on the area in your body where help is needed. If you have swollen ankles, you would focus your mind and thoughts on your ankles.

Now visualize in your mind's eye the affected part. Let's say it is a tumor. All other parts of your body should seem to be non-existent as the only thing you see and feel is the area in question. Imagine healing taking place. You can do this by visualizing white blood cells attacking the tumor and removing it from your body. They may even take on the form of hungry piranha gobbling up diseased or infected tissues. You can visualize blood flowing to the affected part bringing in healing oxygen to neutralize poisons, or perhaps visualize a knife cutting diseased tissue out, or the body's heat consuming it. In your visualization, picture the destruction or removal of affected tissues and

toxins and the regeneration of healthy tissue. As the mind produces these images, the body responds. Tell yourself you are getting healthier. "See" your immune system gaining in strength.

Continue to visualize for about five or ten minutes. Combined with the induction process, the whole process should take only ten or fifteen minutes. You can go longer if you wish. To finish, tell your body to continue the healing or cleansing process throughout the day, then open your eyes. That's all there is to it. Do this at least once a day, every day. Don't do it early in the morning or late at night when you are coming from or going to bed, as you will be too sleepy to concentrate and your mind will either wander or you will fall asleep. Do it sometime during the day when you are fully awake.

As you direct your mental energies to a specific area of your body, you may feel energy build up in that area. The feelings may be a like a soft vibration, or tingling sensation, or an increase in heat. Anticipate these feelings and encourage them. Some areas of the body respond to visualization better than others. It is easier to feel the energies on the skin and muscles where we have numerous sensory nerve endings than on internal organs where we do not.

For those people who are new to meditation and self-hypnosis, such feelings may be hard to imagine. Here is an exercise you may like to try to practice your visualization skills. Sit comfortably in a chair as described above with feet flat on the floor. Go through the deep breathing exercises and relaxation of the body from head to toe. With your mind focused on your feet, visualize energy flowing into your feet. The energy accumulates in your feet, building up heat. Imagine the feel of the heat on the bottoms of your feet. See and feel your soles getting hotter and hotter. You will feel the heat. When you have had enough, simply tell your mind that it is enough and open your eyes. With some people the heat on the soles of the feet can get so intense that it brings discomfort.

Positive Mental Attitude

If you cultivate a positive mental attitude about everything in life, you will become happier and healthier. You will accomplish more in life, be troubled less by mental and emotional problems, and be able to handle stress better. You will have more friends. Have you ever wondered why some people are popular and liked by everyone while others don't seem to have many friends? It's attitude! People like to be around positive people. Negative people only like to be around other negative people so they can support or justify feelings and actions.

Some people say it is not good to be optimistic all the

time as that could lead to disappointment and consequently depression. Such comments come only from depressed people who won't allow themselves to be positive, and want everyone else to be miserable like themselves. They try to discourage those who want to think positive.

The one thing negative people overlook is that optimistic people, being positive, almost always accomplish their goals. And in those cases where they don't, they are optimistic enough to realize some failure is part of the process and that striving for a goal is often just as beneficial as achieving it.

The first step in developing a positive mental attitude is not letting little things bother you. Many people will get upset and angry if someone pulls in front of them on the highway as they fight traffic. Why let this bother you? There is nothing you can do about it. It will always happen; getting angry will not pull the car out of your way, neither will pounding on the car horn or yelling obscenities. Accept the fact that things like this will happen every time you get behind the wheel. Expect it. When it happens, think nothing of it; it is a part of driving and part of life. Doing so will prevent you from getting angry and becoming stressed over it. Apply this concept to all aspects of your life because you will encounter people and situations other than when driving where people can make you angry. Don't let them.

If there is a situation that annoys you that you can't change, ignore it. Stand back and think about it before reacting. Would a negative reaction on your part solve the problem or perhaps make it worse? Responding negatively to any action always makes things worse. The answer is to ignore it and let it go, or respond positively. This way you avoid confrontation and further needless stress.

Sheldon and Sheila Kay Lewis in their book *Stress-Proofing Your Child* relate the following experience:

Several years ago our son Ezra came home from school in a very agitated state, his face red with anger. "That kid!" he shouted. "I can't take that kid anymore." When we asked him what happened, he said a classmate who sat behind him constantly taunted him, calling him names. When Ezra turned to tell the boy to be quiet, the teacher scolded Ezra for turning around and talking.

"What do I do about this kid?" he asked in despair. "He keeps bothering me."

"You may not be able to stop him from bothering you." we said. "But maybe you can learn to ignore him."

"Right," he scoffed.

Ezra was taught that when something or someone agitated him, to learn to relax by taking slow, deep breaths, closing his eyes, and picturing himself in a peaceful setting.

Ezra sat there with his eyes closed for a few minutes. Then he opened them. The lines on his face had softened, and the muscles of his arms and legs looked relaxed.

"Now let's try a game. It's an acting game. You play yourself, and we'll play this boy who's been bothering you. Tell us some of the things he says to you."

Ezra did. "Now as we yell these things at you, pretend that our words are the water from a waterfall. Don't let the words in and don't react to them. Just breathe and let the words slide off you."

Ezra agreed. For the next few minutes we hurled epithets at him. "Hey, kid! Hey, you! Hey, Ezra! Hey, what's your problem, kid? You're stupid. You're a jerk."

Throughout, Ezra maintained a grin. "This is fun," he said.

The next day, when Ezra arrived home from school, we asked, "How was school?"

"Fine."

"How was the kid today?"

"Oh, he was the same," he answered cheerfully. "But I ignored him."

There were two possible solutions to Ezra's problem. One was for Ezra to make an effort to become friends with the boy so he would stop being mean to him. If this were not possible, his other option was to simply ignore him. The first solution in most cases would be the best option. However, sometimes we encounter people who are so negative that it is very difficult to deal with them. In such cases we need to ignore them and not let them bother us. Once we have made up our minds not to react to such people, we can look at the situation from a different perspective. Their actions appear childish and ignorant. You can feel good about your mature attitude for not reacting in a like manner.

We face potentially stress-causing situations and people all day long. The better we handle these situations, the less stress we have and the better off we will be. When confronted with agitating people, a positive response and smile may turn them around. Say to yourself, "Smile, it's contagious!" You may have noticed if someone is grumpy and has a bad attitude others pick up on it and become negative too. The opposite is also true. If you have a friendly smile and positive attitude, yours will spread to those you come in contact with. And it is surely much more pleasant to be surrounded by cheerful, smiling people than grumpy, negative ones. In a sense, heart disease, cancer, and other degenerative diseases can be contagious. Not that they are caused by infectious organisms, but by our reactions to other people's actions. The many negative people we face each day can cause continual stress which, in turn, can cause or open the door to disease. Don't let others give you heart disease, think positive!

Your outlook on life and the work you do also affects your health. Dissatisfaction with your job can create a great deal of stress that can lead to a host of ills. Several years ago, a Northwestern Mutual Life Insurance study found that half the workers in high-stress jobs frequently suffered headaches, colds, indigestion, bronchitis, and pneumonia. Douglas LaBier, director of the Center for Adult Development in Washington, D.C. agrees. "Quite often people have backaches, headaches, or stomach problems during the work week," he says. "Then on the weekend, the symptoms 'mysteriously' disappear, only to return again on Monday morning." And UCLA researchers have discovered that people with a ten-year history of workplace stress also face more than five times the risk of developing colon and rectal cancers compared to those who enjoy their work.

But suppose you hate your job and can't afford to quit? University of Chicago psychologist Mihaly Csikszentmihalyi maintains that a job must offer variety and challenge to be fulfilling. But he adds, "Whether a job has variety or not depends more on a person's approach to it than on actual working conditions."

Csikszentmihalyi once interviewed a man who worked long hours as a welder in a dreary plant in South Chicago. "The plant was hot as an oven in summer, and icy in winter. The clanging of metal was so loud you had to shout just to be heard," Csikszentmihalyi recalls. "Yet despite these stressful conditions, this man was quite happy with his job."

Why? Csikszentmihalyi explains: "Over the years he had mastered every phase of the plant's operation and was the only one who could fix any piece of machinery. He loved being called on to keep the factory running smoothly." Think positively about work and you will enjoy it more. Look for the benefits and the good things about it and ignore the bad. And definitely don't sit around with other employees complaining about the job or the company. This only breeds discontent.

Take control of your life and your health. Don't let the actions of others control you and wear down your health.

Love and Forgiveness

Growing evidence is linking a belief in God to better physical health. In numerous studies, it has been determined that frequent churchgoers have lower rates of many illnesses, ranging from hypertension and heart disease to tuberculosis and cervical cancer. When doctors examined men over 65 who'd been admitted to a veterans hospital in

Love and Health

Researchers have discovered that stress and the many emotions associated with stress (e.g. anger, frustration, anxiety) actually deplete a key immune system antibody known as IgA. This antibody, more than any other, is the body's first line of defense against bacteria. According to one study, a single, five-minute episode of anger produces a brief increase in IgA. Then, it drops steadily to one-half its previous level, and seven hours later it still has not returned to normal. Conversely, a five-minute period of caring and compassion causes a dramatic increase in IgA, boosting the immune system.

Exciting information continues to be released by the Institute of HeartMath (IHM). Their research has shown that emotions associated with love, such as caring, compassion, and appreciation, can increase our ability to fight disease, while anger and hate (the opposite of love and forgiveness) actually lower our resistance levels. According to Professor Jerry Ainsworth of Southern Connecticut State University, love is one of those emotions that can actually improve your health. "Get and give plenty of love," recommends Ainsworth, who teaches a course called Love and Health at the University.

Research has shown that the heart, the very organ most affected by stress and emotional distress, may hold the key to successful health as well. "When people make a sincere effort to have more caring attitudes toward other people, it really does boost the body's immune system. A Harvard study determined that in 1988, and we've confirmed it many times since then," explains Bruce Cryer, one of the directors at IHM.

Durham, N.C., they found that those who said religion was very important to them were less likely to become depressed. Depression can hinder recovery. The evidence strongly suggests faith in God is linked to a long, healthy life.

Why is this so? There may be many reasons: a healthier life-style, social support, hope, and optimism are some of the positive effects instilled by a faith in God. But perhaps the most important is the emphasis most Judeo-Christian religions place on love and forgiveness. Whether you believe in God or not, cultivation of these two traits can significantly affect your physical and emotional health.

Hate and anger are the opposite of love and

forgiveness. When we forgive we cannot be angry. If we love we cannot hate. It is difficult, if not impossible, to completely avoid getting angry. An occasional flash of temper is harmless if kept under control. A permanent snarl is not. Hostile people are perpetually suspicious, wary and snappish, forever tense and on edge. Hostility feeds on itself. The answer is to mentally pull yourself out of the situation and relax, take a deep breath, and look at the situation in a calm manner. If you can step away from the situation mentally for a moment and think about it, the emotional aspect dissipates. You can think logically and decide to forgive and let life go on. Give in to your anger and you become all the more angry. Resist it by keeping your voice down or your teeth unclenched, and the anger melts away.

This concept has met with opposition by those who hold to an older theory which assumes that if you express your anger, you get it out of your system; if you don't express anger, you just keep it inside which could cause further problems. Dr. Aaron Siegman, a stress researcher at Baltimore's Veterans Administration hospital, sees this as smacking of an outdated Freudianism. "The psychoanalysts thought the anger was like physical energy," he says. "They thought it couldn't be dissipated—the only choice was to express it or to repress it. But anger is not like physical energy," he says. "An angry person who chooses to divert his attention will no longer be angry. We have a lot of evidence to show that."

There is, according to Dr. Siegman, a distinction between suppressing the outward expressions of anger and repressing anger itself. The difference is that people who repress their anger don't get rid of it, they hide it and let it brew inside (and may deny they are angry when they really are). Sometimes they may even be unaware of it. The person who recognizes anger, but consciously decides that the matter isn't worth the fireworks and calmly talks it out or lets it fade away, does not build up stress. The result is that the anger neither festers nor explodes, but gradually loses its steam.

When you feel yourself getting angry, stop long enough to ask yourself some questions: Is this really serious enough to get worked up over? Is getting angry going to make any difference? Will anger solve the problem or make matters worse? Often, just asking yourself these questions is enough to cool the anger.

Simply because you do not openly react to a negative situation does not mean you have let it go. Repression of anger can be just as bad as blowing up. When anger is repressed, it is still present but hidden from view. It boils and stews inside. Anger is continually fueled by repeatedly running the incident through your mind. In this case, you

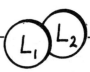

Vitamins L₁ and L₂

Vitamins are essential for good health. Most of us are aware of the benefits of many of these vitamins such as vitamin C, used to build the immune system and fight colds. Two of the most important vitamins for good health are vitamins L_1 and L_2. You won't see them sold in stores or listed on vitamin bottles, for they don't come in bottles—you create them yourself. They are Love and Laughter.

must make a conscious effort to forgive and forget. Once you truly forgive someone, you can't be mad at them anymore.

At times, ignoring a problem will help you cope with it as illustrated in the story of Ezra and his troublesome classmate. Sometimes, however, simply ignoring a problem isn't enough. When someone has done something to annoy you, particularly if it is someone you know, you need to forgive them so that negative feelings won't return. If you can't forgive other people, you will never be able to develop the positive frame of mind necessary to have good health. So do it for your own sake. You will become a much more pleasant person to be around, you will like yourself more, and you will be happier. Keep in mind that no one is perfect; we all make mistakes and do things that annoy or bother others even without knowing it. Don't expect people to be perfect; forgive them for anything they do that might upset you in any way. The act of forgiving is a sign of love.

Love yourself and others, forgive others for their mistakes and shortcomings, and trust and respect others. Go out of your way to be helpful and friendly to people. It is amazing how a smile and friendly tone of voice can bring out similar reactions in others. When we help others, we feel good about it. It produces a kind of euphoria that brightens our spirits and enhances our immune system, thus strengthening our resistance to disease.

Instinctively we know that when we help others, we feel good. But researchers have actually documented health improvements when we help others. After a study using 3,300 volunteers, Allan Luks, executive director of Big Brothers/Big Sisters in New York City concluded that taking care of others improves your health. Those who volunteered regularly were ten times more likely to report being in good health than those who helped others only once a year or didn't help at all. In a recent interview, Luks pointed to three criteria that seemed to lead to this health advantage: helping others consistently (an average of two hours a week), having personal contact with those helped, and helping strangers rather than helping only family or friends. Benefits included emotional uplifts (called the "helper's high"), reduction in awareness of chronic pain, fewer colds, and improved eating and sleeping habits.

Luks found that 1 percent of the volunteers had less uplifting experiences. These people tended to use volunteering as an escape from their own problems. Others overdid their helpfulness. But the great majority of volunteers, including the disabled and the homebound, discovered a powerful health tonic.

 **ADDITIONAL RESOURCES**

Healing and the Mind. Moyers, Bill. New York: Doubleday, 1993.

The Healing Power of Humor. Klein, Allen. Los Angeles: Jeremy Tarcher, 1989.

Healing Yourself: A Step-By-Step Program for Better Health through Imagery. Rossman, Martin L. New York: Pocket Books, 1989.

The Healer Within. Locke, Steven and Colligan, Douglas. New York: Mentor, 1986.

Healing Visualizations: Creating Health Through Imagery. Epstein, Gerald, M.D. New York: Bantam Books, 1989.

How to Hypnotize Yourself and Others. Copelan, Rachel. New York: Harper and Row, 1981.

You Can't Afford the Luxury of a Negative Thought: A Book for People with any Life-Threatening Illness— Including Life. Revised Edition. McWilliams, Peter. Los Angeles: Prelude Press, 1995.

Humor and Aging. Nahemow, Lucille; McCluskey-Fawsett, Cathleen A. McGhee, Paul I. San Diego, CA: Academic Press, 1986.

Mind/Body Medicine: How to Use your Mind for Better Health. Goleman, D. and Gurin, Joel. New York: Consumer Reports Books, 1993.

Living, Loving and Learning. Buscaglia, Leo F. New York: Ballantine Books, 1982.

Mind, Music and Imagery. Merritt, Stephanie. New York: Plume Press, 1990.

The Relaxation Response. Benson, Herbert. New York: Outlet Books, 1993.

Sound Health. Halpern, Steven. New York: Harper and Row, 1985.

Stress Management. Gordon, James S. New York: Chelsea House, 1990.

Chapter 16

HOW TO SURVIVE IN A TOXIC WORLD

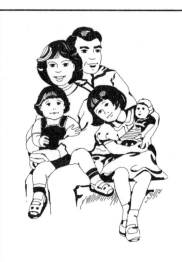

Health is physical, mental, and social well-being, not merely the absence of disease.

There is no quick holistic fix. We're so used to the quick foods, quick weight loss diets, quick beauty, and quick self-help advice that are part of our hurried, achievement-oriented lives that we expect a quick cure when we're sick. We see illness as something to get rid of so we can get back to work as soon as possible, rather than viewing it as a warning signal. Holistic medicine...focuses on creating health, not simply curing illness.

—M. Barry Flint, executive director of the Institute for the Advancement of Health

Sheila had discovered a good sized lump in her right breast a month before getting a mammogram. Earlier when she was 24, she found a lump in her breast that turned out to be benign. "I was not really concerned. My mother had several benign tumors removed; my younger sister has had them too. I am premenopausal, had a child in my mid-twenties and nursed her for 11 months, and have been a vegetarian since high school. I'm 46 years old and very active and healthy."

Two days later the report came back: "highly suspicious."

The physician explained that the lump in Sheila's breast had microcalcifications and that she should make an appointment to have it biopsied as soon as possible. "My heart quickened. I visualized my death. I have known for a long time that dying is part of living, and I am not afraid to die. I have known people who ask themselves, 'Why me?' when they face a life-threatening situation. I found myself asking, 'Why not me?' Maybe my time had come."

The doctor explained that the microcalcifications were tracs of hardened calcium, which show up on mammograms as small, white specks. Most often she said, they're harmless, but sometimes they can be an early sign of cancer. A biopsy was scheduled.

Following the biopsy, the pathology report confirmed that a small part of the lump was, indeed, cancer. The good news was that the cancer appeared to be contained. The surgeon advised that a mastectomy would be the best course of action. The surgery was scheduled a few weeks later and Sheila's right breast was removed.

The last thing on Jonathan's mind in the summer of 1992 was cancer. Most of his energy was spent training for the Pike's Peak Ascent, a grueling marathon to the top of the famous Colorado mountain summit. Jonathan kept himself physically active by jogging regularly. He ate a near vegetarian diet and, at the age of 46, considered himself in the prime of health.

"One morning in June while I was lying in bed, I felt lumps in my groin." Jokingly he said, "I hope this isn't cancer."

A paramedic since 1977, Jonathan recognized the lumps were swollen lymph nodes and monitored them for two months. "I knew there was a problem because they felt hard. Lymph nodes are normally soft and spongy," he says. He made an appointment with an internist who told him the enlarged nodes might indicate lymphoma, a terminal form of cancer that invades the lymphatic system and interferes with immune function. The doctor advised him to get a biopsy.

With the Pikes Peak Ascent just a month away, Jonathan postponed the biopsy because it would have prevented him from training and running in the race.

"I wasn't stressed out about it—I didn't really believe it was cancer—and I wanted to run the race before I found out information that might change my life," he recalls. A few days after the race, Jonathan went in for a biopsy. "The next day the surgeon told me over the phone I had lymphoma."

Jonathan was advised to get a bone marrow biopsy and a CAT scan to determine how widespread the disease was. The test results showed he had stage IV lymphoma, which meant the cancer was diffuse throughout his lymphatic system. However, it was low-grade, meaning the cancer was slow-growing. Exercise and diet apparently had slowed the growth of the disease. Other than enlarged lymph nodes, Jonathan didn't exhibit any symptoms usually associated with lymphoma such as night sweats, fatigue, and weight loss.

He was encouraged to start chemotherapy immediately. He decided to get more opinions. He visited experts at Memorial Sloan Kettering in New York City. Doctors there told him he needed a bone marrow transplant if he wanted a normal life expectancy. "I left there shell-shocked," Jonathan says. "Bone marrow transplantation has less than a 50 percent cure rate. Sloan Kettering has a 10 percent mortality rate from the procedure itself, and their lymphoma specialist told me I must have one to stay alive and that I'd better get my affairs in order.

"By that point I was burned out, and I decided not to do any of the conventional therapies. For me it was a quality-of-life decision," says Jonathan. "I read that people develop cataract, heart tissue damage, lung cancer, and leukemia as a result of chemotherapy and bone marrow transplants, and I realized the treatments could wreck my life. Besides, there's no guarantee the cancer won't come back after treatment."

Since his decision three years ago to refrain from conventional treatments, Jonathan remains healthy. He has turned to alternative medicine for his health care, including acupuncture, herbs, diet, and mental readjustment. These methods have kept his condition from getting worse. Although not totally free from the disease, today Jonathan continues his life, without symptoms, active, and with a positive outlook.

Both Sheila and Jonathan were conscious of their health. Both ate little or no meat, were physically active, and considered themselves in good health. So why did they get cancer? Their diet did not protect them. Exercise did not protect them. Although these things undoubtedly helped, alone they will not protect anyone from the consequences of toxic accumulation. Toxins are found not just in our foods but all around us.

Simply because people may say they are vegetarians does not mean they have a good diet. You can eat donuts, coffee, soda pop, chips, white flour, and processed foods and still call yourself a vegetarian. Many vegetarians eat poorly. Eating vegetables tainted with pesticides and petroleum based waxes is not healthy. Just cutting out meat doesn't make your diet healthier if you eat a lot of junk food or foods tainted with toxins.

Many people aware of the importance of good nutrition try to eat wisely, but are still exposed to high amounts of toxins either in the diet or environment. A diet high in fruits and vegetables could also be high in harmful pesticides.

Sheila described herself as physically active, but that can be defined in different ways. Being physically active does not mean she exercised regularly.

If you have been eating and living as most people do, your body is overloaded with toxins. Switching to a clean diet will help, but it may not be enough to cleanse your body. Exercise, sweat baths, and other detoxification methods are all needed in order to thoroughly clean the body. Toxins have built up for years, probably all your life. It takes time and effort to expel these deep seated poisons. You may feel a world of difference by just adjusting your diet. But degenerative conditions caused by toxins may continue, perhaps at a slower pace until, like Sheila, trouble strikes. The ten-step detoxification program outlined in this chapter uses all of the detoxification methods described in this book. Adherence to this program will clean your body thoroughly. It may take several months, even years, depending on your health and commitment to change, to clean all of the toxins from the tissues and rebuild new healthy body.

I visited the isolated Hunza Valley in Pakistan many years ago to find out for myself if the people were as disease-free and lived as long as Dr. Robert McCarrison reported in the early part of this (20th) century. In a world which seems to be constantly on the verge of being overwhelmed by disease, the residents of the Hunza Valley were a refreshing contrast. There were no jails, hospitals, policemen, or doctors. Why? Because the people were healthy and well-balanced mentally and socially, in a high Himalayan Valley where the corrupt foods, customs and manners of civilization could not easily reach them, and where they had to live off of the simple foods they grew on rich, glacier-watered soil. Cancer, heart disease, diabetes, kidney disease, arthritis were unknown by the residents of Hunza while I was there.
—Bernard Jensen, Ph.D.

TEN-STEP DETOXIFICATION PLAN

In order to gain the most and the quickest results from detoxification, you need to combine the programs described in this book. Depending on your state of health, your rate of progress will vary. You may notice marked improvement within a matter of days, or it may take months to recognize improvement. Many health conditions have been progressing for years, even decades. You cannot expect such chronic conditions to right themselves in a matter of only a few weeks or months. It takes time to dig out deep-seated toxins, remove diseased tissues, flush them out of the body and rebuild with clean healthy cells. Broken bones don't heal overnight and, likewise, diseases and degenerative tissues don't change in a day.

Continued exposure to toxins will hamper and even stifle progress. Follow the programs precisely. Don't cheat! It will only slow down your progress. Look for all sources of toxins that you come into contact—food, water, air, chemicals, cleaning agents, detergents, soaps, cosmetics. Exposure to toxins from any source will slow progress.

The steps below list the programs you should take in sequence. The steps described below aren't done one at a time but overlap to some extent. Some of the programs can be performed at the same time and others should be done separately. Use common sense when following these steps. The Natural Foods Diet should be done before and along with all the other detoxification programs.

The first four steps—positive mental attitude, healthy diet, exercise, and oxygen cleansing—should be things you do daily for the rest of your life. Steps 5 and 6, fasting and heat therapy, are things you should do on a regular and frequent basis, but obviously not every day. Steps 7 through 10 should be done only periodically.

Step 1: Attitude

The very first step you need to take in order to successfully detoxify and improve your health is to develop a positive frame of mind, as discussed in Chapter 15. You must believe and have faith that you can be healed and truly want to be healed in order to do so. This is vital to the success of the entire program! And that is why it is listed first.

If you *truly* want to get better, which means you don't have any hidden or subconscious desires to have ill health in order to manipulate others or get sympathy, and if you honestly believe that natural therapies *will* work, rather than *can* work, then they *will* work for you. If you believe this and commit yourself to keep on the program,

PCB's

If there were a competition for the world's most toxic substance, PCB's would be right in there along with DDT, dieldrin, dioxin, and the others. A few parts per billion can cause birth defects and cancer...

PCB's were first introduced by Monsanto, a company whose motto, "Without chemicals, life itself would be impossible," seems ludicrous in view of what PCB's are doing to human fertility. It wasn't long after Monsanto began producing PCB's that it became apparent that these chemicals posed major problems for human beings. Three years after production began, the faces and bodies of 23 out of 24 workers in the Monsanto plant had become disfigured. But that didn't stop Monsanto. Since then, more than 750,000 tons of these deadly poisons have been produced. They can be found today in every river in America, in the snows of the Arctic and Antarctic and probably in the tissues of every single fish in the waters of this planet.

—John Robins, *Diet for A New America*

you will gain better health.

Most people who fail to achieve positive results on natural healing programs do so because they were not fully committed. They only "hoped" it would work, and after a few days, if they don't see their tumors magically melting away or degenerative arthritic joints quickly healing, then they gave up. Some people love the life-style of fast food and leisure more than they do health, and although they would like better health, they are not motivated enough to change their habits. They would rather sit back and wait for a pill to come along and take care of the problem.

The techniques in this book work! They have been confirmed through the years by thousands of case histories and people like you who have tried them. If you approach this program with the attitude that you will benefit, then you will.

Step 2: Diet

The second step toward detoxification is diet. Diet is a central element in any detoxification program. What goes into the mouth determines to a large degree the status of our health. A healthy diet should be maintained throughout the program and throughout life. Many people heal themselves through wise dietary choices and, once they feel better, go back to eating poor-quality foods. What happens? Illness returns. Eating a healthy diet is not just a temporary thing you do just to get over a particular condition. It should become a life-long habit.

Eating healthfully may be difficult at first for some. We grow accustomed to the foods we normally eat. When you switch to a healthier diet, the foods are unfamiliar and they may not taste as good to you as your old foods did. But give it time. As you get used to eating this way, you will come to enjoy these foods more and even prefer them. As your body cleanses itself, you will be able to taste the chemicals and additives in foods you had once relished. They will not have the power over you they once had, and you may not even like them.

Commit to sticking strictly to the Natural Foods Diet for at least six months and preferably for the rest of your life. This means eating all organic produce. Eat organic meat, dairy, and eggs in moderation (once or twice a week at most). Eat only whole grain breads and cereals. Eliminate all packaged or prepared foods and refined sugars, and limit your use of vegetable oil.

Step 3: Exercise

The third step is to get regular exercise. This is not a leisurely ten-minute walk every day, but a serious aerobic exercise program. Aerobic exercise is any type of exercise that gets your heart to beat faster and your lungs to pump more air for an extended amount of time. Twenty to 30 minutes should be the minimum amount of time you devote to this. You need to stimulate blood and lymph circulation to deliver oxygen and other nutrients throughout the body and to flush out toxins.

Walking is the easiest exercise to start with. Begin with a mile a day, five to six days a week. If you have difficulty walking, set a goal of walking 20 minutes a day—even if you have to stop every block to rest. Gradually increase your time and distance. Work up to at least two miles a day or 30 minutes of brisk walking. Keep in mind not to overexert yourself. Remember that as you walk, you should be able to carry on a conversation at the same time. If you cannot talk while walking, ease up a little.

You should carry on an exercise program for the rest of your life. Try different types of activities such as dance aerobics, tennis, swimming, martial arts, or rebounding. Look for community education classes and enjoy them; perhaps you will find new activities you will like and develop new friendships. Remember that movement is life, stagnation is death.

Step 4: Oxygen Cleansing

Oxygen cleansing or therapy is very important in our modern toxic world. Oxygen levels have decreased in the atmosphere and pollution has increased. Our bodies are oxygen starved. Oxygen is essential to the process of life and is nature's natural cleanser and healer. Increasing our oxygen intake will enhance cleansing and reverse degeneration.

You should increase the amount of clean oxygen you absorb through your lungs. The ways to do this are with deep breathing exercises, as described in Chapter 8, and using an ozone generator. Ozone generators not only increase the oxygen that gets to your lungs, but neutralize harmful environmental pollutants, making the air you breathe cleaner. You should have one at home or at your work.

Hydrogen peroxide solutions are the best way to get significant amounts of oxygen inside of the body. This will bring cleansing reactions faster than any other method of oxygen delivery. Follow the procedure given on pages 113-114. After the initial cleanse, you can continue taking hydrogen peroxide at a reduced rate indefinitely.

Before doing any serious oxygen cleansing, you need to have been on the Natural Foods Diet for at least 3-4 weeks. This is necessary in order to provide your body with the vitamins and minerals it needs to manufacture antioxidant enzymes which prevent oxygen-derived free-radical chain reactions.

Since our environment is seriously oxygen depleted, you can gain benefit from oxygen therapy by using it on a continual basis. This can be from a variety of methods—deep breathing, baths, ozone generators, hydrogen peroxide drinks, etc.

Step 5: Fasting

Fasting is the primary mechanism nature has given to us for cleansing and detoxification. Overeating, even of clean, healthy foods, shortens life and encourages toxicity.

Fasting should be done on a regular basis. Some people fast one day a week. Others 1-3 days at a time, each month. Still others will do more extended fasts of 7-10 days or more, once or twice a year. Preferably, you should fast at least once a month (1-3 days duration) with one or two extended fasts each year.

Fasting should begin only after you have been eating the Natural Foods Diet for at least 3-4 weeks. The reason is that many people who have been eating convenience or prepared foods are marginally malnourished to begin with. Fasting will only deplete their already limited supply of nutrients. The Natural Foods Diet will build up your nutrient reserves so that you can endure the fast without experiencing any deficiency. This is very important. Some people try fasting without being properly prepared and they get sick, not a healing crisis sick, but early stage nutrient deficiency symptoms. Most people with adequate nutrient stores in body tissues can fast without suffering any nutrient deficiencies for 30 days, even if they only consume water.

For fasts of short duration of one or two days, water is the preferred liquid. For longer fasts use juice or herbal teas. In a short fast the body has ample vitamin and mineral reserves and cleansing is accelerated. For fasts of three days or more, the body begins to reserve nutrients and cleansing slows down. Taking juice on longer fasts provides additional nutrients that restimulate cleansing.

Fasting is new to most people in affluent societies where food is plentiful, and is a little difficult at first. Once you get used to it, fasting is no big deal. Start with a 24-36 hour water fast once a month. After a few months, instead of the water fast, do a three-day juice fast or a three-day monofoods fast. If you do the monofoods fast, eat only one type of food, such as grapes, carrots, apples, or melon (whole, juiced, or dried), along with plenty of clean water. A month or so later, do a seven-day juice or monofoods fast. Monofoods fasts are easier because you actually are able to eat something and have roughage go through your digestive tract. Next, try a seven-day juice fast. Use any fruit or vegetable juices using organically grown produce. You may also use herbal teas. When you feel you are ready, you can do a 14-day juice fast.

Make it a habit to fast at least once a month. This should be done for the rest of your life. Every year you should go on one 7 to 14-day juice fast, preferably in the spring or early summer, just as fruit and vegetables are coming into season and the temperature is warming. This way you will have fresh produce, and the decrease in body temperature caused by the fasting will not be as troublesome as it can be during colder months.

Enemas during fasting can have a very cleansing action and remove all sorts of disgusting debris. Enemas can be done every day of a fast or less often if you prefer. They are not absolutely necessary when you fast.

Step 6: Heat Therapy

Heat is another one of nature's wonder cleansers that cultures all around the world have used for centuries. Heat helps to unclog pores, remove toxins, kill harmful germs, oxygenate the body, and stimulate metabolism and healing.

Heat therapy consists of raising the body's temperature. This can be done any number of ways, as described in Chapter 10. When using a bath to generate heat, you should add $1/2$ to 1 cup of 35 percent food grade hydrogen peroxide to the bath water. This will detoxify the tap water as well as oxygenate your body.

Sweat baths should be done on a regular basis. Once or twice a week is good. It should be a part of your regular health maintenance program. Always drink lots of distilled or filtered water before and after treatment to keep body fluids normal. You don't want to run the risk of dehydration. Drinking a cup of hot diaphoretic (i.e. sweat inducing) herbal tea immediately before and during a sweat bath will help to raise the body's temperature, which is the purpose of heat therapy.

Before engaging in heat therapies, you need to have adequate minerals stored in the body. Sweating removes minerals along with toxins. If you are minerally deficient, sweat therapy may compound the matter. To make sure your mineral level is adequate, you should be on the Natural Foods Diet for at least 3-4 weeks before doing any heat therapy.

Step 7: Colon Cleansing

The colon is our primary source of autointoxication and ill health. Having a clean, healthy colon is vital to good health.

Colon cleansing can be accomplished with the diet by eating whole natural foods. Foods rich in fiber and nutrients stimulate regular elimination and the growth of friendly bacteria. The Natural Foods Diet will do this.

The bowels can be stimulated on their own to expel toxic accumulations. There are many formulations sold at health food stores for this purpose. The Ivy Bridges formula is one of the best and, because you mix the ingredients yourself, it is also one of the cheapest. Most anyone could benefit by taking this cleansing drink every day for one to three months, then continuing every two or three days thereafter for as long as necessary.

When the body has been abused by years of eating processed foods, meat, and other animal products, the colon may be in serious trouble. Such foods lead to chronic constipation, diverticulitis, colitis, and other degenerative conditions. Removal of encrusted waste and the regeneration of damaged tissues are facilitated by colonic irrigation. This can be done by way of an enema.

Although most people can benefit by having enemas, they aren't necessary for everyone. If you have normal bowel movements (one for every meal eaten), are not overweight, eat a diet rich in fiber, and have no major health problems, then you probably do not need to use enemas.

When chronic colon problems are present, the Ivy Bridges formula should be taken daily for about three months. Enemas may also be done, once or twice a week until symptoms subside and bowel movements become regular. This may take a long time. Someone who has suffered from serious chronic constipation and who has a deformed or spastic bowel may need several years of treatment to clean out impacted waste and rejuvenate tissues.

Step 8: Kidney Cleanse

The kidneys are one of the major organs of elimination. They must be healthy and working properly in order to filter toxins out of the blood and maintain the body's fluid and electrolyte balance. The kidney cleanse as described in Chapter 12 will be most effective after many of the previous steps have already been initiated. It is absolutely essential that you follow the Natural Foods Diet before and during the cleanse. So many processed foods and drugs contribute to poor kidney health that by eating them while you cleanse will only thwart your efforts. The kidney cleanse program should last for about six weeks the first time it is done. After that, do it for three weeks at a time, every six to 12 months. The more natural your diet is after the initial cleanse, the less often the cleanse is needed.

Step 9: Liver Cleanse

The liver cleanse as described in Chapter 13 should be done after the kidney cleanse. Detoxifying the liver will dump large amounts of toxins into the system and a healthy kidney is necessary to filter this debris out and effectively remove it. The liver is your body's main detoxification organ. Its health is vital to your health. It has hundreds of functions, and dysfunction of any one can cause health problems and even death. Do the liver cleanse three to four times within a one month period. After that, do it once every six to 12 months.

Coffee enemas will also support the cleansing of the liver. They can be done as desired as a part of your normal colon cleansing.

Step 10: Herbal Detoxification

Herbal detoxification can either be very powerful or have little or no noticeable effect. The key to making herbs effective is to prepare your body beforehand. Experience has demonstrated that those people who eat clean, natural foods and have a relatively healthy lifestyle benefit most from the use of herbs. Apparently, a body overtaxed with toxins is so busy trying to fight disease and maintain life and so nutrient depleted, that the healing compounds in the herbs are often not fully utilized and pass through the system without much effect. A body which is fed adequate amounts of vitamins, minerals, and other nutrients is more capable of utilizing the healing compounds in herbs. Being on the Natural Foods Diet and cleansing the body through other methods first will enhance the effectiveness of herbal detoxification.

Chapter 14 listed several detoxifying herbs. Follow the labels on each herb. Herbs are not drugs, and usually do not react as quickly as drugs. They work on strengthening body systems, allowing the body's natural processes to do their work. For this reason, most cleansing herbs should be used for an extended period of time from one to six months (six days a week). It may take this long, or even longer, for degenerative body systems affected by the herbs to build up the strength to function at a more normal level.

Many health problems people experience are directly related to parasites. Parasites can either cause health problems or make existing health problems worse. In areas where circulation is poor, oxygen is deprived, or pH is out of balance, tissues begin to deteriorate. This sets up an environment suitable for parasitic invaders. Parasites naturally migrate to those areas where the immune system has been depressed. This is why parasites are often found in diseased tissues. They are not necessarily the cause of the disease, but they are opportunistic and make a bad situation worse. Everybody, even those in "clean" modern societies, like the North America and Western Europe, are exposed to parasites. Parasite cleansing is important, because even a healthy body can become infected. The herbal parasite cleanse should be done by everyone at lease one or twice a year, every year.

LOW STOMACH ACIDITY

Another very important factor that may have significant bearing on the success of any detoxification program is the ability of the stomach to secrete adequate amounts of hydrochloric acid. Hydrochloric acid is essential to digestion. Low stomach acid or hypochlorhydria, as it is called, will affect the amount of nutrients that are digested and ultimately absorbed. People with hypochlorhydria are more than likely subclinically malnourished. They may eat enough food, or even overeat, but their bodies still cannot get enough of certain nutrients to supply the building blocks necessary for the complete manufacture of enzymes, hormones, and antibodies, as well as facilitate tissue repair.

Some of the major nutrients that are seriously affected by low stomach acid are iron, calcium, and vitamin B_{12}. The malabsorption of calcium, for example, can be a direct cause of osteoporosis. You may eat tons of calcium-rich foods or take calcium supplements, but if the stomach does not secrete enough acid, the calcium will not be completely absorbed and you will still be calcium deficient. The same is true with other nutrients. The importance of this in regards to detoxification is that the body needs these nutrients in order to clean and heal itself. Detoxification is ineffective if the body cannot get the nutrients to facilitate the cleansing process and rebuild healthy tissues.

It is essential that a person be on the Natural Foods Diet for some time before beginning any of the detoxification programs in order to build up the necessary nutrient reserves. But if someone is not producing enough stomach acid to properly digest food, he or she can be eating a balanced diet and still be deficient in many essential nutrients. To gain the greatest benefit from the detoxification programs in this book, this person must improve his or her digestion. It is estimated that as many as 40-50 percent of the population have some degree of hypochlorhydria. Most are unaware of it.

Besides malabsorption of essential nutrients, low stomach acid allows more undigested food mass to pass into the intestines and colon, contributing to fecal compaction and constipation, which leads to numerous other health problems. Some of the conditions often associated with low stomach acid include: allergies, diabetes, eczema, gallbladder disease, osteoporosis, anemia, under and overactive thyroid, lupus, chronic hepatitis, rosacea, and arthritis.

Lab tests can determine hypochlorhydria through hair mineral analysis, stool specimens, or radiotelemetry (directly measuring gastric acidity by swallowing a miniature radio transmitter). An iridologist (i.e., one who studies the iris for indications of bodily health and disease) can identify underacidity by simply examining markings in the iris of the eye. Physical signs that suggest low stomach acid include allergies, food sensitivities, weak and easily broken fingernails, hair loss (in women), and excess gas.

It is important to know if you have hypochlorhydria as it may affect the degree of success of some of the detox programs described in this book. If you suspect you have low stomach acid, you can compensate for it by taking digestive supplements. Many companies make such supplements. You want one that contains either or both betaine hydrochloride or glutamic acid hydrochloride. Digestive enzymes that should also be included are pepsin, bromelain, papain, and pancreatic enzymes. Other enzymes or vitamins may also be present, but these are the most important. You should also take an antioxidant complex (see page 176 for details) and a liquid mineral supplement which contains a full spectrum of trace minerals. The latter two supplements are taken because if you have low stomach acid, you are probably in need of them. The hydrochloric acid and enzymes should be taken at each

meal to help digest the food. The antioxidants and minerals should be taken as indicated on the label. Continue these supplements throughout the detoxification process. Other vitamins and supplements are not necessary because the Natural Foods Diet will supply you with what you need.

ASSISTED DETOX PROGRAMS

This book focuses on detoxification programs that you can do yourself. There are other methods of detoxification that require assistance from a qualified health care practitioner.

Nutritional counselors, naturopaths, or holistic physicians can guide you in a detox program suited for your particular set of circumstances. The programs described in this book will not harm you. They will only make you stronger and healthier. As you have learned, this process may cause a healing crisis which, to most people appears to be a "sickness" or a "negative reaction" to cleansing programs. The healing crisis may be severe, but it is a healing process and not a degenerative process. Although these programs can be self-administered, it is best to use them under the direction, guidance, and encouragement of a qualified holistic health care practitioner. This is especially true when a cleansing crisis hits. An experienced health care practitioner can give reassurance and assistance to help you through these trying periods.

Some individuals have specific health needs which may be best approached a little differently than what is listed here. A competent health care practitioner can be helpful in guiding you.

There are many types of therapies that aid the body towards detoxification and health that require a trained health care practitioner. Some of the most important are briefly described below.

Colon Hydrotherapy

Colon hydrotherapy is the cleaning of the colon by a trained therapist. The use and benefits of colonics was addressed in Chapter 11. Enemas and herbal laxatives can be self-administered. But colonics must be performed by a therapist. They use equipment to flush bowels and massage techniques simultaneously to loosen and break off encrusted debris to achieve thorough cleansing benefits.

Bodywork

There are many types of bodywork which include therapeutic massage, reflexology, chiropractic, acupuncture, and shiatsu.

Therapeutic massage is a wonderfully relaxing means to stimulate blood and lymphatic circulation and cleanse the body. Massage helps to release toxins from body tissue and put them in the bloodstream for elimination. This influx of toxic material may cause mild cold-like symptoms such as a runny nose or muscle soreness. Drinking lots of water after a massage is important to help the body quickly flush out these toxins and reduce cleansing symptoms.

Biological Dentistry

This is a must for anyone who has amalgam (metal) dental fillings or root canals. Amalgam fillings are a prime source of deadly toxins. They are made from a combination of mercury, copper, silver, cadmium, iron, and other metals which are highly toxic. Entire books have been written on the dangers of metal fillings and the health benefits of having those fillings removed. If you have amalgam fillings, it would be wise to see a "mercury-free" dentist and have them replaced with a less toxic material. Most dentists still use amalgam fillings and do not practice mercury-free dentistry. You need to find a dentist who specializes in this type of work.

Chelation Therapy

Chelation therapy is administered intravenously to cleanse heavy metals and other toxins from the blood. It is most noted for reversing the process of atherosclerosis and other cardiovascular problems. It is relatively painless and takes about three hours, after which the patient is allowed to go home. The complete therapy usually requires 20-30 visits at a rate of about 1-3 per week. It must be performed by a medical doctor experienced in chelation therapy.

Oxygen Therapy

Oxygen in one form or another can be administered with assistance using a hyperbaric chamber, intravenously, orally, or rectally. The advantage of assisted oxygen therapy is that a trained health care practitioner can monitor the patient's progress and administer dosages in amounts that can have dramatic effects. Like chelation therapy, it must be given by an experienced medical doctor.

A TIME TO HEAL

Don't expect cleansing to be accomplished overnight. You have taken a lifetime to accumulate the toxins in your body. They won't be miraculously flushed out of the tissues in a few weeks. Just as it takes time to heal a serious injury or get over a severe sickness, toxins and degenerative cells are removed and replaced gradually. This process may last one or two years or even more depending on the health, age, diet, and lifestyle of the individual. A person who is relatively healthy will pass over the healing process quickly. Younger people progress faster than older people because they usually have fewer years of toxic buildup and are better able to respond to healing. Regardless of your age, the higher the quality of food you eat, the quicker your body will cleanse itself of toxins and the sooner you will recover from disease, provided you are able to digest and assimilate food properly.

Risk Factors for Cardiovascular Disease

Total Cholesterol
Below 150 optimal
Below 200 mg/dL desirable
200 to 239 mg/dL borderline high
240 mg/dL or higher high

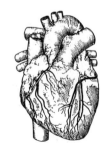

Hypertension
90 to 104 mm Hg mild
105 to 114 mm Hg moderate
115 mm Hg or higher severe

LDL
Below 130 mg/dL desirable
130 to 159 mg/dL borderline high
160 mg/dL or higher high

HDL Cholesterol Ratio
3.2 mg/dL optimal
Less than 5.0 mg/dL less than average risk
5.0 mg/dL average risk
Greater than 5.0 mg/dL high risk

Obesity
BMI* greater than 27.8 for men
BMI greater than 27.3 for women

Triglycerides
Below 100 mg/dL optimal
250 mg/dL or higher risk

* See page 122 to figure your Body Mass Index (BMI).

When the diet is improved, remarkable things begin to happen to the body and the mind. The body discards harmful toxins and diseased tissue, rebuilding with new healthier tissue. Bodily functions improve—digestion, nerve impulses, circulation, respiration all work more efficiently. We begin to feel healthier, have more vitality, experience less illness, become more alert, have a better memory, and are happier. This is how the body was designed to function. The body always tends toward health and always will, unless burdened by accumulating toxins and low-quality foods. Good food is the medicine for obtaining and maintaining good health.

After beginning the detox programs described in this book, many people notice immediate improvement in a matter of days. For most, it may take several months before significant change occurs. Improvement is usually gradual and often goes unnoticed. When we are constantly troubled by pain or discomfort, it is continually on our minds, but when the pain is absent, we tend to forget about it. One way you can determine if progress is being made is to ask others, especially if they haven't seen you for some months. They will tell you how good you look, how much thinner you are, how energetic you appear, and how much happier you seem to be. Others always see improvements first.

Before starting any of the programs in this book, you should have taken the health assessment profile described on pages 36-37. This profile evaluates your functional age which can provide you with a measurement of the status of your health. Other tests, such a blood pressure and cholesterol level, can also provide clues to health, and are important, but they require special equipment or medical assistance. Since this is a self-help book, the health assessment profile is designed to give you a simple evaluation that you can do yourself. It should not be taken as a replacement for a competent medical examination. Its primary purpose is to provide you with a measurement to which you can compare yourself and monitor your progress.

Continue to evaluate your progress by taking the health assessment every six months or so. Compare your results with your first assessment. There should be improvement. Your body should be growing functionally younger (or at least retard the aging process) as you clean poisons out of your system and rebuild with strong, healthy tissues. As you take charge of your own health through cleansing and living a healthier lifestyle, you will gain the benefits of improved health.

 ## ADDITIONAL RESOURCES

Beating the Odds. Marchetti, Abbert, M.D. Chicago, IL: Contemporary Books, 1988.

The Chelation Way. Walker, Morten, D.P.M. Garden City Park, NY: Avery Publishing Group, 1990.

The Complete Guide to Mercury Toxicity from Dental Fillings. Taylor, Joyal. San Diego, CA: Scripps Publishing Co., 1988.

The Healing Powers of Chelation Therapy. Trowbridge, John, P. M.D. and Walker, Morten, D.P.M. Stamford, CT: New Way of Life, 1992.

It's All in Your Head. Huggins, Hal, D.D.S. Colorado Springs, CO: Life Science Press, 1986.

Massage for Common Ailments. Thomas, Sara. New York: Fireside, 1989.

Reclaim Your Health. Frahm, Anne E., and Frahm, David J. Colorado Springs, CO: Pinon Press, 1995.

Spontaneous Healing. Weil, Andrew, M.D. New York: Knopf, 1995.

INDEX

Stress, 8, 23, 128, 149, 159, 183-195
Stress-Proofing Your Child, 192
Stroke, 72
Sudden sniffing death (SSD), 14
Subclinical malnutrition, 33, 42
Sucrose, 64
Sugar, 63-65, 182
Supergerms, 34-35, 155
Sulfites, 11
Sweat therapy, *See* Heat therapy
Synthetic chemicals, 7

T
Tapeworm, 178
Tenenbein, Milton, 14
Tetracycline, 155
Thiamin, 21, 182
Thyroid, 23
Tincture, 162, 174
Tobacco, 13, 25
Toxic accumulation, 23
Trace minerals, 137
Trans fatty acids, 67
Triglycerides, 47
Tryptophan, 10
Tuber, 46

Tumor, 22

U
Underfeeding, 92
Underweight, 122
Uranium, 12
Urea, 164
Uremia, 158
Uremic poisoning, *See* Uremia
Uric acid, 123
Urinary system, 158-159
Uva ursi, 162

V
Vancomycin, 34
Varicose veins, 30
Vegetable glycerin, 162
Vegetarianism, 52
Virus, 12, 21, 179-180
Visual impairment, 30
Visualization, 190-191
Vital capacity (VC), 108, 110
Vital energy, 38, 90, 92, 110
Vitamin B_1, *See* Thiamin
Vitamin B_3, *See* Niacin
Vitamin B_6, 162, 182

Vitamin B_{12}, 55, 66, 182
Vitamin C, 22, 119, 182
Vitamin E, 119
Vitamin K, 147, 151
Vitamins, 43, 44-46, 54-55, 91, 182

W
Walford, Roy L, 36
Wallach, Joel, 30
Warburg, Otto, 109
Water, 8, 11-13, 43-44, 71-73, 137, 158, 161
  distilled, 72
  filtered, 72
  groundwater, 8
  wastewater, 11
Weight control, 148
Werbach, Melvin, 181
Wicker, Henry, 169
Wigmore, Ann, 103
Worldwatch Institute, 7
Wormwood, 179

Z
Zinc, 45, 54